Physical Therapy Services
in the
Developmental Disabilities

Consulting Editor

Leila Green, M.S., R.P.T.
*Assistant Clinical Professor, Programs in Physical Therapy
Medical College of Wisconsin
Supervisor of Physical Therapy
Kiwanis Children's Center of the Curative Workshop
of Milwaukee, Wisconsin*

With a Foreword by

Margaret Jones, M.D.
*Professor of Pediatrics
University of California
UCLA Center for Health Sciences
Los Angeles, California*

Physical Therapy Services in the Developmental Disabilities

Seventh Printing

Edited by

PAUL H. PEARSON, M.D., M.P.H.
*C. Louis Meyer Professor of Child Health
University of Nebraska College of Medicine
Director, Meyer Children's Rehabilitation Institute
University of Nebraska Medical Center
Omaha, Nebraska*

and

CAROL ETHUN WILLIAMS, R.P.T.
*Former Physical Therapy Consultant
Mental Retardation Branch
Division of Chronic Diseases
United States Public Health Service
Washington, D.C.*

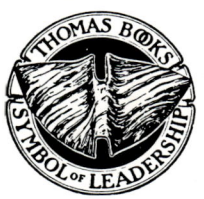

CHARLES C THOMAS • PUBLISHER
Springfield • Illinois • U.S.A.

Published and Distributed Throughout the World by
CHARLES C THOMAS • PUBLISHER
BANNERSTONE HOUSE
301-327 East Lawrence Avenue, Springfield, Illinois, U.S.A.

This book is protected by copyright. No part of it may be reproduced in any manner without written permission from the publisher.

© *1972, by* CHARLES C THOMAS • PUBLISHER
ISBN 0-398-02377-8
Library of Congress Catalog Card Number: 78-180820

First Printing, 1972
Second Printing, 1975
Third Printing, 1976
Fourth Printing, 1976
Fifth Printing, 1977
Sixth Printing, 1978
Seventh Printing, 1980

With THOMAS BOOKS *careful attention is given to all details of manufacturing and design. It is the Publisher's desire to present books that are satisfactory as to their physical qualities and artistic possibilities and appropriate for their particular use.* THOMAS BOOKS *will be true to those laws of quality that assure a good name and good will.*

Printed in the United States of America
N-1

This book is dedicated to all who work for the welfare of children.

CONTRIBUTORS

Berta Bobath, F.C.S.P., S.A.A.O.T. (Hon), Principal, The Western Cerebral Palsy Centre, London, England.

Karel Bobath, M.D., D.P.M., Consultant Physician, Harperbury Hospital, Herts., England and Honorary Consultant Physician, The Western Cerebral Palsy Centre, London, England.

Bryant J. Cratty, Ed.D., Professor, Department of Physical Education and Director, Perceptual-Motor Learning Laboratory, University of California, Los Angeles, California.

Nancy M. Fieber, B.S., R.P.T., Assistant Instructor of Child Health and Senior Physical Therapist, Meyer Children's Rehabilitation Institute, University of Nebraska Medical Center, Omaha, Nebraska.

Duane Kliewer, B.S., R.P.T., Instructor of Child Health, Chief of the Physical Therapy Section, Meyer Children's Rehabilitation Institute, University of Nebraska Medical Center, Omaha, Nebraska.

Helen A. Mueller, Lecturer at the Schools for Speech Therapy, Universities of Zurich and Fribourg; Speech Consultant to the Cerebral Palsy Centers of Switzerland; Teaching Staff (courses in neurodevelopmental treatment) for the Children's Hospitals of the Universities of Berne, Switzerland; Munich, West Germany; Innsbruck and Vienna, Austria; Speech Therapist for the City School for Cerebral Palsy Children, Zurich, Switzerland.

Paul H. Pearson, M.D., M.P.H., C. Louis Meyer Professor of Child Health and Director of the Meyer Children's Rehabilitation Institute, University of Nebraska Medical Center, Omaha, Nebraska.

Shirley A. Stockmeyer, B.S., M.A., Associate Professor of Physical Therapy, Sargent College of Allied Health Professions, Boston University, Boston, Massachusetts.

E. Jack Trembath, M.B.B.S., Research Associate Professor of Pediatrics and Associate Director for Health Programs in the Meyer Children's Rehabilitation Institute, University of Nebraska Medical Center, Omaha, Nebraska.

Dorothy E. Voss, B.Ed., Assistant Professor of Physical Therapy, Northwestern University Medical School, Chicago, Illinois.

Carol Ethun Williams, B.S., R.P.T., Formerly Physical Therapy Consultant, Mental Retardation Branch, Division of Chronic Diseases, U.S.P.H.S.; now in private practice, Miami, Florida.

FOREWORD

In this book, it is good to see emphasis placed on evaluation of developmental progress early in infancy. Enough detail is given in the various presentations of modes of intervention to provide the therapist with a working knowledge of each approach described. Though the title suggests that the book is directed to the physical therapist, perusal of the volume reveals detailed modes of evaluation and management which should be of equal interest to the occupational therapist, the speech pathologist, and nurses and physicians concerned with developmental disabilities. In respect to the infant and very young child, members of all these disciplines should be familiar with the developmental reflex continuums which are so clearly described by the various authors. The chapter on feeding and prespeech by a speech therapist provides practical detailed information of special value to all.

In the field of developmental disabilities, the need for the therapist (physical, occupational, or speech) to be skilled in the teaching of parents and others as a way of extending her effectiveness is aptly and amply stressed. The need for the physical therapist to confer with other disciplines is also appropriately stressed. For the infant and very young child, consideration of assigning only one therapist to carry out treatment recommendations for each child was suggested by one author, while other therapists would serve as consultants. Our experience has supported this approach.

In addition to knowledge about motor development, therapists and those dealing with infants and young children need to be familiar with other aspects of normal child development. As indicated by the author of the chapter on residential treatment, sensory and intellectual training are equally important. Sensory input (vision, hearing, kinesthetic and tactile sensations) first enables the infant to come in contact with his environment. The physical therapist needs to be concerned with sensory input as well as with "handling and positioning." Motivation for initiation of voluntary movement, often being with visual, auditory, or sensory input. Normal reinforcement of movement surely is directly related to success in accomplishing the goal toward which the movement is directed.

Until now, teachers have been involved with learning problems mainly at kindergarten level and above. Increasing knowledge of the tremendous amount of learning achieved before kindergarten age is leading them to take a new look at the infant. By watching therapists in their skillful but frequently frustrating attempts to motivate young children to perform some motion, and by observing the teacher trained in normal child development and experienced with very young children, the special skill of the teacher in motivating the child becomes evident. In order to accomplish the most, the person working with the infant and young child, as well as with the older child, needs to know not only the appropriate intervention but the level of the child's understanding and his personality characteristics. She needs also to be sensitive to the moods of the child and aware of his level of fatigue. The role of teacher is just beginning to become defined. She will need to have a background in normal child development, a fondness for young children, and an ability to handle them. An appreciation for the need to utilize such activities as diapering, potty training, and feeding as training experiences is important. In addition, she must be willing and able to seek and utilize consultants regarding each individual child's needs.

The inclusion in the book of suggestions for the child with minimal physical handicap should prove valuable not only to the physical therapist but also to the physical education teacher. Throughout the book, the many excellent illustrations serve to make the contents more explicit. Authors have been careful to document their contributions, providing good bibliographies. Not included in the references are two which may be of special interest. Prone boards as described by J. U. Bauman,* which as-

---

*Baumann, J. U.: *Operative Behandlung der Infantilen Zerebral Paresen*. Stuttgart, G. T. Verlag, 1970.

sist in developing weight bearing and head, arm, and hand control for children who do not use long leg braces as well as those who do, have been more useful than the conventional standing boxes in our experience. Another reference relates to music therapy. Nordoff and Robbins,[†] one a musician and the other a teacher, collaborated on a book for the nontechnician describing techniques for both group and individual training for handicapped children. A demonstration of their approach in working with a group of severely involved cerebral-palsied children at St. Brendan's Clinic in Dublin, Ireland, was so spectacular as to make one wish that a film had been made of the performance.

The area of training the atypical child is a most exciting one. New approaches are being developed and more are needed. Knowledge gained from such efforts can be expected to bring information useful for the "normal" population in addition to providing assistance for the atypical children.

MARGARET JONES

[†]Nordoff, P. and Robbins, C.: *Music Therapy for Handicapped Children.* New York, Rudolf Steiner, 1965.

PREFACE

> Envy wears the mask of love, and laughing sober facts to scorn,
> Cries to Weakest as to Strongest, "Ye are equals, equal born."
> Equal born? Oh yes, if yonder hill be level with the flat.
> Charm us, Orator, till the Lion look no larger than the Cat.
> —Alfred Tennyson

The decade of the 1960's showed a tremendous increase in general interest in those who are "unequal born," the child with mental retardation, cerebral palsy, myelomeningocele, or other conditions now being called the developmental disabilities. Stimulated by such voluntary organizations as the National Association for Retarded Children, United Cerebral Palsy Associations, Inc., the National Foundation—March of Dimes, and the Easter Seal Society to name but a few, and given visible leadership by the Kennedys and fueled by an infusion of federal and local funds, the 1960's saw valiant attempts made to overcome decades of neglect for these forgotten citizens.

While most of the attention was focused on mental retardation, and rightly so in terms of sheer numbers, there was also an awakening of interest in those conditions requiring physical rehabilitation. As a result, the pediatrician and family physician, as well as the orthopedist dealing with handicapped children are being required to make more and more decisions which involve the use of the allied health professions and the physical therapist in particular.

The great majority of physicians and physical therapists now in practice were not exposed during their training to many of the techniques now in use and to the more optimistic attitudes accompanying them. The editors, therefore, have attempted in this book to provide information on physical therapy services for children with developmental disabilities which would orient and guide the physician to more effective use of the physical therapist and provide for the interested physical therapist an introduction to the newer treatment concepts and techniques.

Traditionally, the greatest use of physical therapy in the developmental disabilities of children has been in the assessment and treatment of cerebral palsy. Increasing recognition that below normal intelligence was not a valid reason for exclusion from treatment has gradually resulted in greater acceptance into the clinical practice of physical therapy of other physical handicaps such as arrested hydrocephalus, myelomeningocele, Down's anomaly, and even simply motor delay secondary to severe mental retardation. Recently, some physical therapists have expanded their areas of interest to include diagnostic and remedial procedures for those children with perceptual-motor and visual-motor disabilities. Since many of the numerically large group of mildly retarded have these more subtle, yet serious, functional handicaps, the physical therapist's contribution to the management of children with developmental disabilities should increase considerably in the future.

Physical therapy is one of the youngest of the health professions. During World War I the United States Army employed women as "restoration aides" to care for the tens of thousands of war casualties. Over the years more formalized training programs developed and the scope of their activities broadened along with the growth of physical and rehabilitative medicine. Perhaps because their origins were in rehabilitative care, physical therapists in this country, when treating cerebral palsy, have tended to borrow from techniques developed from orthopedic surgery, post-traumatic paraplegia, poliomyelitis, and so forth. In classic training, this would involve manual muscle testing, range of motion measurements, electrical diagnostic procedures, sensory tests, measurement of respiratory function and assessment of functional and daily living skills; treatment procedures included passive stretching, range of motion exercises, muscle reeducation and strengthening.

The lack of success from these essentially "peripheral" approaches to the treatment of symptoms of central or developmental origin may account in part for the lack of enthusiasm on the part of many physicians for physical therapy in the early treatment of cerebral palsy. It seems clear that there should be a basic difference in the requirements, both diagnostically and therapeutically, for those conditions arising from damage to the developing fetal or infant brain and those resulting from injury to more peripheral structures under the influence of a developed or normally developing brain.

Temple Fay (1946) was perhaps the first to take a *central* developmental approach to the treatment of cerebral palsy. Based on the neurophysiologic principle that normal postures and patterns of movement are arrived at through a series of ontogenetic developmental steps, he recommended the use of the amphibian crawl as a "necessary step in the long series of levels, through creeping, crawling, and scampering, to eventual standing and walking." It should be pointed out that Fay (1946) presented this recommendation as simply "an additional technique of training for certain cerebral palsy types. . . ."

The major systems of physical therapy chosen for inclusion in this book are the Bobath or neurodevelopmental approach, the Kabat or proprioceptive neuromuscular facilitation, and the Rood or sensorimotor approach to treatment. Critics have questioned the scientific basis for these systems (Mead 1968). Nevertheless, they have gained advocates among those working with cerebral palsy and the other developmental disabilities. The Bobath approach, in particular, is rapidly gaining international acceptance as the most effective approach to the treatment of cerebral palsy, especially in the very young child (Ellis 1967, Kong 1966). Their techniques, and to a lesser extent, the Rood techniques, are particularly attractive to those working with the mentally retarded and the very young since they do not require that the patient be able to consciously cooperate or be particularly attentive. The proprioceptive neuromuscular facilitation techniques employ passive, active, and resistance motions requiring more understanding and cooperation on the part of the patient.

For the physician, one of the sharpest criticisms that can be directed towards any therapy is that it is based on incorrect interpretations of physiologic principles. There is no doubt that the theories offered in support of these lines of therapy may be difficult to justify on known neurophysiologic grounds. Nevertheless, as pointed out by Sedgwich Mead (1968) in his 1967 presidential address to the American Academy of Cerebral Palsy, "Neurophysiologic doctrine is a most perishable commodity and it is a mistake to pin one's hopes on a current interpretation."

Ellis (1967) argues that particularly "in the case of the Bobaths' method of treatment, a theoretical explanation had to be found for the method of treatment which was successful in practice. Our knowledge of the function of the higher levels of the central nervous system may still be inadequate to explain observed facts."

Commenting on the very early treatment of cerebral palsy, Dennis Browne (1966) put forward two principles:

> (1) When the outcome of doing nothing is uncertain, all cases should be treated without exception. This applies just as much to cerebral palsy as to congenitally unstable hips or to scoliosis of the newborn. Most of these correct themselves spontaneously, but if they are left to see which will and which won't, there is a residue of disasters.
> (2) In any congenital abnormality, the earlier treatment is started, the better the results.

It can also be pointed out that while there is no doubt that the basis of these lines of therapy may be difficult to justify on present neurophysiologic knowledge, explanations which are not accepted as dogma in themselves may be the stimulus for fruitful investigations, debate, and discussion and lead to better understanding. There is a wide gap between dogma and a questioning eclecticism. At the same time, to deny available methods when the outcome of doing nothing is uncertain will, as Dennis Browne says, leave a residue of disasters.

The editors take full responsibility for the selection of those systems of treatment included and for those omitted. Space limitations combined with personal judgement, or bias, dictated the selection of the material included. On this point, some criticism could be made for including a chapter on speech therapy in a book on physical therapy services. The decision to include Miss

Mueller's chapter was dictated both by the desire to familiarize the American reader with her work as well as the possibilities this chapter contains for direct application by physical therapists.

PAUL H. PEARSON
CAROL ETHUN WILLIAMS

REFERENCES

Browne, D.: Very early treatment of cerebral palsy. *Develop Med Child Neurol, 8:*473, 1966.

Ellis, E.: *The Physical Management of Developmental Disorders.* Little Club Clinics in Developmental Medicine, No. 26. The Spastics Society, Medical Education and Information Unit. London, Heinemann, 1967.

Fay, T.: Observation on rehabilitation of movement in cerebral palsy problems. *W Virginia Med J, 42:*77, 1946.

Kong, E.: Very early treatment of cerebral palsy. *Develop Med Child Neurol, 8:*198-202, 1966.

Mead, S.: Presidential address. The treatment of cerebral palsy. *Develop Med Child Neurol, 10:*423-426, 1968.

ACKNOWLEDGMENTS

We first wish to thank the contributors to this volume for their patience with the editors and their editing. The considerable contributions of Mrs. Leila Green and Mrs. Nancy Fieber in the editing process also must be acknowledged. We are equally indebted to Judy Welk, artist and friend, who prepared the illustrations for Chapter Ten. Last, but not least in importance, was the cheerful forbearance of Miss Kathy Moore who typed and retyped the manuscript.

P.H.P.
C.E.W.

CONTENTS

	Page
Contributors	vii
Foreword—MARGARET JONES	ix
Preface	xiii
Acknowledgments	xix

SECTION ONE
MANAGEMENT

Chapter

One. GENERAL PRINCIPLES IN THE MANAGEMENT OF THE DEVELOPMENTAL DISABILITIES—*Paul H. Pearson* 5
    Introduction 5
    General Principles of Management 7
    Summary 13

Two. THE PHYSICIAN AND THE PHYSICAL THERAPIST: THEIR ROLES IN THE DEVELOPMENTAL DISABILITIES—*E. Jack Trembath and Paul H. Pearson* 17
    Introduction 17
    Assessment 19
    Planning the Treatment Program 21
    Specific Disabilities 23
    Summary 26

SECTION TWO
THE THERAPIES

Three. CEREBRAL PALSY—*Karel Bobath and Berta Bobath* 31
    PART 1
    Diagnosis and Assessment of Cerebral Palsy
    Background Information 31

xxii *Physical Therapy Services in the Developmental Disabilities*

Neurophysiologic Basis of Motor Development	41
Some Basic Concepts of Brain Function	41
The Relationship of Automatic to Voluntary Movement	43
The Development of Normal Motor Abilities	44
Sequential Development of Motor Activity	48
The Neurologic Picture in Cerebral Palsy	64
Tonic Reflex Activity	64
Abnormal Muscle Tone	76
The Type of Disturbance of Reciprocal Innervation	81
Characteristic Types of Cerebral Palsy	83
Diagnosis and Assessment	101
Early Diagnosis	101
Assessment	104

PART 2

The Neurodevelopmental Approach to Treatment	
Theoretical Considerations	114
Principles of Treatment	117
The Planning of a Treatment Program	121
Techniques of Treatment	126
The Use of Reflex-Inhibiting Patterns	126
Techniques of Facilitation	134
Techniques of Proprioceptive and Tactile Stimulation	170
General Management	173
The Link-up of Physical Therapy with Occupational and Speech Therapy	173
The Importance of Play	175
The Management of the Child Outside Treatment Sessions	177

Four. A SENSORIMOTOR APPROACH TO TREATMENT—*Shirley A. Stockmeyer* 186

Contents

Basic Concepts	186
The Contribution of Physical Therapy Treatment and the Total Development of the Child	186
Duality of Sensorimotor Functions as a Basis for a Therapeutic Approach	187
The Influence of Sensory Factors in Total Development	188
General Treatment Procedures	192
The Development of Mobilizing Responses and Their Role in Coordinating Movement	197
The Development of Stabilizing Responses and Their Role in Coordinating Movement	201
Combining Mobility and Stability Functions	210
Treatment of Specific Problems	212
The Child Whose Sensorimotor Activities Are Normal but Delayed in Relation to His Chronological Age	213
The Child Whose Movements Are Slow, Stereotyped, and Difficult to Initiate	214
The Child Who Is Hypotonic and Lacks the Reflex Basis for Movement and Posture	215
The Child Who Lacks the Controlling Influence of Stabilizers	216
The Hyperactive Child Whose Sensorimotor Activity Is Dominated by Tactile Avoidance Responses and a Low Threshold for Environmental Stimuli.	217
Five. PROPRIOCEPTIVE NEUROMUSCULAR FACILITATION: THE PNF METHOD—*Dorothy E. Voss*	223
Guide Lines from Animal Behavior	224
Guide Lines from Human Behavior	228
Unique Features of the PNF Method	232
Assessment of Motor Performance	235
The Problem	252
General Suggestions	253

	Primary Problems and Suggested Procedures	261
	Closing Comment	279
Six.	FACILITATING FEEDING AND PRESPEECH—*Helen A. Mueller*	283
	The Approach	283
	Sensorimotor Evaluation	285
	Feeding Behavior	286
	Breathing, Voice, Phonation	291
	Basic Principles of the Technique	293
	Facilitating Feeding	294
	Facilitating Prespeech	305
Seven.	THE USE OF MOVEMENT ACTIVITIES IN THE EDUCATION OF RETARDED CHILDREN—*Bryant J. Cratty*	311
	Phase I: Impulse Control	312
	Phase II: Body-Image Training	319
	Phase III: Perceptual-Motor Competencies	324
	Phase IV: Seriation	332
	Phase V: Pattern Recognition	333
	Phase VI: Decision Making and Problem Solving	335
Eight.	IMPROVING THE PHYSICAL FITNESS OF RETARDATES—*Bryant J. Cratty*	338
	Program Guide Lines	339
	Equipment and Facilities	340
	Game Modifications to Promote Fitness	345
	Suggested Exercise	348
	Summary	350

SECTION THREE
PROGRAMS

Nine.	PHYSICAL THERAPY IN A CHILDREN'S REHABILITATION CENTER—*Nancy M. Fieber and Duane Kliewer*	355
	Who Are the Developmentally Disabled?	356
	Physical Therapy Evaluation	359
	Developmental and Functional Assessment	360

Neurodevelopmental Evaluation of Postural Reflex Mechanisms and Tone	365
Evaluation of Muscle Strength	368
Evaluation of Musculoskeletal Status in Terms of Range of Motion, Limb Measurements, and Postural Deviations	369
Evaluation of Specific and Integrative Sensory Functions	370
Evaluation of Perceptual-Motor Skills	372
General Suggestions	374
The Treatment Program	376
Setting Goals	376
Types of Programs	377
Role of Physical Therapy at Different Ages	379
Programming for the Child with Perceptual-Motor Disability	396
A Good Home Program	404
Coordination Between Services	406
The Schedule and Service	409
Organization of Space and Equipment	409

Ten. PHYSICAL THERAPY IN RESIDENTIAL FACILITIES—*Carol Ethun Williams* ... 420

Introduction	420
Administration of the Physical Therapy Department	422
Program Planning	422
The Physical Therapy Department	444

Physical Therapy Services
in the
Developmental Disabilities

SECTION ONE
Management

Chapter One

GENERAL PRINCIPLES IN THE MANAGEMENT OF THE DEVELOPMENTAL DISABILITIES

PAUL H. PEARSON

Introduction

THE PURPOSE of this chapter is to discuss general principles in the medical management of the handicapped, but with particular emphasis as it relates to physical therapy for the child with mental retardation, cerebral palsy and the other developmental disabilities.

Management is probably the least understood part of the care of the handicapped. To do it well requires wide experience, sound professional knowledge, a particular appreciation of the contributions to be made by the educational and social as well as the health disciplines, and the ability to organize and coordinate these various needs. Above all, it requires a basic humility leavened by concern for the fellow human we are trying to assist. Without this, the problem of professional omnipotence as it relates to both the patient and one's colleagues can raise barriers to effective management. While treatment for a specific condition can be carried out in relative professional isolation, management of the person who is handicapped requires both interprofessional collaboration and the application of human management principles.

The discussion will be centered on management of the child who is handicapped, although the principles can be applied with equal validity to the handicapped adult. It is during infancy and childhood that the factors of growth and development as they react with a constantly changing emotional, physical, and social environment make effective management as difficult as it is crucial. Historically, attention, especially in the medical profession, has been centered on treatment of the handicap, forgetting, as Sheridan (1965) puts it "the child who happened, as it were, to be attached to the handicap. . . ."

All too often when discussing such a child we start off by describing his handicaps rather than his capabilities, forgetting that treatment and training, indeed the whole management program, must be based on what the child can do rather than what he cannot do. Indeed, to focus on the child's deficits will often limit one's expectations and therefore influence what is done for the child. The diagnosis may in that case become the prognosis.

This myopia can be overcome if we accept as the goal of management the *maximum normalization of the child and his family*. This concept of *normalization* (Nirji 1969) for the handicapped individual is, as Dybwad (1969) states, a concept "elegant in its simplicity and parsimony. . . . It can be readily understood by everyone. . . ." But, like most basic ideas it has far-reaching implications when placed in practice.

As Dybwad points out, it entails programming on three levels. First, it entails teaching the deviant individual within the limits of his abilities so that his every act of daily living approaches that of his normal counterpart. This, as mentioned earlier, requires an accurate assessment of ability rather than disability. Secondly, it is concerned with our interpretations of the deviant person to others; that is, our methods of communication, verbal and visual, should serve to maximize his similarities and minimize his differences to others. This will have a circular effect on those working with the physically and mentally deviant and in turn on the deviants' self-perception. If our words and our actions indicate a concern for a child, not a spastic limb, and an expectation for development, limited though it may be, the effect on the handicapped individual and his family cannot help but be to strive towards those goals we set.

The third level of programming for normalization involves moving public attitudes towards greater acceptance of deviancy per se. "The deviancy . . . will be diminished to the degree that ordinary citizens gain a broader perception of normality and become accepting of a wider range of variation in the performance, appearance, and capability of fellow human beings" (Dybwad 1969).

General Principles of Management

The cardinal principle in effective management of the problems of the child who is handicapped is that the program must be concerned with both the child and his family. At the same time, this need to be concerned with the family as well as the individual can create serious problems unless the program, while centered around the family, is kept sharply focused on the needs of the person who is handicapped.

It has often been said that the ultimate prognosis for any handicapped child is as much dependent on the functional effectiveness of the family in dealing with the problems such a child creates as in the child's own capabilities. Although this may somewhat overstate the case, it is clear that the family is of central importance in management, both in terms of direct reduction of the disability and in the broader sense of dealing with the consequences of that disability. The interfamily relationships are directly affected by the presence of a handicapped child and the way in which they are affected will have direct relevance to the success in achieving the goal of maximum normalization for both child and family. The family "serves as a funnel for the communication of ideas, concepts and values which are culturally significant; it can maintain a continuous and stable background against which the progress towards maturity and independence can be achieved without loss of security" (The Carnegie U. K. Trust 1964).

The family is the principle, and often the least utilized, source of help to the child who is handicapped. The long-term nature of these problems and the need to utilize a diversity of health, educational, and other social services are factors which become monumental unless the family is maintained as an effective, functional unit (Begab 1966). Direct involvement of the family as *therapists* in a specific program developed by the professionals for their child is in itself an effective way of mobilizing the family's energies towards constructive efforts. Thus, by taking advantage of the parents' very real need to be doing something to help their child, the demands on scarce professional time can be reduced while at the same time greatly increasing the treatment time for each child.

To do this well requires, first, that the professional accept the concept that nonprofessionals can be taught specific therapeutic techniques; second, that the parent receives adequate, ongoing instruction and supervision; and, third, sensitive support from the professionals. This use of parents as therapists for their own child can be utilized most effectively in physical therapy but also has its place in speech and occupational therapy. It has the further advantage of showing the parents that they have a significant role in their child's treatment which need not be entirely abrogated to the experts.

A word of warning, however, is due on this point. The degree to which parents can be utilized effectively in treating their own child will, of course, vary widely. The responsible professionals must at all times be aware of the capabilities of the parents for such involvement. Before shifting the burden of treatment and training back to parents, particularly with those who have come to depend heavily on professionals, careful consideration must be given to the family's resources, both internal and external. Their tolerance will depend both on their physical, temporal, intellectual, and emotional resources and on their child's combination of problems.

The elderly parent or one with physical handicaps of his own may not be able to handle a heavy or badly handicapped child. A working mother or one with a large family simply may not have adequate time or energies to invest in a strenuous home therapy program. Other parents will not be emotionally capable of such direct involvement with their child. All parents will require professional support and understanding, for they feel quite keenly the added responsibility of contributing directly to their child's treatment. "If I don't do it properly, I will be responsible for his failure to make progress." This also throws added responsibilities onto the professionals to provide realistic objectives so that the parent does not blame himself unnecessarily for the child's failure to reach stated goals.

The importance of keeping the program goals sharply focused on the "child attached to the handicap" can be and often is overlooked. Particularly in dealing with conditions for which there is no absolute cure, therapeutic defeatism may threaten professional omnipotence and it becomes easier to shift the *focus* of efforts to the needs of the family which arise from the presence of the disabled child. The physician's concern for the child is displaced by his concern for the family (Dybwad 1964). This is particularly true in the case of the child with severe physical or mental handicaps where our ability to substantially improve function may be limited, forgetting as it were, "that the physician is just as responsible for alleviating as for curing . . ." (Powers 1953).

This phenomena may also account for the disproportionate amount of effort often expended in diagnostic and assessment procedures, with little being done therapeutically as a result. All too often after the initial and often repeated diagnostic procedures, the major concern, particularly as it pertains to treatment, becomes focused on counseling the parents—not on what might be done for their child, but on how to "accept their burden." Difficulty in obtaining any help for their child simply provides frustration to compound their natural feelings of guilt and sorrow. How much more effective if we focus instead on what can be done to ameliorate the child's handicaps and provide programs which take advantage of his capabilities, limited though they may be, thus providing some measure of relief for the *cause* of the family's emotional problems (Pearson 1965).

This same point must be made in the discussion of the second general principle for successful management. Because most of these problems are lifelong, they require long-term planning with periodic reassessment and programmatic updating. While this principle may seem an obvious one, it is often overlooked or carried out in a haphazard or desultory manner. For various reasons, many clinics seem to utilize the greater part of their energies in carrying out exhaustive diagnostic and assessment procedures while giving only minimal attention to planning an effective, ongoing program with the family (Wolfensberger 1965). Thus, the assessment becomes largely an academic exercise of interest to the professionals involved but of little value to the handicapped child and his frustrated family who must continue shopping in hopes of obtaining real help for their child's very real problems.

The corollary to this principle is that in children, all planning must evolve from a knowledge of growth and development, physical and intellectual, emotional and social. The basic principles of good child health care are as important in working with handicapped children as in normal children (Holt 1966). We do well to remember that children with cerebral palsy are not born with deformities; rather, they have deformity-producing tendencies resulting from their abnormal patterns of posture and movement. As growth takes place, these tendencies are likely to be fulfilled unless we provide preventive or ameliorating therapy.

Intellectual and emotional development are greatly affected by the kind of sensory and motor experiences provided. The child who is physically handicapped and cannot explore his environment may be just as impoverished as the deprived child left to lie in his crib all day. Emotional deprivation may also occur if the mother withdraws from the mentally retarded child who fails to provide necessary feedback for her, or if physical contact with an abnormally stiff or floppy baby is repugnant to her. The need to provide optimum sensory stimulation for the normal child is well recognized. In the handicapped child it becomes not only more critical, but often requires specifically directed kinds of stimulation to compensate for sensory, motor or intellectual deficits or to circumvent abnormal reactions to normal sensory input.

It follows from this that diagnostic assessment and treatment must be carried out at the earliest possible age. The handicapped or retarded child has limited abilities with which to compensate for previous experiential deficits. Equally important in the child with severe motor delay or with cerebral palsy is the need to prevent the establishment of abnormal movement patterns by means of treatment techniques which will facilitate development of potential ability in a more normal way (Bobath 1967). All too often, valuable treatment time is lost when treatment is not started until the appearance of deformity signals the unquestioned need for referral to the appropriate specialist.

It is a pediatric maxim that the child is not a small adult with miniaturized versions of adult needs. Thus a sound understanding of normal child development is required in order to appreciate the problems arising from the interplay of the handicap with the maturing organism. The child's environment is changing as he grows with the result that the handicap will have different significance for the child, his family, and society at different life stages (Holt 1966).

The physically handicapped infant or toddler is unaware of or may show a remarkable ability to bypass a defect which is of major concern to his parents. By school age, problems of peer acceptance may be paramount, for contrary to popular belief, the retarded person is often acutely aware that he is not "equal born." The mildly retarded child may escape notice of parents and professionals until the school years, require specialized educational and vocational services during that time, and as an adult, if character and emotional development are adequate, escape further notice from the community in which he may marry and support a family.

The need for periodic updating of the program is more obvious in the rapidly developing child or growing youth but is of equal importance in the handicapped adult. The frequency of reassessment may only be less in adults.

The third general principle is that effective management requires true interdisciplinary collaboration and coordination. This is probably the most difficult principle to put into practice and the least understood. Yet, without it, the handicapped child and his family can become confused wanderers adrift between "circumscribed islands of service" (Thelander 1964). This is a particular problem between the health and education professions where there is often an ocean of mistrust and misunderstanding.

The problem is further complicated by the question of who among the various professions will provide the necessary central point of reference or supervision to insure both program coordination and continuity of services.

There is no simple rule which will accomplish true interdisciplinary coordination, unless it is the golden rule. It requires first and foremost an understanding and appreciation of the contributions the other disciplines can make. In addition, it is absolutely essential that all participants find a means of communicating about their objectives and their activities. This means of communication must be explicitly provided for with the recognition that it takes energy, time and resources. The problem of communications, while greatest between medicine and education, also exists between closely related disciplines where the same words, for example, may have quite different meanings.

With effective communication, the groundwork for cooperation can be laid. Since true cooperation yields a product which is greater than the sum of its parts, it requires that those who participate learn certain basic principles and techniques. The mere wish to cooperate is not sufficient. As one health official said, "When it comes to cooperating, what I want to know is, who is going to be doing the *co-ing* and who is going to be doing the *operating?*" This is the real nut of the problem since the "co-ing" and "operating" roles will have to be different at different times and for different needs. In addition, these roles are not necessarily reciprocal between any two people or agencies in any given situation. All concerned must understand the need for a shifting of authority and emphasis at different times and at different life stages depending on both the kind and degree of handicap present and the availability of services to meet these needs.

The pediatrician or family physician involved in the management of the very young child with spastic cerebral palsy and mild mental retardation, for example, must know how to utilize physical therapy along with occupational, speech, and drug therapy. Later he may consider the need for orthopedic surgery or bracing. Since he is the only member of this team primarily concerned with the whole child, it is important for him to integrate each of these therapies so as to realize the maximum benefits of each. Concurrently, he may counsel the family or refer them to various social and welfare agencies for counseling or for financial and other assistance. During this period, he is the one professional most apt to be familiar with the child and the family in terms of their needs and resources and therefore able to provide the continuity needed for adequate supervision and coordination (Pearson and Meneffee 1965, Pearson 1968).

By school age, these medical problems may have become relatively stable so that the child's prime needs, and therefore the program emphasis, become educational. At this time the physician must recognize that the child's basic right to receive training and education to the degree commensurate with his potential must not be subordinated to an overemphasis on a medical program. The educator must also bear in mind that it is particularly in the severely handicapped child that a sound medical program can provide the foundation on which to build the educational and other necessary life services (Pearson 1965). Success in terms of helping the child to achieve his maximum potential will then depend on the degree to which each professional is able to consider the whole child while bringing to bear his own expertise to alleviate specific handicaps.

Summary

We must keep in mind that the needs of the handicapped child are almost always multiple, complex, and changing (Fig. 1-1.). A number of interrelated dimensions of needs and relevant factors must be incorporated in meaningful ways if these needs are to be met effectively.

First, there is the particular combination of handicaps present and their relative degrees of severity. The child with severe cerebral palsy but with little or no intellectual deficit has both similar and markedly different needs compared to the severely retarded child with little or no neuromuscular deficit. All will have both generic and specialized needs in health, physical and emotional, in education, including training in activities of daily living, and in social or vocational areas.

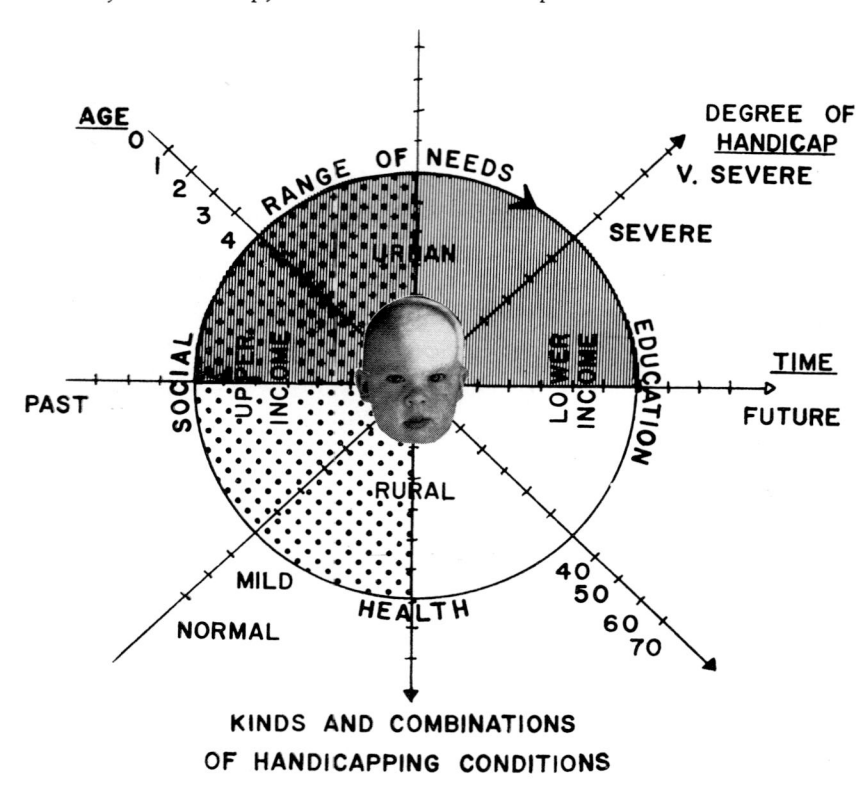

14   *Physical Therapy Services in the Developmental Disabilities*

Figure 1-1. Various dimensions of the problem.

Second, there is the setting in which the child is found, with its many important implications for optimal management. The type of community, the availability of services, and the resources of the family, emotional, intellectual and financial, will all be determining factors in any planning. The child with multiple handicaps secondary to maternal rubella in the first trimester of pregnancy born into a well-to-do family living near a major urban university presents quite a different problem in management when compared to the child with the same handicaps born to a poorly educated family living on a farm in a sparsely populated rural area.

All the above factors are relevant and interacting with respect to any given child and possess dynamic and fluid properties. The child will grow older and the nature of his needs will change with time. In many cases, the setting in which the child lives will change, and all the service agencies relating to his various needs will change.

If we are to successfully assist the child to achieve the optimal development commensurate with his abilities, we must (1) begin the management program as early as possible, (2) keep the program objectives sharply focused on the unique needs of the individual child, (3) involve and utilize the child's family in a meaningful way, (4) provide long-term and continuous planning based on sound principles of child development, and (5) require coordinated interdisciplinary cooperation in the provision of services.

BIBLIOGRAPHY

Begab, M.: The mentally retarded and the family. In Philips, I. (Ed.): *Prevention and Treatment of Mental Retardation*. New York, Basic Books, 1966.

Bobath, B.: The very early treatment of cerebral palsy. *Develop Med Child Neurol, 9*:373-390, 1967.

The Carnegie U. K. Trust: Handicapped Children and Their Families. Reports to the Carnegie United Kingdom Trust on the Problems of 600 Handicapped Children and Their Families. Dunfermilne, 1964.

Dybwad, G.: Action implication, U.S.A. today. In Kugel, R. and Wolfensberger, W. (Eds.): *Changing Patterns in Residential Services for the Mentally Retarded*. President's Committee on Mental Retardation. Washington, D.C., 1969.

Dybwad, G.: *Challenges in Mental Retardation*. New York, Columbia, 1964.

Holt, K.: The handicapped child. *Proc Roy Soc Med, 59*:134-150, 1966.

Nirji, B.: The normalization principle and its human management implications. In Kugel, R. and Wolfensberger, W. (Eds.): *Changing Patterns in Residential Services for the Mentally Retarded*. President's Committee on Mental Retardation, Washington, D.C., 1969.

Pearson, P.H.: The forgotten patient: Medical management of the multiply handicapped retarded. *Public Health Rep, 80*:915-918, 1965.

Pearson, P.H., and Menefee, A.R.: Medical and social management of the mentally retarded. *GP, 31:78-91, 1965*.

Pearson, P.H.: The physician's role in diagnosis and management of the mentally retarded. *Pediat Clin N Amer, 5*:835-859, 1968.

Powers, G.P.: The retarded child and his family as a challenge to pediatric practice. *Pediatrics, 12:*210-266, 1953.

Sheridan, M.D.: *The Handicapped Child and His Home.* National Children's Home, Highbury Park, London, New Jersey, 1965.

Thelander, H.E.: Redevelopment in pediatrics. *Amer J Dis Child, 108:*316-319, 1964.

Wolfensberger, W.: Embarrassments in the diagnostic process. *Ment Retard, 3:*29-31, 1965.

Chapter Two

THE PHYSICIAN AND THE PHYSICAL THERAPIST: THEIR ROLES IN THE DEVELOPMENTAL DISABILITIES

E. Jack Trembath and Paul H. Pearson

Introduction

Physical therapy is playing an increasingly important role in the overall management of the child with developmental disabilities. Coincidentally, the broad nature of developmental disabilities and the evolution of roles played by allied health professionals has brought about a blurring of classic boundaries and a changing accent on the nature of the help and assistance the therapist may provide. This is why the field of developmental disabilities is today offering a wider challenge to the skills and imagination of the physical therapist.

The spectrum of handicaps which are present in the developmental disorders, such as cerebral palsy and mental retardation, offers to the physical therapist the opportunity of a wide variety of problems, where emphasis may range from diagnostic evaluation of the young child, to teaching management techniques to parents, to the imaginative application of knowledge in treatment. At the same time, to make optimal use of their professional skills, both therapist and physician must understand the limitations and the attributes of the therapist's art.

Because of the serious shortage of therapists skilled in treating children with developmental disabilities, it is equally important that both physician and therapist be aware of ways to extend treatment time beyond the traditional one-on-one, therapist-child relationship. Probably the best method will be through the education of the parents and parent surrogates in the application of specific therapeutic methods to meet the daily needs of children with handicaps. This means the physician, the physical therapist, and the mother or mother surrogate must all be involved in the handling and management of the child. This is the essence of good therapy!

The central therapeutic emphasis in working with these children should be on the transmission of motor and sensory information, and its integration and useful application by the child. The therapist or parent-therapist at all times must monitor and correct the child's application of this sensory-motor information much in the same way any teacher does with educational information given to children in the school classroom (Halpern 1969). The teaching characteristics of the physical therapist, therefore, become basic to any physical therapy program with children. This educational emphasis is a somewhat different use of the physical therapist, who in the past has been used primarily as a technician. To place the attention of any professional within a limited sphere of a specific technical ability is to limit the scope of modern management.

Developmental disabilities are distributed in many functional areas. The distribution is not uniform and the involvement of the physical therapist in the general rehabilitative process will vary with the degree and kind of handicap which the child may present. Integrated therapy programs today will require not only the services of the physical therapist but those of an occupational and speech therapist. The occupational therapist will emphasize the visual-motor, visual-perceptual and fine motor coordination and the speech therapist will be concerned with the neurological basis of language development and communication problems.

It is probably most helpful to see them as supporting disciplines since many children with developmental disabilities at all levels will require the combined efforts of these professionals. For example, a child with borderline intellectual functioning with visual-perceptual problems and poor static balance skills will require the effective use of both disciplines. At the upper end of the continuum, the severely retarded, bedridden, spastic quadriplegic will require assistance with activities of daily living as well as corrective positioning for the prevention of contracture and deformity. The child with motor apraxia or with difficulty in the organization of complex motor acts may readily be identified through the analysis of the complex act of speaking with the cooperation and involvement of the speech therapist. The physical therapist, occupational therapist and speech therapist can also assist the psychologist's assessment of children and further the definition of the overall problem through their own testing and study of perceptual-motor function.

Assessment

Since treatment, to be successful, starts with a base line for guidance, it will be important for the physical therapist to know both *what* the child can do and *why* he can do some things and cannot do others. This requires an assessment of the child's development in terms of the evolution of the postural reflex mechanisms and the degree to which they are interfered with by abnormal postural reflex activity in association with abnormal postural tone (Paine et al. 1964, Bobath and Bobath, Ch. 3). In addition, for the child with motor delay secondary to intellectual deficit, the assessment of the availability of motor activities *developmentally* becomes important. This information enables the physical therapist to include in the treatment program training in these motor activities as they become available (Halpern 1969). It also permits training of the neuromotor prerequisite necessary for the next level of motor development.*

Thus, the physician seeing an infant with developmental disability must determine to what extent the lack of coordinated motor function stems from the stage of development or is the result of abnormal neurologic reflex patterns and abnormal muscle tone since this becomes important both in terms of management and prognosis.

In the case of simple mental retardation, early recognition is generally dependent on the identification of a delay or deviation in the motor milestones. That is, the established motor developmental norms are the guide lines for the physician in the early

---

*(See Ch. 9, sect. on "Role of Physical Therapy at Different Ages.")

recognition of possible intellectual deficit. At the same time it must be recognized that many routine postnatal checkups depend heavily on the mother's history which is often unreliable. Often the routine outpatient visits consist of an evaluation of the child against the physician's personalized, internalized norms supported in the main by pragmatic hopefulness.

Although many pediatricians become quite skilled at early recognition of developmental deviation, such "eyeball observations" and testing of deep tendon reflexes will not provide all the developmental information that is needed. Unless the physician routinely includes in his assessment such standardized methods as those of the Denver Developmental Screening Test (Frankenburg and Dodds 1966) or the motor development screening examination of Milani-Comparetti and Gidoni (1967), the recognition of the child with motor and mental retardation will often be postponed considerably beyond the time when a diagnosis might have been made. It is an accepted fact that the earlier treatment is started in any congenital defect, the better the results will be (Browne 1966).

Where cerebral palsy is suspected the average static central nervous system examination simply will not provide the necessary type of information to plan an adequate treatment program. This has made it necessary for physicians and indeed the well-trained physical therapist working with young children to incorporate the methods of André-Thomas, Yves Chesni, S. Saint-Anne Dargassies (1960) and Pieper (1964) into a systematic functional assessment of neuromotor status.

With this information, the aims of treatment then will be to counteract the development of abnormal tone and postural reaction, to facilitate the development of normal postural reaction with functional patterns of movement which will later be incorporated into self-help skills such as ambulation, feeding, dressing, and prevent the development of deformity. The child's progress may then be followed by noting the sequential acquisition of the normal mechanisms, the disappearance of abnormal postures, tones, and abnormal reflexes.

Planning the Treatment Program

Inclusion of the physical therapist in the treatment program of a child with developmental disabilities is extremely important. Ideally, this should be done as soon as there is a reasonable presumption that the child has any abnormality of neuromotor integration, even as early as two or three months of age in the case of cerebral palsy (Kong 1966).

If the therapist is not developmentally oriented or has had little experience with infants, the physician must take time to work out a systematic developmental program and provide the therapist with guides to information on child development. If this is not done, the most that can be accomplished is in maintenance of range of motion and prevention of deformities and contractures. At the same time much therapeutic time is being lost. "Treatment can at best help the child to develop his full potential abilities. If treatment is started before abnormal patterns have become established, it can help him organize his potential ability in the most normal way" (Bobath 1967).

Differences of opinion exist as to how specific the physician should be in his instructions to the therapist. Unless he is quite knowledgeable about physical therapy and can maintain very close supervisory contact with the progress of treatment, he is better off to provide the therapist with the necessary information concerning the child's problems, his developmental status, any necessary restrictions, and the specific goals he wishes to reach. A well-trained therapist can then utilize those techniques he feels will bring about the desired result. Some physical therapists may ask for very specific instructions from the physician. In this situation, the physician should satisfy himself that he is not dealing with an individual with limited knowledge or experience in the treatment of young children with neurodevelopmental problems.

The physician should also make certain that the physical therapist spends a major portion of each treatment session teaching the mother the special ways to handle her baby and how to carry out at home the essential treatment techniques needed by her child. The importance of this approach is easily demonstrated when one considers the relatively small fraction of time the therapist can spend with any one child. In addition, and of equal importance, is the fact that particularly in the severely handicapped retarded child, the mother often cannot "come to the child"; that is, acceptance and therefore physical contact is often very difficult for her.

Handling is physical handling, the actual normal contact of the adult caretakers with the child throughout the day. As much of the physical therapy—especially if the neurodevelopmental approaches are utilized—is performed on the floor in a play situation, this direct involvement should become a rewarding experience for the mother as she watches the child acquire, even if slowly and ever so laboriously, some of those so easily acquired yet little understood patterns of behavior and motor development which are accepted as a matter of course in the normal child.

If the mother is in daily physical and emotional contact with the child on a program with short-term goals which are attainable, she begins to understand that although the child may not be progressing rapidly, he is progressing; furthermore, she realizes that realistic goals have been set. This is in contrast to the parent who is sent away from the office with the remark that the child is mentally retarded or has "some cerebral palsy" and told to come back for reevaluation in six months. This whole hiatus of time is left for the mother to stew over an unacceptable diagnosis given in the most indifferent terms.

Most mothers can be taught specific handling and physical therapy techniques which apply to their own baby and become proficient in a suprisingly short time (Ethun 1966, Fieber and Kliewer, Ch. 9). The therapist needs to provide the mother with a specific list of instructions, usually including some simple line drawings to illustrate positional aspects, which are to be carried out daily at home. These are then modified and updated as the child progresses through various stages of development. Although initially time-consuming, this approach makes it possible to reduce the frequency of clinic visits and thus enables the therapist to treat many more children.

The importance of the home program cannot be stressed enough. In fact it seems safe to say that unless the mother can provide a knowledgeable extension of the therapist's efforts through a daily home program, the ultimate results will be little affected by the physical therapy given in the clinic setting. Incorporating the mother into the treatment program not only greatly increases the treatment time for each child but should provide considerable psychological benefits to the parent as well. At the same time, as pointed out in the previous chapter, the physician should be aware that any conscientious parent will feel the weight of responsibility for treating their own child and will require considerable reassurance and support on this point.

Specific Disabilities

There are many defined conditions in which the physical therapist has worked in the past, such as central nervous system dysfunction with residuals, muscular dystrophy, poliomyelitis and meningomyelocele. The latter disorder probably illustrates more readily the need today of interaction between teams of disciplined professionals, each with an interest in aspects of the condition and each primarily directing their attention toward the preparation of the child for effective use of education and, by this means, interaction with his environment.

The physical therapist's role has been in the prevention of contractures, maintenance of a full range of motions, the use of the maximum muscle power and the education of a braced child towards the erect posture and a practical gait. If these are not possible, it should be remembered that a child may participate well in an educational process, provided that the alternative of transfer activities and wheelchair life are correctly taught to the child.

Children with chronic neurological handicaps are in the growing process and the normal progression towards independence should be recognized and guidance provided by all therapists. By the adoption of a correct teaching approach, the physical therapist prepares the child for his subsequent educational experiences.

A common condition of mental retardation with a diagnostic anomaly is Down's syndrome. Despite the fact that this is usually not associated with gross neuromotor dysfunction, the physical therapist can provide assessment of the motor development as well as programs for motor training and physical fitness. During infancy this will involve teaching the parents ways to facilitate and challenge the child toward ambulation and other gross motor skills. In older children, directed play activities leading to improved body-image, left-right orientation, and fine motor coordination can be carried out. Explaining the process of motor development and anticipating stages of change are important both for the child's development and hopefully the attitudes of the parents.

Parents are often told the diagnosis of their child when confronted with his slow development, but are given little direct assistance. A program can be arranged in which they actively participate in the developmental training for their child. This personal involvement cannot be too greatly stressed if the parents are to realize that although the developmental norms and guide lines for the average child do not apply to their child, significant gains are still able to be made at a relatively slower rate. This should encourage them and strengthen their desire for good rehabilitative services for their child. One should avoid both the Scylla of over-encouragement and overinvolvement with the Charybdis of disinterest.

In no area are the professional lines more blurred and the roles more overlapping for physicians, physical therapists, educators, psychologists, occupational and speech therapists than in the apraxias of movement in which children are incapable of the volitional planning and execution of motor tasks. Associated often with mild mental retardation, these children, in order to function, in an education program, will need the assistance of all the helping professions in the acquisition of good posture, equilibrium, visual-motor, visual-perceptual, auditory and verbal skills.

The whole process of normalization (Nirji 1969) for these children should commence with efforts to overcome these apraxic movements. These are the old-fashioned stigma of the "funny-looking kid" which, associated with minor skeletal or physical anomalies, often distinguishes a handicapped and mentally retarded child from his peers. Even if the congenital anomalies are not subject to remedial efforts, a sustained effort should be made to incorporate all disciplines early in the correction of the associated neuromotor problems. This again represents a challenge to the physical therapist. Here a broader knowledge of child development, physical abnormality and remedial therapy is required.

Cerebral palsy and mental retardation have been inextricably mixed, although the degree of mental retardation, if any, can be primary or secondary to a specific muscular involvement such as a dyskinetic type. Of particular interest is the milder involvement in cerebral palsy where the functional impairment is slight and the child must be carefully explored and evaluated for motor, intellectual and visual-perceptual problems.

Again it cannot be stressed too strongly that the teaching process ideally should include those people in direct contact with the child. It is not possible nor will it be in the near future for us to have sufficient physical therapists to provide care on a one-to-one basis for handicapped children. The ideal primary therapist is still the parent. It has been our experience that the parents manage their children well. Nothing is more saddening or more useless than to see the physical therapist working with the child while the parent is sitting in a chair reading a magazine. This often is not by parental desire but is the result of an unconscious surrendering by the parent and an assumption by the therapist of primary responsibility for the child's development.

If at any time it is decided to place a severely handicapped child in a residential facility it should be done only with the greatest of care. It is the severely retarded, multiply handicapped child who is most likely to be placed on a back ward, kept in a crib and given little more than nursing care, becoming more and more immobile from the resulting contractures and severe deformities. This restriction of mobility is a restriction of environmental interaction resulting in a further depression of functional abilities. Instead, treatment must be directed towards training these patients to be mobile and self-sufficient in activities of daily living, including work, play and educational activities where possible.

The provision within a residential facility of a special ward for these children should be an obligatory requirement. This ward should meet the absolute requirements of the normalization process. It should be staffed by trained sympathetic nurses-aides, supervised by skilled and experienced nurses with the consultation and assistance of physical therapists and occupational therapists. The quick flush-feeding and the depersonalized neglect which has so often in the past resulted in the grossly deformed, contracted spastic wreckage seen in the back wards of residential institutions should be prevented on moral, medical and esthetic grounds. Early intervention is all that we have to offer. It should be energetic and sustained.

In those cases where deformities have already developed, consultation with the orthopedic surgeon should be sought. As pointed out by Brown (1963), "Treatment by the orthopedist may be for relief of pain or it may be for correction of deformities by either conservative or surgical means. By appropriate treatment, more efficient nursing care and body hygiene can be achieved for bedridden patients and for those with severe involvement. In others, the orthopedist can make an important contribution to rehabilitation." In the majority of cases where surgical procedures are carried out, it will be necessary to follow with intensive physical therapy as well as education of the staff on the wards regarding day-to-day handling.

It can be said that within a residential setting, one may judge the effectiveness of the rehabilitation program by the availability of the physical therapist for staff-training programs on the wards for severely handicapped children. If the physical therapist's role is limited to the rehabilitation unit or as a pair of hands in post-surgical cases, then the role is indeed a very limited one. Above all, it should be pointed out that the principal service the therapist may be able to provide is in the prevention of such severe contractions and deformities.

Summary

The physical therapist has a crucial role to play in the treatment of the child with developmental disabilities. This role, however, requires that the therapist have a sound knowledge of neuromotor maturation and development. It is a knowledge of the sequential acquisition of developmental motor skills which sets the guide lines and goals for intervention. This role also requires that the therapist act as a teacher of motor development for the child, the parents, and the parent surrogates including the aides, teachers' assistants, and all who will have direct daily care of the child. Only if physicians utilize physical therapists in this way will they be able to develop the range and quality of physical therapy services needed in the management of the developmental disabilities.

BIBLIOGRAPHY

André-Thomas, Chesni, Y., and Saint-Ann Dargassies, S.: *The Neurological Examination of the Infant.* Little Club Clinics in Developmental Medicine, No. 1. The Spastics Society, London, Heinemann, 1960.

Bobath, B.: The very early treatment of cerebral palsy. *Develop Med Child Neurol,* 9:373-390, 1967.

Brown, S.W.: Orthopedic surgery in the mentally retarded. *J Bone Joint Surg* (American) 45-A: 841-855, 1963.

Browne, D.: Very early treatment of cerebral palsy. *Develop Med Child Neurol,* 8:473, 1966.

Ethun, C.A.: Physical management of the handicapped child. *GP,* 34:20-86, 1966.

Frankenburg, W.K., and Dodds, J.B.: Denver Developmental Screening Tests. University of Colorado Medical Center, Denver, Colorado, 1966.

Halpern, D.: Personal communication, April 17, 1969.

Kong, E.: Very early treatment of cerebral palsy. *Develop Med Child Neurol,* 8:198-202, 1966.

Milani-Comparetti, A., and Gidoni, E.A.: Routine developmental examination in normal and retarded children. *Develop Med Child Neurol,* 9: 631-638, 1967.

Nirji, B.: The normalization principle and its human management implications. In Kugel, R. and Wolfensberger, W. (Eds.) : *Changing Patterns in Residential Services for the Mentally Retarded.* President's Committee on Mental Retardation, Washington, D.C., 1969.

Paine, R.F., Brazelton, T.D., Donovan, D.E., Drorbaugh, J.E., Hubbel, J.P., Sears, E.M.: Evolution of posturoreflexes in normal infants and in the presence of chronic brain syndromes. *Neurology,* 14:1036-1048, 1964.

Pieper, A.: *Cerebral Function in Infancy and Childhood.* Philadelphia, Lippincott, 1964.

SECTION TWO
The Therapies

Chapter Three

CEREBRAL PALSY

Karel Bobath and Berta Bobath

PART 1
DIAGNOSIS AND ASSESSMENT OF CEREBRAL PALSY

BACKGROUND INFORMATION

Definition

Cerebral palsy is the result of damage or maldevelopment of the brain, occurring in utero or in earliest childhood. The lesion is nonprogressive and acts on an immature brain, interfering with its normal process of maturation. The term "cerebral palsy" comprises a group of conditions of great variety. With respect to the motor handicap, all cases have in common an impairment of the coordination of muscle action with an inability to maintain normal postures and balance and to perform normal movements and skills. Although the most striking deviation from the normal is usually seen in the child's motor behavior, associated sensory and perceptory disturbances are not rare.

Incidence

Phelps (1950, 1955) estimated that seven infants born each year in every 100,000 of the population were likely to suffer from cerebral palsy. More recent surveys indicate that the incidence is probably higher; thus Asher and Schonell (1950) give a figure of 1.7 per thousand, Woods (1957) of 1.9 per thousand infants who reach the age of five-years-plus. This latter figure is confirmed by a more recent survey undertaken by Ingram (1964) in Edinburgh which gives a figure of 1.99 per thousand.

Classification

The classification of cases has proved very difficult and so far no satisfactory scheme has been evolved. The reasons for this are not far to seek. There is still insufficient correlation of clinical and laboratory data with anamnestic and autopsy findings. Furthermore, cerebral palsy has many causes and too little is known about the causative factors to make etiology a useful guide to classification. The difficulty is increased by the well-known fact that most cases are of a mixed type and do not fit readily into any clear-cut scheme. It seems best, therefore, at this stage of our knowledge to use a purely descriptive scheme of classification. The scheme proposed here combines distribution of the disability with the type of abnormal postural tone found.* The abnormal postural tone is a factor common to all types of cerebral palsy.

DIPLEGIA. The whole body is involved, the lower limbs more so than the upper ones. The distribution is fairly symmetrical. Head control and speech are usually not affected, although some children may show some impairment of eye coordination. To this group belong predominantly spastic children though some may show some distal athetosis.

QUADRIPLEGIA. The whole body is affected, but the upper parts more so than the lower ones, or at least equally to the lower parts. The condition is usually very asymmetrical in distribution. These children usually have poor head control and show involvement of speech and eye coordination.

To this group belong many spastic or rigid cases and most of the athetoid group of children. Cases of choreo-athetosis, of ataxia and of a hypotonic type also are seen in this group. Some of the children of the athetoid group show marked fluctuations of postural tone between hypo- and hypertonia. This group may perhaps be classified separately as "dystonic cerebral palsy." A small group with athetoid quadriplegia shows fluctuations of postural tone between low and normal although it remains basically low. Many cases are of a mixed character.

---

*The term "postural tone" is used here in preference to the term "muscle tone" to give expression to the functional significance of muscle tone, that of maintaining posture.

In very mildly affected children of this group, involuntary movements may be just twitches or sudden jerks, involving especially the proximal parts, neck, trunk and shoulders.

Pure ataxia is very rare in cerebral palsy. It is usually associated with spasticity, athetosis, or both. The ataxia may be of the motor type, presumably due to damage to the cerebellum or its connections, or of the sensory type, caused by damage to subcortical structures subserving proprioceptive functions. Hypertonus is then usually moderate and affects predominantly the flexor groups of muscles.

In very young babies a temporary and transient state of cerebral hypotonia as a result of brain damage is not uncommon. These children may in time develop a spastic or rigid type of hypertonus or they may later on become athetoid or dystonic. In a few cases this early flaccidity may persist; this seems especially so in children with considerable intellectual impairment.

HEMIPLEGIA. One side of the body is affected. Postural tone is generally of the spastic type, although some children may develop some additional distal athetosis later on, around the sixth or seventh year. Hemiathetosis seems to be very rare.

PARAPLEGIA. Both lower limbs are affected, the upper parts are free of involvement. However, most of the paraplegias are, in fact, diplegias in whom the arms are so slightly affected that this may not be easily detected. A pure case of paraplegia should be carefully investigated with regard to the family history; it may be of hereditary origin and may belong to the familial type of paraplegia.

MONOPLEGIA. Monoplegias are also very rare in cerebral palsy, one limb only being involved. Most cases are, however, hemiplegias in whom the arm is only slightly involved. A scheme of classification may perhaps be tabled as in Table 3-I.

Etiology

It is generally agreed that about 60 percent of all cases are of perinatal origin, 30 percent caused by prenatal, and 10 percent by postnatal factors. Thus, Brandt and Westergaard-Nielsen (1958) who analyzed the history of 628 children, found that prenatal and

TABLE 3-I
SCHEME OF CLASSIFICATION

	Spastic	Rigid or Plastic Hypertonus	Fluctuating Hypertonus (Athetoid)	Hypotonus	Mixed
Diplegia	++	+	—	±	—
Quadriplegia	++	++	++	+ permanent ++ transient	++
Hemiplegia	++	+	±	—	+
Paraplegia	±	±	—	—	—
Monoplegia	±	±	—	—	—

Code: ++ = Frequent
+ = Occasionally
± = Rare
— = Never

perinatal factors were responsible for 87 percent of all cases and postnatal factors for the remaining 13 percent.

> Prenatal cases accounted for 54 percent of all cases of symmetrical diplegias, and 41 percent of all cases of asymmetrical diplegias (probably the quadriplegias of above classification.)
> Perinatal factors accounted for most cases of the athetoid group.
> Prematurity (27%) and neonatal factors (23%) were the most frequent single causes of cerebral palsy.

We give below some comparative figures which may point towards the relative significance of some etiological factors. They are of 190 consecutive cases in our files from which we could obtain reliable birth histories by personal interview. Of these 190 cases, 33 showed normal birth histories and 5 had acquired cerebral palsy in early childhood. Of the remaining 152 cases, 36 were born prematurely. They, and the remaining 116 cases, showed the birth histories as in Table 3-II.

It will be seen from Table 3-II that the factors at birth most frequently responsible for cerebral palsy in this group of 152 children were asphyxia, forceps delivery, prematurity and prolonged or precipitate labor.

The number and the percentage of cases in the present series attributed to these four conditions as well as the figures given by Asher and Schonell (1950) are shown in Table 3-III.

TABLE 3-II
BIRTH HISTORIES

	Premature		Full term Abnormal Labor
Blue or white asphyxia oxygen given (2 jaundiced)	17	36	(10 precipitate labor, 4 prolapsed cord, 1 jaundiced)
Forceps delivery (breech presentation)	1	37	(7 asphyxiated, 2 prolapsed cord)
Rhesus incompatibility (1 asphyxiated)	2	8	
Toxemia of mother	1	9	(3 jaundiced)
Neonatal jaundice	4	3	
Prolapsed cord	0	2	
Caesarian section	0	7	(2 asphyxiated)
Precipitate labor	3	6	
Prolonged labor	3	8	(4 breech presentation)
Premature only	5	0	
Totals	36	116	

Associated Defects

Associated handicaps are those affecting vision, hearing, speech, and proprioception. Intellectual impairment, emotional and social disturbances, and epilepsy also are not infrequently met with in this condition.

DISTURBANCE OF VISION. Disturbances of coordination of eye movements are frequently seen, especially among the quadriplegias, but also in some diplegic children. Guibor (1953) estimates that 50 percent of all children have some defect of eye movements. Internal or external squint, either alternating or fixed, and lack of accommodation are common. Many children are unable to move their eyes independently from the head. Some children of

TABLE 3-III
FACTORS MOST FREQUENTLY RESPONSIBLE FOR CEREBRAL PALSY

Causal Factor	No. of Cases	Present Series (152 cases)	Asher and Schonell
Asphyxia	62	40%	38%
Forceps	38	25%	24%
Prematurity	36	24%	No comparable figures
Prolonged and precipitate labor	30	20%	15%

the athetoid group with strong neck retraction experience difficulties in looking down.

A strong asymmetrical tonic neck reflex in a spastic or dystonic child may fix the eyes laterally towards the "face side" and prevent the child from moving them across the midline to the other side. The lack of head control and inability to move the eyes freely and independently from the head will make it impossible or difficult for the child to focus properly and to scan a line in attempting to read. The impairment of conjugate movement of the eyes with a resulting impairment of stereoscopic vision alone may have a profound influence on the child's ability for spatial orientation. (Abercrombie 1960, 1963, 1964).

Total blindness is rare in cerebral palsy. It may be caused by retrolental fibroplasia or optic atrophy. It must be differentiated from delayed maturation of the retina in early infancy. Defects of the visual fields are not uncommon, especially in hemiplegic children (Tizard 1953) due to damage to the optic radiation.

Disturbance of Hearing. The most common disturbance of hearing are high frequency deafness and auditory imperception or agnosia. High frequency deafness is most frequently met with in certain types of athetosis due to neonatal jaundice, but is not rare in spastic conditions. Fisch (1955) estimates that about 20 percent of all children with cerebral palsy have some hearing defect. It is most important to test these children in earliest infancy and to correct any hearing loss at a very early age, if one is to prevent any delay in the development of speech. It seems that unless a child develops inner speech at least by the age of seven or eight years of age, he will have missed the critical period and efforts to develop it will be unsuccessful.

Disturbance of Speech. Many children have a dysarthria—a pseudobulbar palsy of a spastic, athetoid or mixed type. Pure motor or sensory aphasia is rare. Luria and Yudowich (1959), in developing earlier research by Vigotski, have emphasized that the acquisition of speech is an important factor in the development of the capacity for abstract thinking and symbol formation. In the more intelligent child the motor deficit by itself does not seem to affect the acquisition of internalized speech and speech comprehension even in cases of dysarthria. However, in the patient with a double handicap, the inability to verbalize may affect the discrimination of words and retard the development of internal speech. The relationship of speech to the development of intelligence is a very complex and difficult problem which will require further research and investigation. In some cases the inability to speak is apparently due to apraxia of the speech apparatus of the mouth, throat, and larynx.

OTHER ASSOCIATED SENSORY HANDICAPS. Other associated sensory handicaps are a corporeal or spatial agnosia, or both. The corporeal agnosias may involve parts or the whole of the body. Hand or finger agnosia is not uncommon and has been studied especially in hemiplegic children. The involvement of the whole body will result in a more or less severe impairment of the child's percept of his own body, "the body-image," and secondarily, to a disturbance of the child's orientation in space. These may not be wholly due to cortical damage, probably of the parietal lobes, but may be the direct result of the motor deficit. A child, deprived by his motor handicap of touching and feeling his own body, of getting his hands or fingers to his mouth, of acquiring eye-hand coordination and the ability to grasp and manipulate objects, will not be able to develop a proper concept of his own body, nor be able to explore his environment. His physical handicap alone may, therefore, result in a profound retardation of his mental and intellectual development.

MENTAL RETARDATION. Mental retardation or mental subnormality is frequently very difficult to assess with any accuracy. Normally, intelligence tests are given to assess the inborn capabilities of an individual, and insofar as a test is successful in attaining this aim, it is considered to be of predictive value. This is almost impossible if the child is severely affected and can neither communicate nor manipulate objects. Care must be taken in every case of cerebral palsy to exclude any of the aforementioned associated sensory or perceptory disturbances.

Schilder (1931) and Bender (1938) among many others have stressed that the mental and intellectual development of a child is a function of learning by exploration and experience of his environment in relation to his ego and his own body. The child with cerebral palsy suffers from a double handicap, as he is not only restricted in mobility but also, in many cases, has specific perceptory disabilities and difficulties of coordinating sensation with motor activity. He is prevented by his abnormal movement patterns from exploring his own body and from coordinating visual and other sensory clues.

By its very definition cerebral palsy is a condition arising from damage to an immature brain. This entails two aspects of great importance for the total development of a child. It means, on the one hand, an interference by the lesion of normal child development with all it entails, both in the physical and mental field. On the other hand, it leads to a more or less severe disturbance of the relationship of the child with his environment, especially his mother, a point that will be enlarged upon later on.

The problem of testing the intelligence of these children is fraught with difficulties and most psychologists of experience tend to adapt existing test material by utilizing flexibility in its administration. In ordinary intelligence testing, only a correct answer is acceptable. The examiner is not allowed to accept an answer unless it is formulated correctly. In testing a child with cerebral palsy, however, it is essential that the examiner should be able to guess the response. However, experience at Harperbury Hospital with this type of patient has taught us to be very careful not to express the results of any of these tests in the form of a formal intelligence quotient (IQ).

It seems preferable to speak of a "functional level at the time of testing," and to look upon the result as a possible "base line." One has to watch the progress of a child in frequent retesting situations at fairly regular intervals. This may in the long run give a truer picture of a child's true potential than an IQ obtained during any one single session even if the examiner uses a battery of tests. Clarke and Clarke (1958) seem to share this view. They rightly consider that any unknown variable such as a slight speech, hearing, or other motor defect may have caused lack of normal experience with resulting depression on the test score.

Opinions about the relative value of the various tests of intelligence in children with cerebral palsy vary considerably. Anyone working with these children should be thoroughly familiar with the use and limitations of the more common tests (Dunsdon 1952, Schonell 1956, Mein 1962).

An assessment of the incidence of mental retardation in cerebral palsy still awaits correct evaluation. Any figures published so far must be accepted with great reservation. Dunsdon (1952) estimates that of 916 children tested 58.6 percent had an IQ under 69, 17.2 percent had an IQ between 74 and 80, and 23.75 percent had an IQ over 85. Floyer (1955) found IQ's under 85 in 75.5 percent of his children.

These figures seem to indicate, therefore, that at most a quarter of the children tested had an IQ within the normal range.

An estimate of the numbers of children and adults with cerebral palsy within a hospital for the mentally subnormal shows great variations from 6-10 percent (Doll 1933) to 23 percent (Kirman 1956). The number at Harperbury Hospital is estimated to be about 12-15 percent.

EPILEPSY. Epilepsy is not uncommon in cerebral palsy and may be of any type—grand mal, pettit mal, Jacksonian. Estimates of the incidence vary from 68 percent (Yannet 1944) to 14 percent (Dunsdon 1952). These seizures, if well controlled, do not offer a serious obstacle to effective treatment. Cerebral dysrhythmias without overt seizures are more frequent and may be responsible for behavioral disturbances, outburst of temper and irritability. If seizures are not properly controlled, they may lead in time to a deterioration of the child's physical and mental condition.

PSYCHOLOGICAL FACTORS. This is one of the most important single factors, for it determines whether a child can come to terms with his disability and is able in time to make a satisfactory adjustment. Disturbances of personality and behavior are complex and depend partly on the primary results of the brain injury and partly on the reaction formations of the child with regard to his environment, especially his parents and family. Most children will experience difficulties of integration, of adaptation to new situations, and anxiety and insecurity when faced with new and unexpected situations. This may assume the character of "catastrophic reactions" as described by Goldstein (1948, 1939).

Most children will show an accentuation of normal dependence associated with emotional immaturity. Generally speaking, they will find themselves excluded from the group of normal children, if only because they are physically incapable of keeping up with the others. The child will, therefore, be thrown much more intensely on the emotional relationship with his family. The attitude of the family will, therefore, have a greatly magnified effect on the child and on his personality.

The effect of mental defect on a child with cerebral palsy is variable. It can produce either a general emotional flattening and indifference to his surroundings or emotional instability and irritability. However, the emotional needs and problems of a mentally subnormal child with cerebral palsy are just as important and pressing as those of a child with normal intelligence. In the setting of a hospital for the subnormal, there is danger of patients withdrawing from surroundings. If these patients are allowed to sit around or lie in cots without any stimulation or occupation, they will suffer in consequence and fall far behind their true potentialities. In the severely handicapped child, careful assessment of his potential is of great importance. He is in real danger of being classed as severely or profoundly retarded, and thus not given the benefit of treatment and proper management.

The correlation of personality structure with a specific physical handicap as a result of an early brain lesion has not so far received the attention it merits. Many athetoid children, for example, show marked emotional instability and at times explosive behavior. It is possible that this is of hypothalamic origin. The spastic child, on the other hand, often shows marked obsessive-compulsive traits, is unwilling to adapt to new situations and prefers a limited routine.

The danger of withdrawal from the environment is a very real one, especially in the unstimulating atmosphere of a hospital ward. Among the patients chosen for treatment at Harperbury Hospital a sizable number showed withdrawal symptoms and it took a considerable time of intense treatment and stimulation to establish contact with them.

Maturation is dependent upon physical, mental and emotional growth. Any breakdown in this development, be it in the physical field only, has its repercussions on the child as a whole. In cerebral palsy, therefore, the interaction of the physical handicap and the intellectual and emotional development will lead to a disturbance in the growth of the total personality. Treatment, especially if started early, by improving the physical abilities of a child, by regulating the relationship between the child and his family, and by stimulating the child, may go a long way towards keeping the child's capabilities as near as possible to his true potentialities.

NEUROPHYSIOLOGIC BASIS OF MOTOR DEVELOPMENT

Some Basic Concepts of Brain Function

The performance of functional skills such as dressing, feeding, walking and writing requires very complex and selective patterns of muscular coordination. These depend on an intact and mature central nervous system and a fully developed background of basic motor patterns such as a normal child acquires during the first three years of life. The child with cerebral palsy has a damaged brain and as a result has both abnormal and primitive patterns of posture and movement which are incompatible with the performance of everyday skills.

An understanding of some basic concepts of the function of the central nervous system with respect to the organization of normal motor activity may explain the nature of the handicap of children with cerebral palsy and offer a rationale for an approach to treatment.

The central nervous system is an organ of integration. Muscles are activated always in patterns in the performance of even the most selective movements. Hughlings Jackson (1958) expressed this idea when he said, "Nervous centres represent movements, not muscles. From negative lesions of motor centres there is not paralysis of muscles, but loss of movements." This explains why a lesion to the brain leads to an interference with the normal process of coordination of movements—that is, an abnormal coordination of muscle action—and not to a paralysis of single muscles.

Magnus (1926) remarked that there exist a great number of

studies of movements but that little attention has been paid to an analysis of posture and postural changes. He explained this by the fact that the eye of the observer is always caught by the moving part and pays little attention to the less obvious and often invisible adaptive postural changes which precede and accompany each movement.

All our movements require constant changes of posture and the maintenance of equilibrium in constantly changing conditions. In fact, postural changes provide the constantly changing background for every movement. These changes are purely automatic and we are not conscious of them. They may be either invisible shifts and changes of postural tone throughout the body musculature or compensatory movements. They represent man's normal postural reflex mechanism. The patterns of coordination of these postural reflexes are typical and common to man, a fact which finds expression in the basic similarity of our motor behavior. We all stand up, sit down, turn over, walk, and run in fundamentally similar patterns.

This is tacitly accepted in our teaching of "typical fractures," based on the fact that under similar conditions of stress, when our normal postural defense reactions fail, we react in the same way and therefore sustain the same type of injury. It will be appreciated that this concept of the postural reflex mechanism looks on posture as something dynamic and constantly changing. In fact, the patterns of postural adjustment to movement are as varied as the movement itself. Postural changes not only accompany a movement but also precede it.

For instance, in standing, we transfer our weight automatically to one leg before making a step. In sitting, we first pull our feet under the seat of a chair and lean forward before standing up. We not only maintain our balance but constantly lose and regain it. In walking, for instance, the body weight is thrown forward over the standing leg. The body is allowed to fall forward and is caught on the stepping leg. In fact, walking has been considered as a constant process of losing and regaining our balance (Purdon 1961). The teaching of static postures, whether sitting, kneeling, or standing, is a wholly artificial process and cannot ensure any carry-over into movement.

The Relationship of Automatic to Voluntary Movement

An *active* movement does not necessarily have to be identified with a *volitional* movement. When trying to define volition, one may perhaps ask oneself, "What is a voluntary movement? What does it entail, and how does it differ from an active movement which is not performed voluntarily and to a purpose?" One may also ask, "Are automatic movements less active than willed movements and do their patterns of coordination differ essentially from those of voluntary movement?" These are different problems which Kinnier Wilson (1925) has tried to answer. In a lecture on "The Voluntary Motor System" he states:

> The word "voluntary" with regard to movement is in constant use but of elusive connotation. Voluntary movements do not constitute a class apart; they are equivalent to "least automatic movements" and all gradations may occur from the "most automatic movements" to the "least automatic." In objective characters they are not to be distinguished from other types of movements, especially coordinated and apparently purposeful, from which the element of volition is nevertheless wanting.

The concept of degrees of volition, of movements being graded from "least automatic" to "most automatic" is a most valuable one. It has proved helpful to explain the effect of a particular approach to treatment which aims at improving the child's patterns of coordination. The fact that the child in treatment responds to handling with automatic reactions, does not mean that the child is passive, nor does it mean that active responses so obtained need necessarily be volitional or purposeful, at least not in the first place.

The techniques of handling used in the neurodevelopmental (Bobath) approach serve to obtain active automatic movements from the child, first the automatic patterns of earliest babyhood and childhood on which voluntary and purposeful movements are gradually built up (facilitation). The child does not, therefore, have to initiate these movements voluntarily, at least not initially. However, once his patterns of coordination have become established, he is encouraged to use them at will. In this way, movements in abnormal patterns, the only ones the child with cerebral palsy knows how to use at will, are avoided, and their strengthening by habitual use is prevented.

These techniques will, therefore, prevent an increase of spasticity or athetosis which usually result from the child's excessive effort and possible anxiety when faced with a task on request. A further great advantage is that active movements in more normal patterns of coordination can be obtained without the child's intelligent cooperation. They can, for instance, often be obtained in play form, an essential when treating babies. It is this aspect of the approach which has made this (Bobath) treatment so eminently adaptable to the needs of the mentally subnormal and uncooperative child.

The Development of Normal Motor Abilities

Before going into some detailed description of the motor handicap of a child with cerebral palsy, it may be useful to study the development of the motor abilities of normal children in some detail. It is important to interpret this development in terms of the gradual appearance of the normal postural reflex mechanism and the elaboration and modification of the early primitive total synergies of movement. This will provide a better understanding of the nature of the motor handicap of children with cerebral palsy which is essential in developing a rational approach to the diagnosis, early recognition, assessment and treatment of this condition.

Essentially, normal child development is characterized by two features which are as follows:

1. The development in a definite sequence of events of a normal postural reflex mechanism (that is, of righting), equilibrium and other protective reactions, associated with a normal postural tone.

2. The increase of inhibition of the maturing brain leading to a gradual breaking up and resynthesis of the early total synergies of muscular coordination in many and varied ways to allow for discreet and selective movements later on.

The Normal Postural Reflex Mechanism

The normal postural reflex mechanism consists mainly of the two types of automatic reactions, righting and equilibrium reactions. The former have been studied by Magnus and Schaltenbrand (1925, 1926, 1927) on a number of babies and young children. They have described the sequence of their appearance during the period of growth and maturation of babies and their gradual modification and partial inhibition and disappearance in childhood. They have related them to the sequence of a development of a child's overt functional activities as described by Gesell and Amatruda (1947), Buehler (1932, 1927), André-Thomas and Saint-Ann Dargassies (1952, 1960), McGraw (1943), and others. Equilibrium reactions have been studied by Weisz (1938), Zador (1938), and Rademaker (1935) among others.

THE RIGHTING REACTIONS. The first reactions to come into play in the growing baby are the righting reactions. These develop from birth onwards, reach their maximal concerted effect around the tenth to twelfth month, and are then gradually modified and inhibited, to disappear towards the end of the fifth year. They safeguard the normal position of the head in space (face vertical, mouth horizontal) and secure the normal alignment of head and neck with the trunk, and of the trunk with the limbs. They guide the child's motor activities throughout the quadripedal stage and are gradually integrated into his volitional behavior. To them belong the following:

1. The neck-righting reaction. This is present at birth. Turning the baby's head towards one side, either actively or passively, may be followed by a rotation of the body as a whole towards the side to which the head is turned. From lying supine the baby turns to his side.

2. The labyrinthine-righting reaction on the head. This comes gradually into play from the fourth to sixth week onwards. Initially this reaction is weak and the baby raises his head intermittently in the prone position. As it gains strength with the maturation of the labyrinths, the baby begins to raise his head from the supine position from the sixth month onwards.

3. The body-righting reaction acting on the head. This reaction serves to right the head in response to some part of the body touching the supporting surface. For instance, righting the head will follow when the baby's feet touch the ground. This reaction interacts with the labryinthine-righting reaction on the head to secure and doubly-secure the normal position of the head in space.

4. The body-righting reaction on the body. This reaction appears around the sixth to eighth month of the baby's life, and modifies the primitive neck-righting reaction by introducing a rotation of the trunk between the shoulders and pelvis. By turning the head to one side the child will now be able to start the movement of the trunk with the shoulder, while the pelvis will follow, or vice versa. It is this rotation within the body axis which gives the baby his first chance to turn over to the prone position when he is about eight months old. Turning over from supine to prone is aided by the child's ability to raise the head when lying prone and to extend his spine and hips.

5. The optical-righting reactions. These are of secondary importance at first but gain quickly in influence as the child grows. In the adult, vision has become the main factor in maintaining the normal position of the head and body, while the other righting reactions have fulfilled their function and have become partially inhibited.

All the righting reactions interact closely, and secure and doubly-secure the normal position of the head in space and the normal alignment of the body and its parts. A simple means of showing their activity in the growing child is to observe how he sits and stands up from the supine position (Schaltenbrand 1925). As long as the righting reaction of the body on the body is active, the child will do this by first turning over to the prone position and by getting up on his hands and knees before sitting or standing up. As the righting reactions are gradually inhibited and disappear, the rotation of the body will become less pronounced, and by the fifth year the child will get up in the adult symmetrical manner. He will sit up straight from lying supine, and then stand up.

THE EQUILIBRIUM REACTIONS. Like the righting reactions, the equilibrium reactions appear in a definite sequence. The first equilibrium reactions can be seen around the sixth month, when the righting reactions are already almost fully established. From then on they gradually modify and inhibit the righting reactions. The equilibrium reactions have complex and varied motor patterns, and probably require for their proper function the full interplay of the basal ganglia, subthalamic nuclei, the cerebellum, and also the cerebral cortex.

They remain with us throughout life, and serve to adjust posture and maintain or regain equilibrium. They are essentially compensatory movements, making the maintenance of equilibrium possible, and are activated by changes of the position of the body in space or by a change of the relationship of body and supporting ground as, for instance, when standing on a moving platform. They can, therefore, be demonstrated in two ways—either by putting a child on a moving platform like the "Rademaker table," or by pushing the child gently from side to side, or forward and backward when sitting, kneeling, or standing on the ground.

The perfecting of all equilibrium reactions lags somewhat behind the child's attempts at more difficult activities. For instance, the equilibrium reactions in the prone and supine positions appear and are perfected at a time when the child can already sit, although he cannot yet sit up by himself. The necessary equilibrium reactions, which enable him to sit up and keep his balance in sitting, appear only when the child tries to stand up.

The first reactions to tipping on a movable table appear in the prone position around the sixth month and in the supine position shortly afterwards. Before that time the baby just rolls off the table when it is tipped without any adaptive and protective reaction. From the sixth month onward, the baby lying prone bends the head and arches the body towards the raised side of the table as a result of a compensatory increase of tone in the muscles of the raised side. The arm and leg of that side are abducted and the hips often rotate towards the lower side of the table. The reaction to tipping when lying supine is identical.

The equilibrium reactions in sitting can be tested by moving the child at varying speeds from side to side or backward and forward. If the child is gently pushed to one side—for instance, the right side—the head moves towards the left; it angulates with the body and tends to maintain as far as possible the normal position in space (Fig. 3-1). The left arm and leg abduct and extend, and the left hip moves forward while the right arm and hand extend, ready to support the body weight if the reaction fails. When the child's center of gravity is disturbed by pushing him backward, his head, shoulders and arms move forward and his legs extend. Pushing the sitting child forward makes his legs flex, his spine and neck extend, and his arms move backward.

The equilibrium reactions to moving the child in the kneel-standing and standing positions are very similar to those in sitting (Fig. 3-2 and 3-3). However, in standing, other reactions can be observed as well. The child may keep his balance by making a few sideways steps in the direction of the weight transfer. If the child is moved backward, he will either step back or will move his head, trunk, and arms forward and dorsiflex his ankles and toes to counteract the transfer of his body weight (Fig. 3-4A).

These are only a few examples of the many typical reactions which can be observed. The variations of these reactions depend upon the range and speed of the movement which disturbs the child's equilibrium. For children with cerebral palsy they are usually absent (Fig. 3-4B and 3-4C).

Righting and equilibrium reactions interact closely and harmoniously. They represent man's normal postural reflex mechanism and form the necessary dynamic background for the performance of any functional skill. They provide what has been called "principal motility" by Schaltenbrand. They can fulfill this function only when postural tone is normal (that is, sufficiently high to give proper support against gravity, but not too high so as not to interfere with any intended movement).

Sequential Development of Motor Activity
The Newborn Baby

Generally speaking, the newborn baby at rest shows a symmetrical attitude in flexion in all positions: supine, prone, verti-

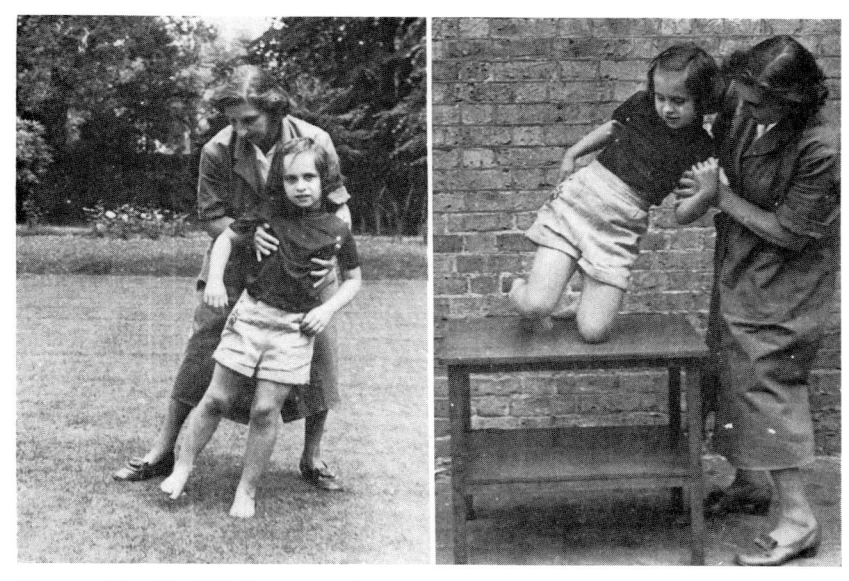

Figure 3-1. Equilibrium reactions in standing.

Figure 3-2. Equilibrium reactions in kneeling.

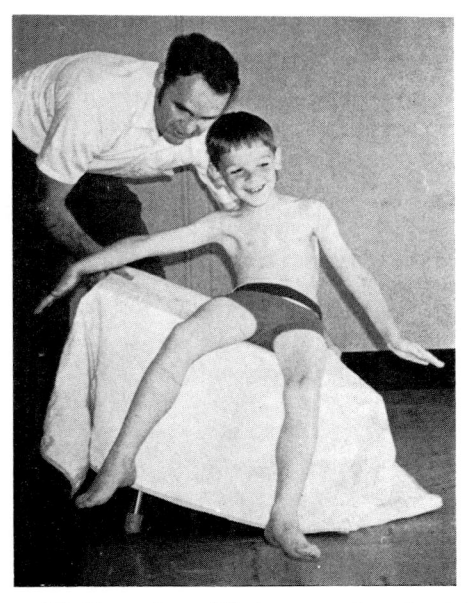

Figure 3-3. Normal equilibrium reactions in sitting.

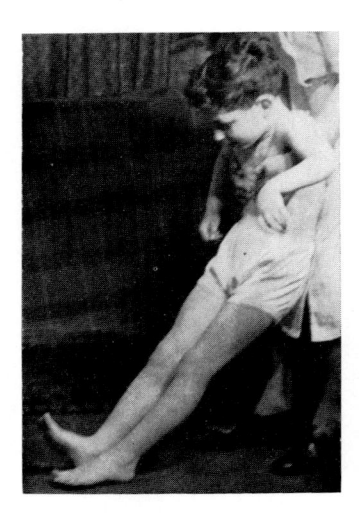

50   *Physical Therapy Services in the Developmental Disabilities*

Figure 3-4A *(Left).* Absent equilibrium in hemiplegic left lower limb.

Figure 3-4B *(Bottom Left).* Absence of equilibrium in sitting. Note: no head-righting, no propping reactions of right arm; lack of trunk stability.

Figure 3-4C *(Bottom Right).* Spastic quadriplegia absence of equilibrium reactions in standing.

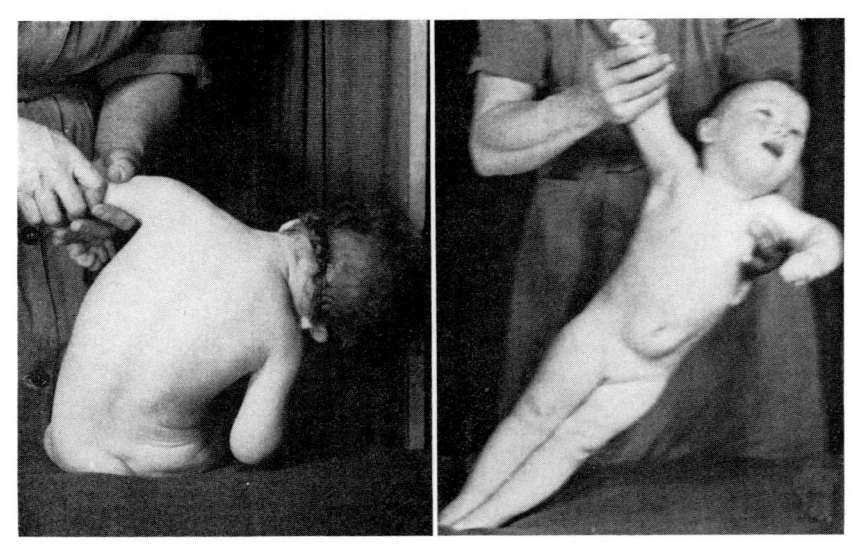

cal, or ventral suspension. This is due to a physiological hypertonus of the flexor muscles of trunk and limbs of symmetrical distribution (Figs. 3-5A, 3-5B, 3-5C, and 3-5D). Head control is inadequate. If pulled to sitting from supine, the head will drop back. When placed in prone, the baby may raise his head for a

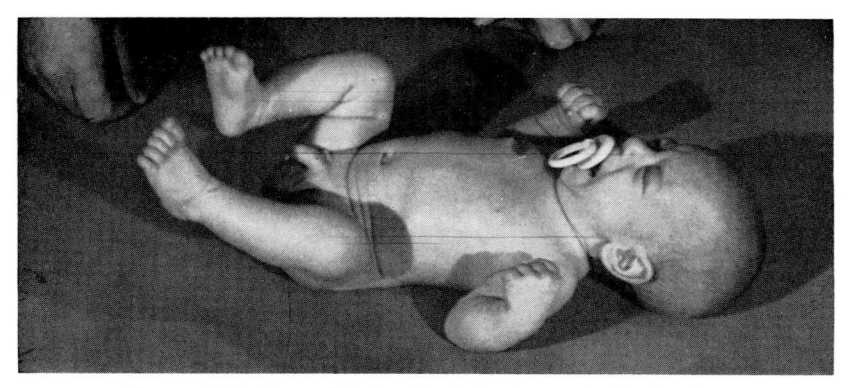

Figure 3-5A. Normal baby. Early flexion attitude. Supine.

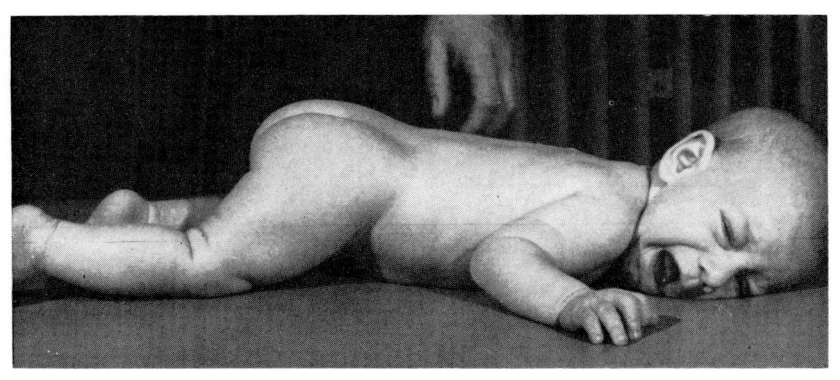

Figure 3-5B. Normal baby. Early flexion attitude. Prone. Note: head turned to side.

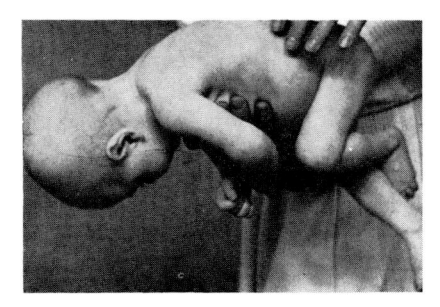

Figure 3-5C. Normal baby. Early flexion attitude.

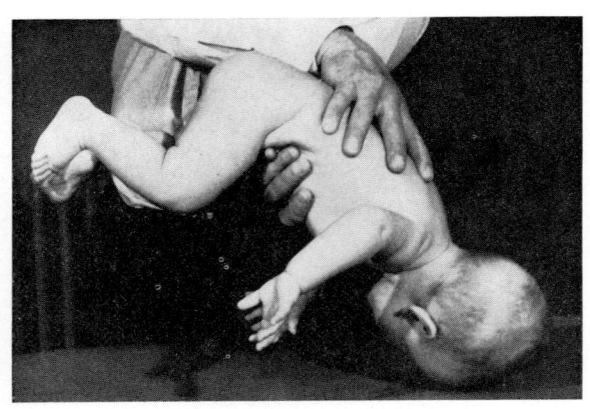

52 *Physical Therapy Services in the Developmental Disabilities*

Figure 3-5D. Early baby attitude of flexion. Physiological absence of head-righting and parachute reaction of arms.

fleeting moment and turn it to one side (Prechtl 1964, Illingworth 1960).

CHART 3-I
NATURAL COURSE OF DEVELOPMENTAL REACTIONS

Type of Reaction	1-4 Weeks	2 Mos	4-6 Mos	7-12 Mos	12-14 Mos	2-3 Yrs	3-5 Yrs	After 5 Yrs
Moro (startle)	+	+	±	—				
Asymmetrical TNR	+	+	±	—			—	
Grasp reflex	+	+	±	—				
Sucking reflex	+	±	±	—				
Neck-righting	+	+	±	±	—			
Labyrinthine-righting on the head		+	+	\multicolumn{4}{c}{Partly and increasingly inhibited by optical-righting reactions.}		
Landau reaction			+	+	+			
Propping (parachute) reaction			+	+	+	+	+	+
Body-righting on-body				+	±	±	±	
Equilibrium reactions								
Prone			+	+	+	+	+	+
Supine				±	+	+	+	+
Sitting				±	+	+	+	+
Kneeling					+	+	+	+
Seesaw reaction					+	+	+	+
Standing					±	+	+	+

Key: + = Present
± = Inconsistent or weak
— = Not present

MORO REFLEX. The arms are fairly firmly fixed to the trunk in an attitude of flexion with pronation of the forearm, the hands fisted, the thumb adducted. Although the arms will resist passive extension and spring back into flexion once stretch is discontinued, they will extend widely and abduct horizontally in the Moro reflex (Fig. 3-5E). This reaction is a complex one, the functional significance of which is not known. It consists of a wide horizontal abduction-extension movement of the arms with opening of the hands and abduction of thumbs and fingers in response to a variety of stimuli such as a sharp blow on the support on which the baby lies, blowing cold air on his abdomen, or raising the baby from supine and letting the head fall back fairly quickly. In this form the Moro reflex persists for about six to eight weeks. It then becomes modified by a less marked extension of the arms. According to Richmond Paine (1960), the last trace of the Moro reflex probably consists of a slight flexion of the thighs on the pelvis which persists up to about six months.

GRASP REFLEX. The fingers, as André-Thomas and Saint-Ann Dargassies (1960) rightly stress, show at this stage not a true grasp reflex, but a "tonic reaction of the finger flexors," a purely propri-

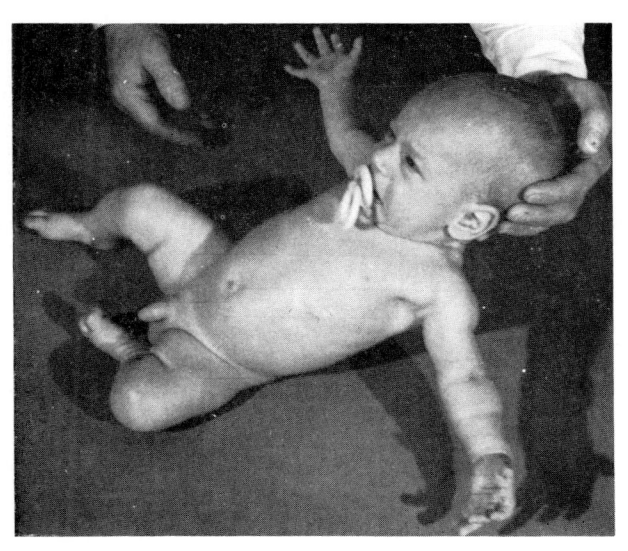

Figure 3-5E. Normal Moro (startle) reaction.

54   *Physical Therapy Services in the Developmental Disabilities*

oceptive response to stretch of the flexor muscles. The lower limbs show alternating flexion and extension, the normal kicking pattern of a baby. They are already considerably modified and quite different from the flexor withdrawal or crossed extension reflexes of spinal animals (Fulton 1951). The hips do not fully extend in kicking but retain their outward rotation, and the ankles remain dorsiflexed.

NECK-RIGHTING REACTION. As stressed before, the neck-righting reaction is the only one of the righting reactions present at birth (Fig. 3-5F). The baby is, therefore, able to turn from side-lying to supine. The labyrinthine-righting reaction on the head is weak, and the baby therefore has poor head control. Equilibrium reactions are absent at this stage. If the baby is placed on a table which is then tilted to one side, he will roll over towards the lower side without any protective reaction (Weisz 1938).

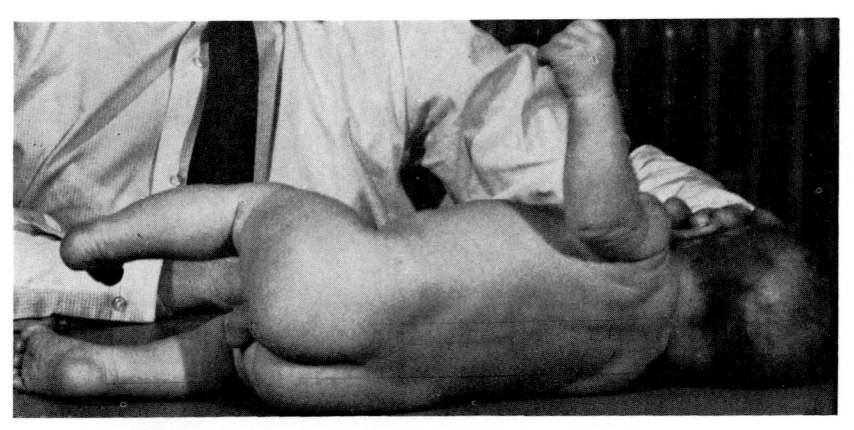

Figure 3-5F. Normal Baby. Normal neck-righting reaction.

ASYMMETRICAL TONIC NECK RESPONSE. This response is never conspicuous in the normal newborn. The position of the arms is only occasionally affected by active or passive rotation of the head. The newborn is flexed and symmetrical, and more definite asymmetrical tonic neck reflex attitudes will appear only towards the fourth or fifth week, at a time when the baby has developed more extensor tone. Even then, however, the response is unpredictable and variable, not sufficiently strong and regular enough to interfere with the baby's random activities, and should, therefore, not be called a "reflex." This is borne out by a study of 108 healthy newborn babies between the first and sixth day by Vassella and Karlsson (1962) which showed that in only nine of them (8%) could the asymmetric tonic neck reflex response be obtained with the regularity of a true reflex.

Other automatic reactions which can be observed at this stage are the following:

1. Primary standing.
2. Early automatic walking.
3. Galant's reaction or the incurvation of the trunk.
4. The placing reaction of the legs.

PRIMARY STANDING. This is obtained by placing the baby with his feet on a table (Fig. 3-6) He will then gradually right himself and assume the standing position (Fig. 3-7). This righting ability gradually disappears during the second month (André-Thomas et al 1960). According to Peiper (1961) however, this does not denote true righting ability, but the assumption of the primary standing posture is the result of a chain reflex starting with the positive supporting reaction of the lower limbs.

AUTOMATIC WALKING. This can be elicited by placing the baby with his feet on a table, the examiner supporting and stabilizing the baby's trunk with both hands (Fig. 3-7). The legs will extend and the baby assumes the standing position. If the body in righting is now tilted slightly forward, the baby will begin to walk with well-coordinated rhythmical steps (Fig. 3-7). His hips and knees remain flexed however, and do not extend fully. Equilibrium reactions of trunk and stability with cocontraction of the trunk muscles, the prerequisite of normal walking, are absent. If support is withdrawn, the baby will, therefore, slump to one side and collapse. This walking persists for a variable period of up to two months (André-Thomas et al. 1960). However, according to MacKeith (1964) primary walking can still be obtained in some babies up to the age of one year by combining the above described maneuver with passive extension of the head.

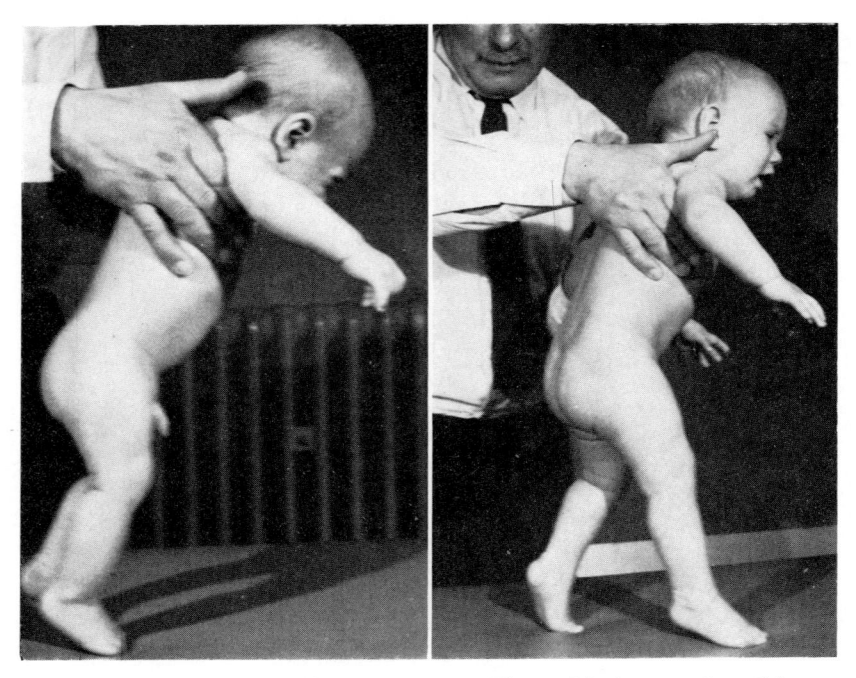

56 *Physical Therapy Services in the Developmental Disabilities*

Figure 3-6. Primary standing.

Figure 3-7. Automatic walking.

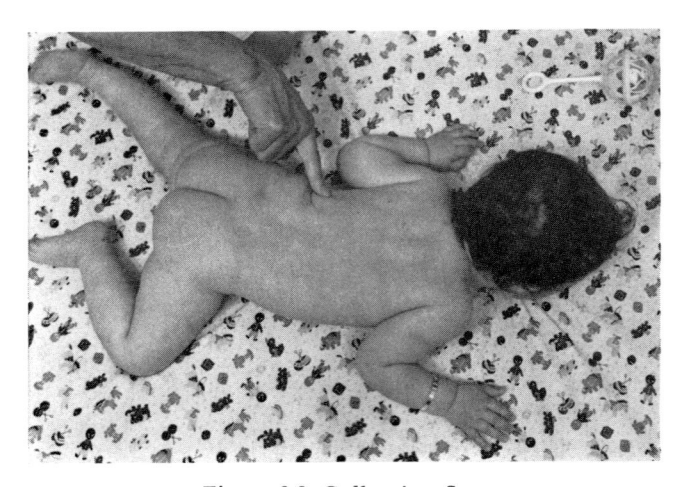

Figure 3-8. Gallant's reflex.

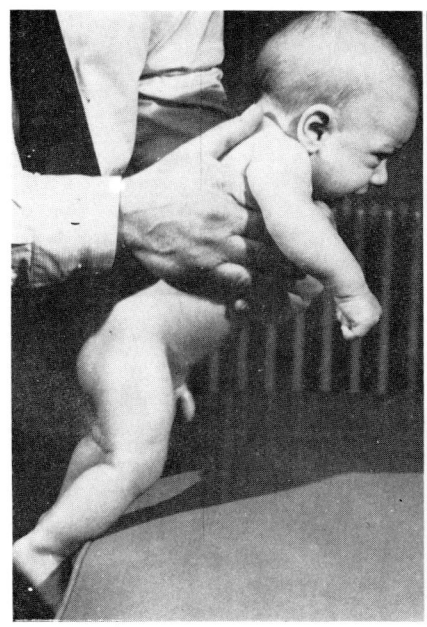

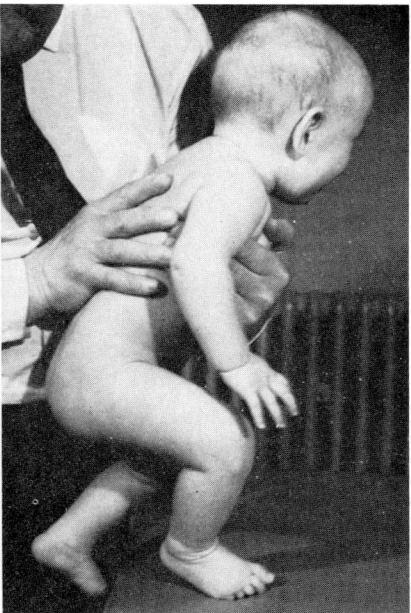

Figure 3-9. Normal baby. Testing for placing reactions of lower limbs.

Figure 3-10. Placing reaction of legs.

GALANT'S REFLEX (the trunk incurvation reaction). The baby is tested in the prone position. The skin of the lumbar region between the twelfth rib and the iliac crest is pricked lightly and repeatedly. The result will be a contraction of the side flexors of the trunk on the stimulated side with a side flexion of the baby's spine (Figure 3-8). According to André-Thomas et al. (1960), this reaction normally disappears during the second month. Ingram (1964) has, however, observed it in babies up to three months. In children with cerebral palsy, especially of the athetoid type, it may persist for much longer. Its retention may cause considerable delay in the development of a symmetrical stabilization of the trunk and of independent movements of the head and trunk, necessary for standing and walking. This instability of the trunk may be further aggravated by the persistence of an asymmetrical tonic neck reflex and may be responsible for the frequently observed scoliosis of the spine.

THE PLACING REACTION OF THE LEGS. This is obtained by lifting the baby into an upright position and bringing the shin into contact with the edge of a table (Fig. 3-9). The baby will flex the leg and bring it first above the table. He will then extend the leg and place it on the surface (Fig. 3-10), This reaction is obtainable after the first ten days (André-Thomas et al, 1960). Zappella et al. (1964) state that the absence of this reaction is closely associated with severe degrees of mental subnormality. This statement can only be accepted with the greatest reservation. It has been found to be absent also in children with severe degrees of extensor spasticity of the lower limbs regardless of the degree of mental retardation.

When examining normal babies, it must be kept in mind that an important feature of their responses is their variability. None of the above described reactions can be obtained always and with absolute regularity. The statement that the newborn is a "pallidum being" (Peiper 1961) cannot be accepted. Although the brain of the newborn is still immature, the influence of higher centers on the early automatic reactions is clearly seen. This is evidenced by the great variability of these responses in the normal baby. In fact, if some of these automatic responses, such as the asymmetrical tonic neck reflex, the plantar extensor response (Babinski), or any other assume the obligatory character of true reflexes, it should be considered as pathological at any age.

From Two to Twelve Months of Age

This is a period of fast development and maturation; in fact, at no time during his life does a child develop at so fast a rate as during the first twelve months. Gradually, the normal postural reflex mechanism matures.

RIGHTING REACTIONS. First to be seen are the remaining righting reactions. They originate in the labyrinthine organs, in the proprioceptors of the neck muscles, in the touch and pressure receptors of trunk and limbs, and in the eyes. Righting by vision, through the optical-righting reactions, becomes predominant in man later on but it is not known when vision becomes the decisive factor in the righting and spatial orientation of the growing

Cerebral Palsy 59

baby. This process probably begins around the sixth month—at a time, that is, when the normal head position and its alignment with the trunk has been fairly well established with the help of the labyrinthine- and body-righting reactions.

In step with the maturation of the labyrinthine organs, the baby gradually improves his head control. This begins around the fourth week in prone-lying first. The baby is then able to raise his head, although at first only weakly and intermittently. From about the eighth week he can control it in this position fairly well. This improving head control can also be observed when the baby is pulled up to sitting from supine by both arms. Although at first unable to raise his head and to assist in this way when pulled to sitting, his head will begin to move forward at about two or three months of age, and from the fourth month onward there will be only a slight initial head lag. From the sixth month, only a slight initial pull is necessary to assist him in sitting up.

Head-raising in prone initiates a process of general extension of trunk and limbs against gravity which gradually proceeds cephalocaudad to reach hips and knees around the sixth month (Fig. 3-11). At this time the baby is able to raise his head well up in prone, and support himself on extended arms in a pattern of total extension against gravity. By this time, however, the baby is also able to raise his head against gravity by flexing it forward

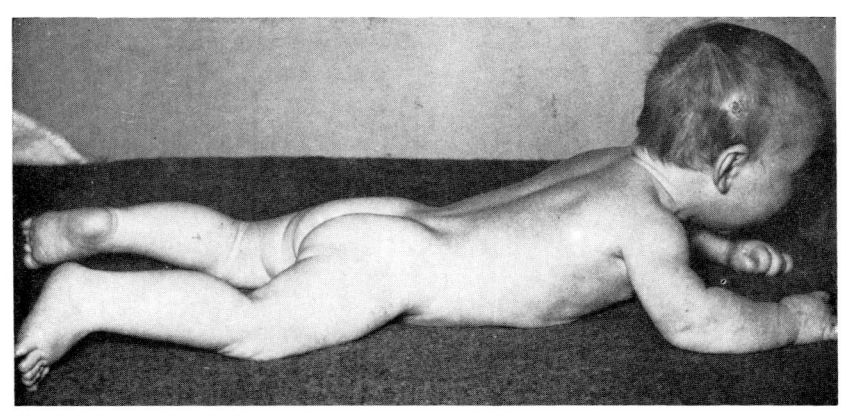

Figure 3-11. Normal baby. Note: primary, primitive extension pattern in prone.

from supine-lying. Up to about the fifth or sixth month the normal baby moves with primitive total patterns of flexion and extension against gravity. He is, therefore, not able at this stage to sit with flexed hips and extended spine until he is about eight months old.

There is also a short-lasting phase when the baby in prone-lying, although able to rest fully extended on extended arms, is unable to move into four-foot kneeling, because he cannot maintain extension of spine and arms when attempting to bear his weight on flexed hips and knees. During the next few months, both the primitive total flexor and extensor synergies are broken up, allowing the baby to kneel, to crawl, and to sit with flexed hips and extended spine and legs.

The ability to raise the head in prone and supine remain throughout life an essential factor of our ability to initiate sitting and standing up from supine or prone.

The body-righting reactions on the body appear around the sixth to seventh month. It breaks up the total pattern of turning to one side of the earlier and more primitive neck-righting reaction. It introduces instead the ability of rotation within the body axis, the shoulders initiating the movement and the hips following or vice versa. This, together with the necessary extension of head and trunk established at this stage, enables the baby to roll from supine into prone, and soon to move from prone into side-sitting and sitting.

EQUILIBRIUM REACTIONS. The first equilibrium reactions appear around the sixth month, thus following and partially overlapping with the righting reactions. They first appear in prone, soon in supine, later in sitting, kneeling, standing and walking. They are of a more complex nature than the righting reactions and are most highly developed in man. It is interesting to note that the first equilibrium reactions appear at a time (six months) when the baby already sits. They appear in sitting when the baby begins to stand, and in standing when the baby begins to walk. This shows the considerable overlap in the development of the basic functional activities in a growing child. This fact must be kept in mind when treating children with cerebral palsy and when facilitating these patterns in their developmental sequence. Equilibrium reactions are gradually perfected over the next five years.

THE MORO REACTION. This, even in its modified form, has disappeared by about six months when the baby is able to sit momentarily without support (Ingram 1955). Its disappearance seems to coincide with the improving head control and the appearance of the protective extension of the arms.

THE LANDAU REACTION. This makes its appearance at about six months of age. It is tested with the baby in ventral suspension, supported by one hand under the lower chest. The baby will first right his head, followed by a symmetrical extension of spine and hips (Fig. 3-12A). If the head is passively flexed, the body flexes as a whole (Fig. 3-12B). One can only speculate about the functional significance of this reaction. It seems that the symmetrical extension of trunk and hips at this stage is an important phase of development which prepares the child for stability in standing. When the Landau reaction attains its full strength, around the eighth month, reciprocal kicking stops (Illingworth 1960).

PROTECTIVE EXTENSION REACTIONS. The protective extension reaction of the arms, also called "propping reaction" (André-Thomas et al. 1960) or "parachute reaction" by Milani-Comparetti (1964) and Paine (1964), appears around the sixth month. At this stage the baby can support his weight in sitting on arms which are extended forward (Fig. 3-13A). From the eighth month onward, he can support himself in sitting, the arms extended sideways, (Fig. 3-13B) and from the tenth to twelfth month onward, with the arms extended backward. At first, weight is taken on fisted hands, although the hands may be open and the fingers extended and abducted until they touch the support. Soon afterwards, however, the hands will remain open.

This reaction can also be tested by tilting the child from the Landau test position, head first down towards the support, when he will take his weight on extended arms. In this form the reaction has also been called "precipitation reflex" (André-Thomas et al. 1960, 1952) (Fig. 3-14).

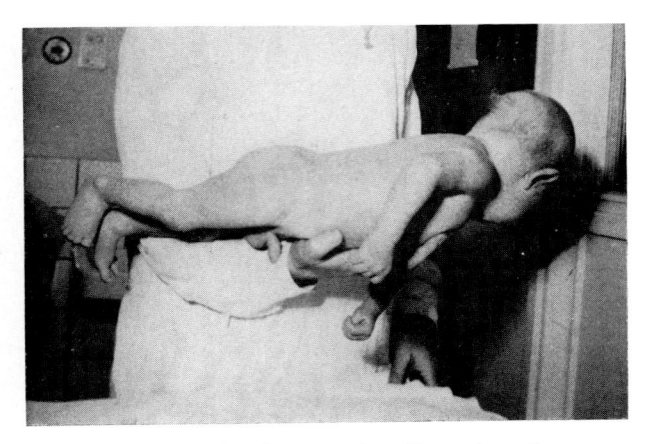

Figure 3-12A. Landau reaction. Extension phase.

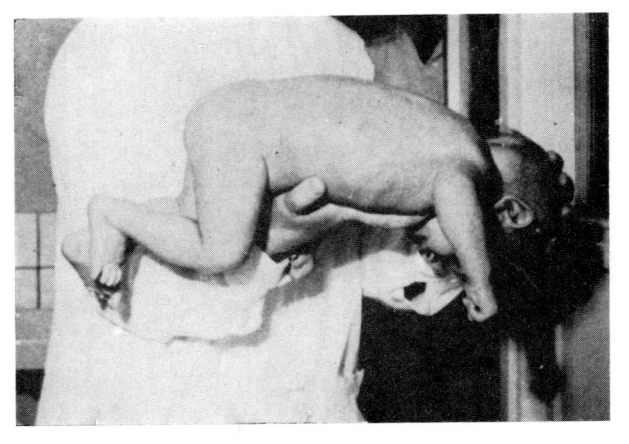

Figure 3-12B. Landau reaction. Flexion phase.

PLACING REACTIONS OF THE ARMS. These appear towards the end of the third month. They are tested by bringing the dorsum of the hands or forearms into contact with the edge of a table. The child will then place his hand, first fisted and later open, palm down, on the tabletop (Figs. 3-15A and 3-15B).

Cerebral Palsy 63

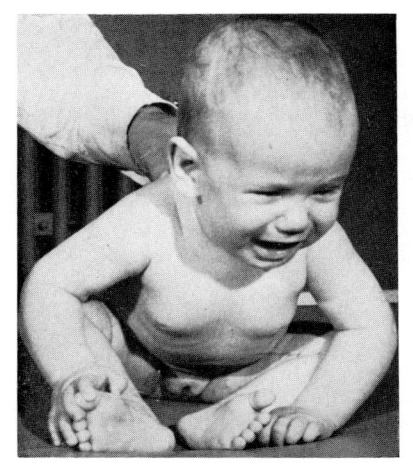

Figure 3-13A. Early propping reaction. Forward.

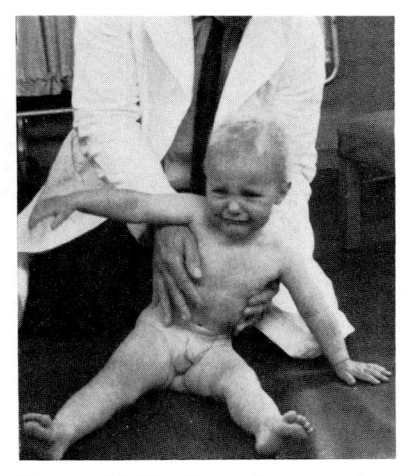

Figure 3-13B. Propping reaction. Sideways.

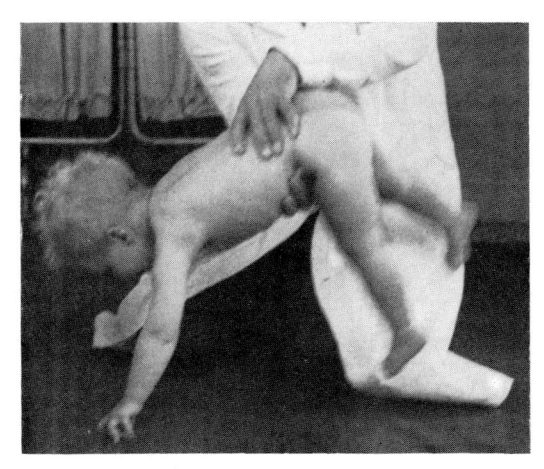

Figure 3-14. Precipitation reflex (parachute reaction).

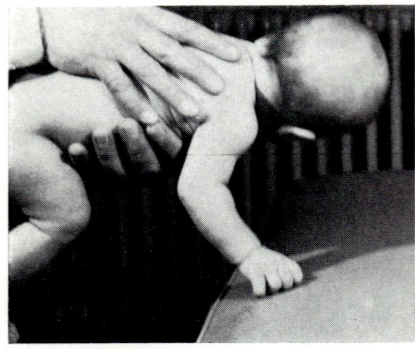

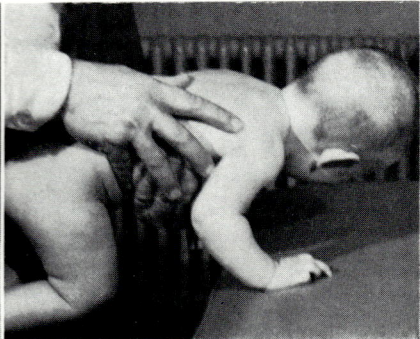

64 *Physical Therapy Services in the Developmental Disabilities*

Figure 3-15A. Placing reactions of arms.

Figure 3-15B. Placing reaction of arms.

THE NEUROLOGIC PICTURE IN CEREBRAL PALSY

In cerebral palsy the lesion interferes with orderly neuromotor development. Essentially this will result in two sets of symptoms as follows:

1. Symptoms of arrest or retardation of motor development. These are seen in an insufficiently developed postural reflex mechanism, resulting in poor head control, lack of rotation within the body axis, and poor equilibrium. Also, they are seen in insufficiently developed inhibition with the retention of primitive synergies of earliest babyhood. This can be seen in the retention of primitive kicking, of the grasp reflex, the Moro reaction (usually in the modified form of the second phase), of the neck-righting reaction, or primary walking and the Galant reflex, among others.

2. Abnormal symptoms—that is, signs of a release of abnormal postural reflexes, the tonic or static reflexes of Magnus (1926) and Walshe (1923). They produce abnormal patterns of coordination in association with an abnormal postural tone.

Tonic Reflex Activity

It is important to appreciate that in experimental animals a lesion which results in hypertonus also produces the abnormal patterns of coordination of tonic reflexes. Decerebration produces an animal which can stand but is unable to maintain the static position against disturbing influences, as it has neither righting nor equilibrium reactions. For this reason, Sherrington (1947) called this state "reflex standing" or "a caricature of standing." Decerebration releases the centers of facilitation and inhibition of the brainstem in animals (Magoun and Rhines 1947) which regulate postural tone by influencing and modifying the spinal reflex mechanism. This will also set free the various tonic or static reflexes with the resultant typical patterns of posture and movement associated with abnormal postural tone. It seems logical, therefore, to assume that hypertonus in all its forms and the abnormal patterns of coordination are co-existent, the expression of one and the same lesion. In other words, the various types of hypertonus and their patterns of coordination are one and the same thing, the expression of a "short-circuiting" of all sensory input into the patterns of released and abnormal postural reflex activity.

The relevant tonic reflexes are as follows:
1. The tonic labyrinthine reflex.
2. The tonic neck reflexes.
   a. The asymmetrical tonic neck reflex.
   b. The symmetrical tonic neck reflex.
3. Associated reactions (Walshe 1923).
4. The positive supporting reaction.

The Tonic Labyrinthine Reflex

The tonic labyrinthine reflex is evoked by changes of the position of the head in space, probably by stimulation of the otolith organs of the labyrinths. It is an abnormal reflex, not found in the normal baby. In the child with cerebral palsy it usually causes maximal extensor hypertonus in the supine position (that is, with the face up) with a relative inhibition of flexor activity. In the prone position, with the face down, it produces minimal extensor hypertonus with a relative increase of flexor hyperactivity. Intermittent degrees of hypertonus of the extensors are obtained by positions of the head between these two extremes—for instance, in sitting.

66   *Physical Therapy Services in the Developmental Disabilities*

In a severe case of established spastic quadriplegia, extensor spasticity in supine may be very strong. The head, neck, and spine are retracted, the shoulders pulled back, the arms abducted and flexed at the elbows. The lower limbs are extended, inwardly rotated and adducted (Fig. 3-16).

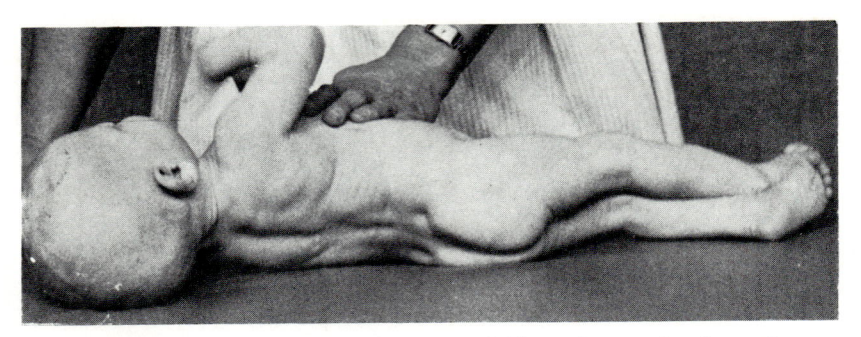

Figure 3-16. Severe quadriplegic. Note: rigid, total extension in supine.

The patterns of extensor hypertonus in the supine position will prevent the child from raising the head. He has difficulty, therefore, in initiating sitting up. The child is unable to bring his arms forward due to retraction of the shoulders. He cannot, therefore, grasp a support to pull himself up to sitting. This difficulty is further enhanced by his inability to flex his hips. He cannot bring his hands together in midline and often cannot touch his body. Retraction of the shoulders will prevent him from turning into prone (Fig. 3-17). The child is, therefore, very severely handicapped and prevented from performing any of the most basic motor activities. This must have a profound effect on both the physical and mental development. It is for this reason that the supine position is one of the worst positions in which to place a child with cerebral palsy, and parents and nurses should be advised to avoid it.

In prone-lying, most children will show maximal flexor hypertonus. In a severe case of spastic quadriplegia, head and spine are usually flexed, the shoulders pulled forward and down, and the arms are usually caught under the body with the hands fisted (Fig. 3-18). Hips and knees are often flexed. If, however, the hips are

Cerebral Palsy 67

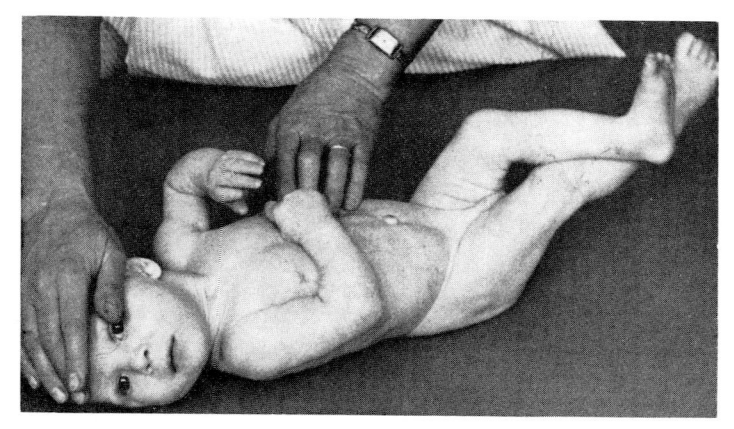

Figure 3-17. Note absence of neck-righting reaction.

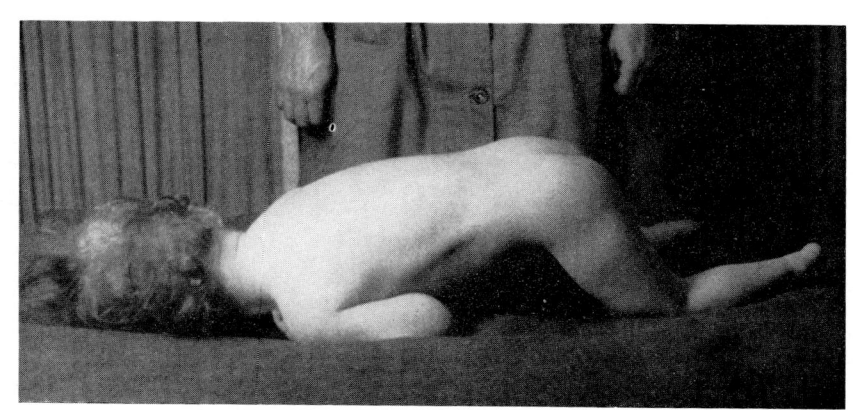

Figure 3-18. Tonic labyrinthine reflex in prone.

extended, the knees are usually extended as well with inward rotation and adduction of the legs. This pattern prevents the child from raising his head. He cannot extend his arms to take his body weight and cannot extend his spine sufficiently to free his arms from under the body. He cannot, therefore, get himself up to kneeling. Lack of rotation also prevents side-sitting and sitting up.

Even in the fully established case of quadriplegia, the clear picture of extension in supine and flexion in prone is *not* the rule.

68 *Physical Therapy Services in the Developmental Disabilities*

A few of these patients, and they are usually the most severe ones, may show severe extensor hypertonus with opisthotonus in supine. They will still show fairly severe extensor hypertonus in prone, although of lesser degree than in supine. The head may still be retracted in prone-lying (Figs. 3-19A and 3-19B) as long

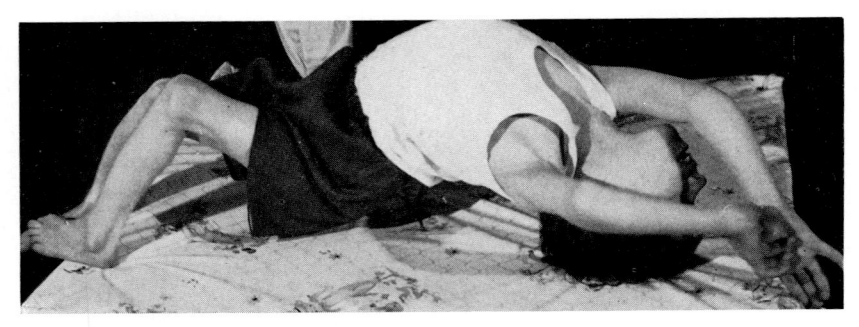

Figure 3-19A. Description in text.

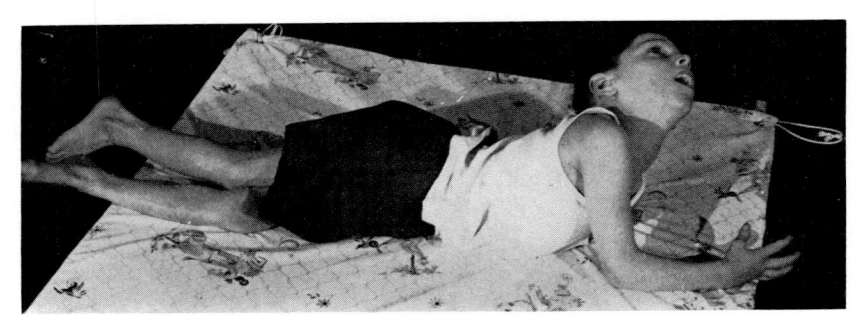

Figure 3-19B. Description in text.

as the child's trunk and legs are stiffly extended. There may then be resistance of the head to active and passive flexion. However, if one flexes the child's hips or knees, or abducts his legs, the head may suddenly flex and the child be unable to raise it.

Other cases, a very few in number, may show flexor hypertonus in prone and supine; this is very much stronger in prone.

In both types of cases one may doubt that the ability to raise the head in supine or prone is the result of normal head-righting or of an abnormal postural tone. However, the normal child from the sixth month on can raise his head in both supine and prone, whereas these children can raise it only in either supine or prone.

The Tonic Neck Reflexes

THE ASYMMETRICAL TONIC NECK REFLEX (Figs. 3-20A, 3-20B and 3-20C). The asymmetrical tonic neck reflex (ATNR) is a proprioceptive reflex obtained from the muscles of the neck and probably also from the receptors of the ligaments and joints of the cervical spine. Turning of the head to one side will increase extensor hypertonus on the side to which the face is turned (the face side) and flexor hypertonus in the opposite side (the skull, or occipital side). In the severe case of cerebral palsy the response may be an almost immediate one, the face limbs extend and the occipital limbs flex. This inequality of distribution of hypertonus will frequently also affect the whole trunk and produce a scoliosis and tilting of the pelvis (Fig. 3-20A). In milder cases there may be some delay in the response due to a lengthy latency period of this reflex. It seems that the latency period of this reflex is inversely related to the severity of the individual case. The effect is usually more clearly seen in the upper limbs than in the lower ones Fig. 3-20B. Sometimes it can be seen only in the arms Fig. 3-20C. In a milder case the response may appear only when the child is excited or tries to do something difficult. Sometimes its influence can only be demonstrated by testing the change of resistance of a limb to passive flexion or extension with the head first towards and then away from the limb.

The asymmetrical tonic neck reflex may prevent a child from grasping an object while looking at it. He may also be unable to bring his fingers to his mouth, his face, or his body. Not infrequently his eyes may be fixed towards the side to which the face is turned and he cannot move them across the midline to the other side. The acquisition of the coordination of eyes and hands is, therefore, impossible or difficult. The asymmetrical tonic neck reflex is usually stronger to one side, generally the right. This seems to be the reason why so many children appear to be left-handed, as they can grasp objects only with the left flexed arm and hand.

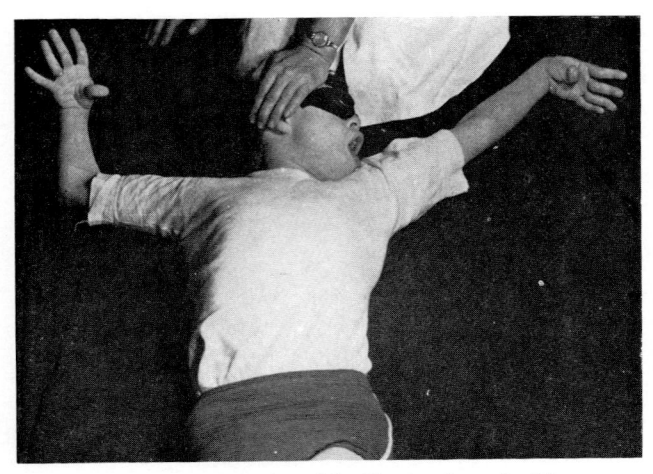

Figure 3-20A. Spastic quadriplegia with distal athetosis. Note: asymmetrical TNR on arms and trunk, with resulting scoliosis and tilting of pelvis.

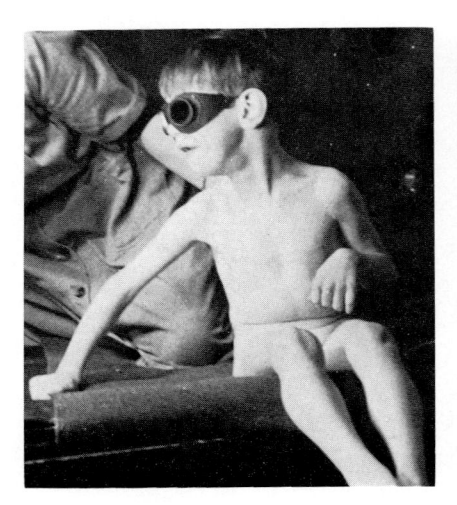

Figure 3-20B. (Left). Asymmetrical TNR in sitting.

Figure 3-20C (Right). Asymmetrical TNR in walking.

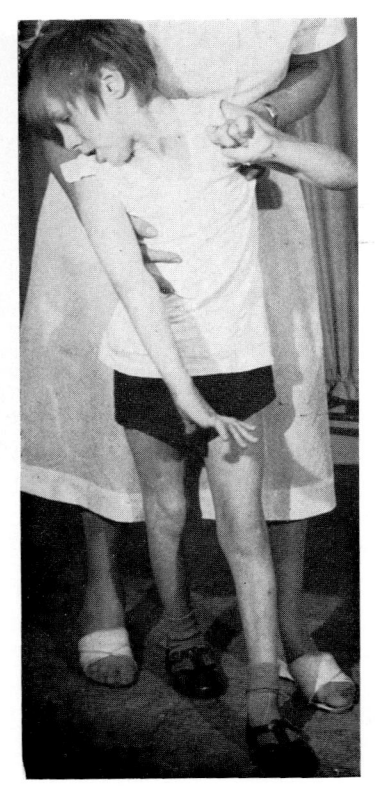

Cerebral Palsy

Under normal circumstances an asymmetrical tonic neck *response* can be seen in babies up to the age of 16 weeks. However, it is very weak, a vestige of the reflex. It never affects the trunk and shows itself only in an occasional assumption of the "fencing position" at rest. The normal baby's activities are not dominated by this response. He can easily move away from this position and can, for instance, suck his fingers regardless of the position of the head. The functional significance of this response is not known but it does not appear to play a significant role in the functional organization of development of the normal child.

THE SYMMETRICAL TONIC NECK REFLEX. The symmetrical tonic neck reflex (STNR) also is a proprioceptive reflex originating in the neck muscles. It is obtained in suitable cases by active or passive raising or flexing of the head. Raising the head produces an increase of extensor hypertonus in the upper limbs and of flexor hypertonus in the lower limbs. The lowering of the head (flexion) has the opposite effect. It is not usually seen in normal babies although they will show a tendency towards better extension of the arms in prone-lying with raised head at some early stage of development.

A child with quadriplegia, when placed on his knees, usually shows a picture of total flexion and is unable to extend his arms. However, if his head is passively raised, the arms may extend in a hypertonic pattern of extension and inward rotation (Fig. 3-21A). If his head is lowered, he may flex his arms and slide forward on extending legs (Fig. 3-21B). The reflex can also be observed in supine, when on raising the child's head forward the arms may flex, while the legs extend, adduct, and may even cross (Fig. 3-21C).

Associated Reactions

Associated reactions, so-called by Walshe (1923) rather than associated movements, are released postural reactions producing a widespread increase of hypertonus in all affected parts of the body not directly concerned with any intended movement. They are released tonic reflexes acting from one limb on the other (Walshe 1923). They can be seen in normal people when they take strenu-

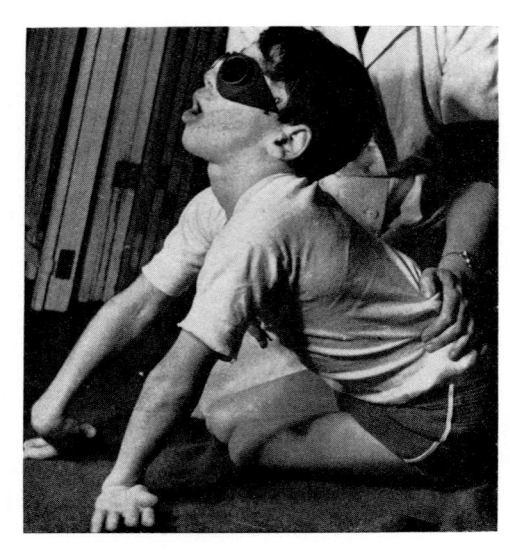

72   *Physical Therapy Services in the Developmental Disabilities*

Figure 3-21A. Spastic quadriplegia with distal athetosis. Symmetrical TNR. With head up, arms in spastic extension; lower limbs locked in flexion.

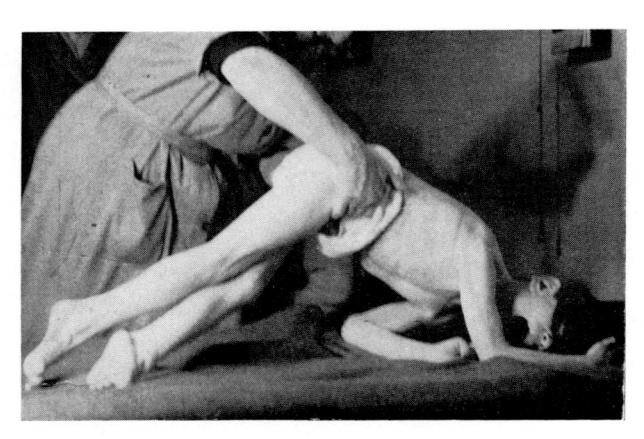

Figure 3-21B. Symmetrical TNR. With head down, legs in spastic extension, upper limbs flexed.

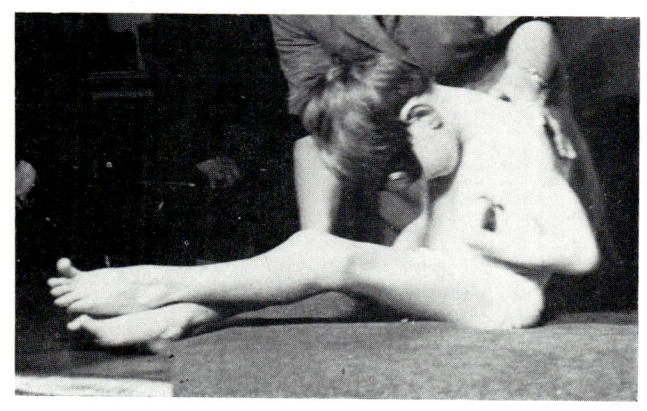

Figure 3-21C. Symmetrical TNR in supine. Head flexed forward. Arms flexed. Legs extended and crossed.

ous exercise—for instance, when lifting a heavy weight. In a spastic quadriplegia the effort to move a limb will increase spasticity throughout the affected parts. If a hemiplegic child from a position of rest (Fig. 3-22A) squeezes an object with the sound hand (Fig. 3-22B), or tries to stand on the sound (Fig. 3-22C) or hemiplegic (Fig. 3-22D) leg, spasticity will increase in the involved side and lead to an accentuation of the abnormal posture.

In treatment, associated reactions must be prevented. One should not make the child use excessive effort of any one part of the body, for one may, in trying to improve the functional use of one part, make the rest of the body worse. For instance, in trying to obtain extension of the spastic arm of a hemiplegic child, one may increase the extensor spasticity of the spastic leg.

The Positive Supporting Reaction

The positive supporting reaction is the result of a twofold stimulus.
 1. The touch of the ball of the foot with the ground.
 2. Pressure with stretch of the intrinsic muscles of the foot.

As a result, hypertonous increases in both the flexor and extensor group of muscles of the leg and more so in the antigravity muscles. This simultaneous contraction of antagonistic

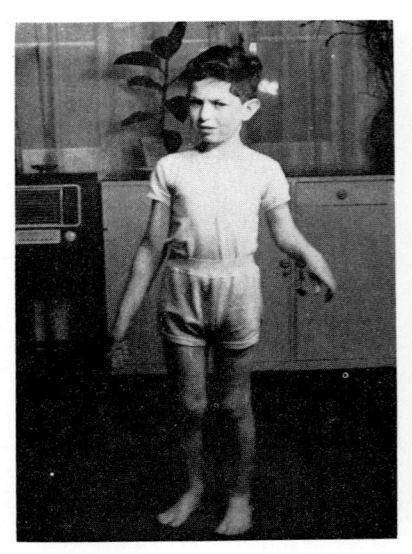

Figure 3-22A. Left-sided hemiplegic. Rest Position.

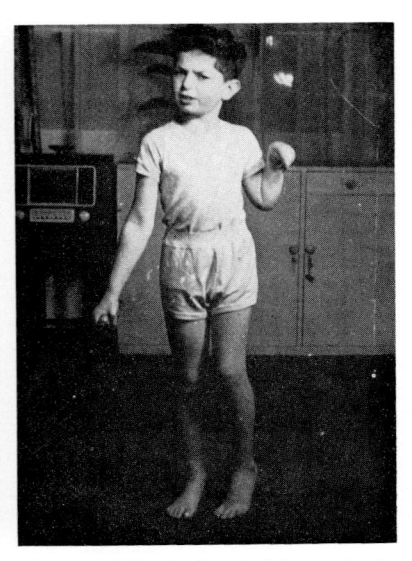

Figure 3-22B. Left-sided hemiplegic. Associated reactions. Note: accentuation of hemiplegic posture of both upper and lower limbs. Note also: head turns towards hemiplegic left side.

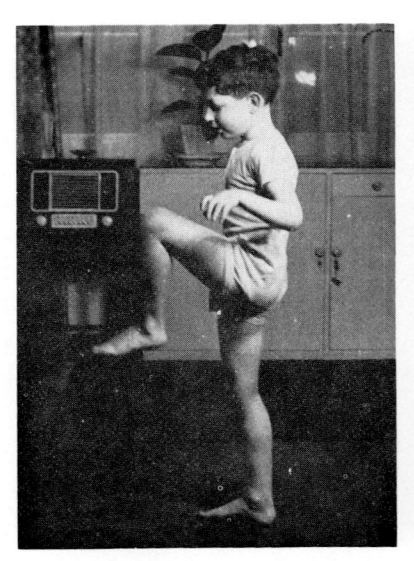

Figure 3-22C. Left-sided hemiplegic. Associated reactions.

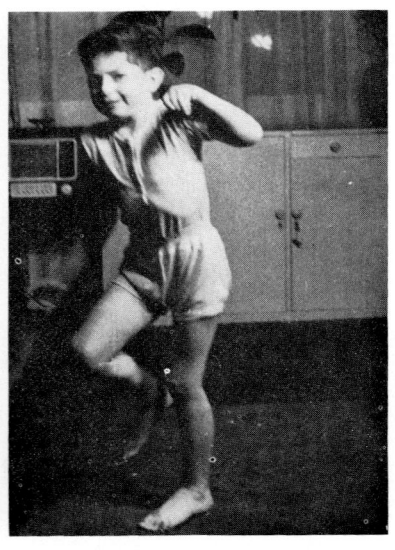

Figure 3-22D. Left-sided hemiplegic. Associated reactions.

muscle groups has been called *cocontraction*. The leg stiffens and becomes a rigid and immobile pillar. The effect persists as long as the two types of stimuli are active. The spastic child walks on tiptoes and as a result of the positive supporting reaction, spasticity in the leg increases every time the child puts his foot down. The child will, therefore, tend to fall backward; weight transfer forward over the standing leg is made very difficult because of insufficient dorsiflexion of ankles and toes.

The Interplay of Tonic Reflex Activity

A knowledge of the individual abnormal postural reflexes may be of great value in analyzing the motor behavior of children with cerebral palsy, and in recognizing the influence of each postural reflex on the coordination of a child's postures and movements. Although these reflexes can only rarely be seen in isolation since the patterns observed are the result of a combination of all of them acting simultaneously, certain distinct patterns which recur in the same circumstances can be traced to the dominating influence of one or the other of these single postural reflexes.

It is comparatively easy to see this in the severely hypertonic patient who shows released tonic reflexes most clearly. Such a patient can only learn to sit up by himself if he has sufficient head control. This will enable him to strike a balance between extensor and flexor hyperactivity. He may also be able to learn to walk if arms and trunk are less involved than the legs. He can, for instance, modify the extensor hypertonus of his legs by thrusting his head and trunk forward, and by semiflexing his hips and knees.

In an athetoid child, tonic reflexes of varying strength appear only momentarily and interfere with his attempts at voluntary activity. In the less severe cases of the athetoid or spastic group, only traces of the typical tonic reflex patterns can be seen, as these children have more varied and adequate postural reactions and are capable of a greater variety of voluntary activity. The abnormal reflexes proper cannot usually be elicited, but their combined influence can often be traced in the child's movement patterns. For instance, even a mildly spastic or athetoid child will walk with his legs inwardly rotated and will put his toes down to the ground first.

In time the primary picture of abnormal coordination of posture and movement produced by the abnormal postural reflexes will undergo secondary changes. In individual cases, especially the milder ones who have greater scope for compensation, these changes may be considerable. Certain individual variations are the result of the interplay of the relevant tonic reflexes and their relative strength. Individual variations are also due to the coexistence of a variety of normal primitive reactions with the abnormal postural reflexes, and depend upon the degree to which the latter interfere with the former. Moreover, changes in the primary picture will result from the child's compensatory efforts. The intelligent child will make use of his abnormal patterns, and he will compensate for the shortcomings of more involved parts by excessive use of less affected ones. This will in time result in an obscuring of the primary picture and in a greater complexity and individuality of the abnormal patterns. It must be admitted, furthermore, that factors as yet unknown may also contribute to the complexity of the picture in the individual case. At the present state of our knowledge, it is often impossible to explain the postures and reactions seen in the individual case in terms of tonic reflexes only. However, a study of the prevailing patterns of posture and movement and their variations in the individual case is of great importance and will give valuable information with respect to diagnosis, early recognition, and treatment.

Other factors, although admittedly of lesser importance, cannot, however, be altogether disregarded. Together with an analysis of the individual patterns of coordination, they will prove of importance in diagnosis, differential diagnosis, and treatment. Two additional factors must be taken into account. They are (1) the type and strength of the abnormal muscle tone, and (2) the type of disturbance of reciprocal innervation.

Abnormal Muscle Tone

All cases of cerebral palsy have in common an abnormal muscle tone. This is classically examined by passively moving a limb and testing the resistance a muscle offers to passive stretch. It is unfortunate that modern neurophysiology has so far not been

Cerebral Palsy

able to explain the different types of abnormality of muscle tone found in cerebral palsy.

Not enough is known about the nature of spasticity. It is considered to be due to a release of the Gamma-system, or very rarely the Alpha-system, from higher inhibitory control (Rushforth 1960, 1962). Presumably, the release of a facilitory mechanism in the brainstem enhances the sensitivity or "bias" of the Gamma-system.

The explanation of rigidity seems to be more difficult. This term is unfortunate as this type of hypertonus is different from the rigidity of Parkinson's disease. It is probably similar to the type of rigidity obtained by decerebration, as described by Sherrington (1947). It is in fact a severe type of spasticity and is perhaps better called "plastic hypertonus." It is characterized by the unchanging resistance a muscle offers to passive stretch throughout its whole range in the direction of either flexion or extension (The Little Club Memorandum, 1959). This phenomenon may be due, at least in part, to cocontraction.

Little is known about the nature of the fluctuating type of muscle tone, found characteristically in the athetoid group of cerebral palsy. The amplitude of fluctuation may vary widely in the individual case, either against a background of a general hypotonic condition, or of a fairly normal postural tone.

A flaccid muscle tone, hypotonia, is usually seen as a transient phenomenon only in cerebral palsy. It then occurs in earliest childhood, followed sooner or later by a spastic or plastic type of hypertonus or by the fluctuating type of tone of the athetoid group.

The assessment of the type and strength of the response of a muscle to stretch may be of some value in the diagnosis and classification of cases. It is, however, of very limited value in the assessment or reassessment of a case, and especially in the planning of a treatment program. For this one may mention the following reasons:

1. Hypertonus and hypotonus as muscular phenomena are quite variable, changing with the child's general condition and excitability and the strength of stimulation—that is, the speed and strength of muscle stretch.

2. Different types of abnormality of muscle tone can be seen in the same child in different parts of the body.

3. One type of muscle tone may change in time in the same affected parts, necessitating reevaluation and reclassification of the case.

4. The distribution and strength of hypertonus in any particular part of the body will change in keeping with the laws of tonic reflex activity; thus, it depends on the position of the head in space or on the relative position of head and trunk.

The assessment of the nature of the abnormal muscle tone and its changes in response to stimulation is regarded as an important factor in the evaluation of a child's condition prior to treatment. However, it is essential that this is done in certain functional patterns, by testing the adaptations of muscle groups to varying attitudes, or, to normal patterns of posture imposed upon them. One is, in fact, testing muscle tone by using postural (functional) patterns rather than the resistance of muscles to passive stretch. The argument for testing in patterns rather than individual muscles has been put forward most cogently by Milani-Comparetti (1965a). When testing in this way, one makes the following observations:

1. If postural reflex activity is normal, quick and immediate, adjustment of muscles to postural changes will result.

2. If spasticity or rigidity are present, undue resistance of muscles to postural changes and delay of adjustment, if any at all, will result.

3. If postural tone fluctuates, as is the case with the athetoid group of cerebral palsy, undue resistance to postural changes, intermittent in nature and alternating with complete absence of resistance will result.

4. If flaccidity is present, undue lack of resistance and hypermobility of joints on changing the children's postural pattern will be observed.

Techniques and Patterns Used in Testing Muscle Tone

IN SUPINE. The following methods are used:

1. Elevation, horizontal abduction and placing of arms by the sides of the child's body, all tested in extension and outward ro-

tation of arms. Test for resistance of extension, outward rotation and supination of arms, and for resistance to extension of wrist and fingers with abduction of thumb.

2. Stretch child's arms out forward as in being picked up and pulled to sitting. Test resistance at shoulders and elbows to forward flexion at shoulders and to extension of elbows.

3. Sit child up from supine. Test resistance at hips to flexion and abduction.

4. Abduct legs with outward rotation in flexion and in extension. Test resistance to abduction, to outward rotation, and to dorsiflexion of ankles and toes; compare degree of resistance with legs flexed or extended.

5. Lift child's head off support, and turn it to either side. Test for resistance to forward flexion, or to side-turning. Note also asymmetrical tonic reflex patterns on arms and legs, i.e. whether the face, arm, or leg becomes more stiff in extension, or the skull, arm, and leg more stiff in flexion.

IN PRONE. The following techniques are suggested:

1. Lift child's head and shoulders off support. Note resistance to extension of neck, shoulders, spine and hips.

2. Stretch child's arms above head with arms extended at elbows and outwardly rotated. Note resistance to elevation, outward rotation and extension of arms and hands.

3. Place child's arms extended in outward rotation beside child's body. Note resistance to extension, outward rotation and any tendency to flexion of spine and hips.

4. Abduct child's legs and legs extended and in outward rotation. Note resistance to abduction and outward rotation, as well as to dorsiflexion of ankles and toes.

5. Bend child's knees with adducted and with abducted legs. Note resistance to flexion and compare degree of resistance with adducted and with abducted legs. Also, note tendency to hip flexion and compare this with adducted and with abducted legs.

6. Test resistance to flexion of hips and knees when putting child from prone onto his knees.

SITTING. Techniques and patterns are as follows:

1. Put child into long-sitting with abducted legs, arms for-

ward. Note resistance to abduction and extension of legs, to dorsiflexion of ankles and toes, to flexion of hips with trunk leaning forward, to lifting of head and to moving extended arms forward, hands to ground.

2. Side-sitting. Put both knees rotated towards one side, extend child's arms on the side towards which his knees are placed and put his hand to the ground for support. Note resistance to rotation and placing legs to one side and to extending child's arms and hands. Change position of legs and arms towards opposite side and note and compare degree of resistance.

KNEELING. The following methods are suggested:

1. From side-sitting place child on his hands and knees. Note resistance to lifting his head, extending his elbows, abducting his arms if they tend to adduct too much, and resistance to getting his hips off his feet (i.e. to about 90° of flexion).

2. Kneel-standing. Lift child's body up by his shoulders so that he supports himself on his knees only. Note resistance to extension of his hips and to lifting his arms up.

STANDING. Techniques are the following:

1. Squatting and standing up. Make the child squat on his haunches, heel down, and help him to stand up, lifting him from under his chest. Note resistance to squatting (i.e. to flexion of hips, knees, and ankles). Also, note resistance to dorsiflexion of his toes in squatting. Then note resistance (i.e. downward pressure of head, shoulder-girdle and trunk) when helping him to stand up.

2. Make the child stand with abducted outwardly rotated legs, heels on ground. Note resistance to abduction and outward rotation of legs, and extension of knees. Compare resistance to extension of knees when hips are extended. Also note resistance to dorsiflexion of toes in standing.

3. Make child stand with body leaning forward and downward, hands on floor, and lift his body up from under his chest wall to stand upright. Note resistance to lifting his head and trunk to extension.

When testing muscle tone by using the above patterns, one may find resistance in the form of severe, moderate, or slight spasticity. Resistance may be transient or sudden, and may then alternate with complete lack of resistance. These changes may be encountered at irregular intervals when repeating the same test (e.g. in athetoids). There also may be lack of resistance in flaccid children.

The findings will give an indication of the child's abilities or difficulties in performing the movements necessary to assure these postures and to maintain them. Treatment can then be planned to improve the child's postural tone and motor patterns.

The Type of Disturbance of Reciprocal Innervation

A study of the law of reciprocal innervation and of the type of disturbance caused by an abnormal interplay of opposing muscular forces may be of great value in differentiating the various types of cerebral palsy and offer valuable additional clues to treatment. It may also explain, at least to some extent, the reasons for the imbalance of opposing muscular forces which the orthopedic surgeon finds so difficult to assess when dealing with the surgical problems of this condition (Jones 1961, Sharrard 1961). This problem is also mentioned by Tardieu (1961).

Sherrington (1913) stressed the importance of reciprocal innervation for the regulation of postural tone in the maintenance of posture and balance and the performance of normal movements. He showed that in a reflex coordination such as the flexor withdrawal reflex, the agonists were excited and contracted while the antagonists were inhibited and relaxed. He called this phenomenon "reciprocal inhibition." He stressed that inhibition was a central phenomenon and that reciprocal inhibition, as studied on spinal animals, was a special case of reciprocal innervation and not likely to occur under normal conditions.

In normal circumstances agonists, antagonists, and synergists are pitted against each other in a far more adapted form of reciprocal interaction than in simple reciprocal inhibition. This is the result of the regulating influence of higher centers in brainstem, midbrain, cerebellum, and cerebral cortex on the spinal reflex mechanism of muscular coordination. The antagonists are inhibited and relax in a finely graded and adapted manner, in step with the contracting agonists, thus exerting a steadying and guiding influence on the movement in progress. Synergistic muscles are made to contract to steady and fix neighboring joints, to lend precision to the movement and optimize mechanical conditions for the interplay of opposing muscular forces in the performance of a skill. Sherrington (1907) also showed that in certain circumstances, especially in the service of postural fixation and control, both agonists and antagonists may be made to contract simultaneously by reciprocal innervation. Palpation of the muscles of the thigh of a standing leg will show this to be the case.

This simultaneous contraction of agonists and antagonists Riddoch and Buzzard (1921) later on called "cocontraction."

In a child with a spastic hypertonus, there seems to be on the one hand a deviation of reciprocal innervation towards an excess of cocontraction, when spastic agonists are opposed by equally or more spastic antagonists. This is especially so around proximal joints. On the other hand, there may also be a deviation towards excessive reciprocal inhibition. The severe tonic inhibition of certain muscles by their spastic antagonists will prevent any attempt at a movement. These muscles will, therefore appear to be "weak."

Both types of deviation can be seen in the same spastic child in different parts of the body. For instance, all the muscles around the shoulder are in spastic contraction with severe depression of the shoulder and fixation of the shoulder-blade. There is resistance of the arm to elevation, to backward extension, to moving it forward, and to horizontal abduction. Another example is the simultaneous spastic contraction of flexors and extensors of the hips, with resistance of the hips to both full flexion and extension. Examples of tonic reciprocal inhibition are the apparently "weak" dorsiflexors of the ankle, seemingly "weak" peronaei in opposition to spastic tibialis anticus and posticus.

In some cases, cocontraction may not be evident until the child attempts to move; the effort will make him stiffen his limbs in a cocontraction pattern with simultaneous contraction of agonists and antagonists. For instance, an attempt to raise the arm will result only in a further depression of the shoulder. It seems as if the stimulation of effort is misdirected into the abnormal pattern of coordination.

These facts seem to explain the relative immobility and fixation of the spastic child. He is fixed in a few typical and abnormal patterns and if movements are at all possible, they require excessive effort and are limited in range and direction.

In the ataxic and athetoid group of patients the abnormal patterns of coordination seem to be towards excessive reciprocal inhibition. Any attempt at a movement will lead to an immediate and excessive inhibition and relaxation of the antagonists. The lengthening group of muscles are, therefore, unable to hold and guide the movement. Lack of the necessary degree of cocontraction is also responsible for the poor supporting action of the synergists. This explains the well-known excessive mobility and lack of fixation and postural control, so characteristic of this group of patients. Their movements are poorly controlled, of extreme range and poorly coordinated.

Characteristic Types of Cerebral Palsy

The various types of cerebral palsy will be considered next, classified in accordance with the three factors previously discussed: type of abnormal muscle tone, deviation of reciprocal innervation and the patterns of posture and movement shown by the individual case. The motor development of each type will be sketched and the early appearance of abnormal postural reflex activity will be described. The influence of the abnormal patterns of posture and movement on the child's functional activities will be analyzed with a description of the change of the primary patterns resulting from it and leading finally to the typical contractures and deformities.

The Spastic Child

The spastic child shows hypertonus of a permanent character, spastic or rigid hypertonus. The degree of spasticity varies with the child's general condition, his excitability and the strength of stimulation. If spasticity is severe, the child is fixed more or less in a few typical postures. This is due to the severe degrees of cocontraction of the involved parts, especially around the proximal joints. Some muscles may seem to be weak as a result of tonic reciprocal inhibition. This applies, for instance, to the gluteus, quadriceps femoris, the dorsiflexors of the ankles and the abdominal muscles. True weakness may, however, develop in some muscle groups because of disuse in cases of long-standing. It will develop also fairly quickly after prolonged and sustained bracing. Spasticity is of a typical distribution, and changes in a predictable manner owing to tonic reflex activity. Movements are restricted in range and require excessive effort.

The severely affected spastic quadriplegic children are usually very insecure and helpless. They are unable to move effectively and to adjust themselves to changes of posture, especially if they are handled quickly when being washed, dressed, picked up, sat up, etc. They cannot right themselves when being placed into uncomfortable positions, and cannot maintain or regain their balance. They are in constant fear of falling if not sufficiently supported and assured. They cannot express themselves with speech or gesture. They may develop obsessive-compulsive traits, be very reluctant to adapt themselves to new situations, and may even become passive and withdrawn. They surround themselves with a protective wall and do not react to stimulation. They have learned that they cannot respond adequately and that any attempt usually results in failure and frustration.

SPASTIC QUADRIPLEGIA. The whole body is involved. The distribution is asymmetrical, one side being more affected than the other. The upper parts are either more involved than the lower ones, or they are at least equally affected. Head control is, therefore, usually poor and speech and articulation are more or less severely involved. If spasticity is severe, the child is helpless and any attempt to move will lead only to a further increase of spasticity as a result of associated reactions. Thus, any attempt at moving will lead to an accentuation of the abnormal postures.

Once spasticity has established itself, the child is unable to right his head, maintain his equilibrium in any position, or to use his arms or hands. In supine he usually shows strong head, neck, and shoulder retraction. Neck-righting is absent and rotation of the head may only lead to the assumption of the fencing position (ATNR). Trunk rotation is prevented by shoulder retraction. The child is, therefore, unable to roll over from supine to side-lying (Fig. 3-16). He lacks rotation within the body axis—the result of the body-righting reaction on the body—and therefore cannot roll over into prone. Inability to raise the head prevents him from initiating sitting up. This difficulty is further enhanced by his inability to flex spine and hips, and to bring his arms and hands forward to pull himself up.

In prone-lying, he is usually unable to raise his head or to use his arms for support, and cannot, therefore, get up or kneel. If the body is lifted up and off the support by the shoulders, shoulders and spine are flexed and the arms pull up in flexion. Hips and knees may either be flexed or, if the hips are extended, the legs are also extended in a total pattern with inward rotation and adduction (Fig. 3-18).

Only a few of these children may acquire some limited righting ability of the head. This is, however, interfered with by tonic reflex activity whenever the child moves his head into a position which favors its occurrence. This will happen, for instance, in sitting when the child tries to raise his head in order to look up. He will then tend to fall backward into extension, not infrequently throwing his arms up and out in a startle reaction.

If the child has a fair measure of head control and is intelligent, he may learn to avoid these danger positions. He may learn a certain equilibrium between flexor and extensor spasticity. He will then lean slightly backward because of insufficient flexion of the hips. He will compensate for this by a kyphosis of the dorsal spine in order to bring trunk and head over the sitting base. The neck will be hyperextended and the head will be held stiffly in a more or less normal position. The sitting base is narrow and precarious due to the flexor-adduction pattern of the legs.

He cannot use his arms for support, being unable to extend them (Fig. 3-23). When trying to raise his head, he is in danger of falling backward, due to the increase of general extension (Fig. 3-24). When looking down, he will slump forward (Fig. 3-25). Balance reactions will be absent or very poor. If, in addition, he

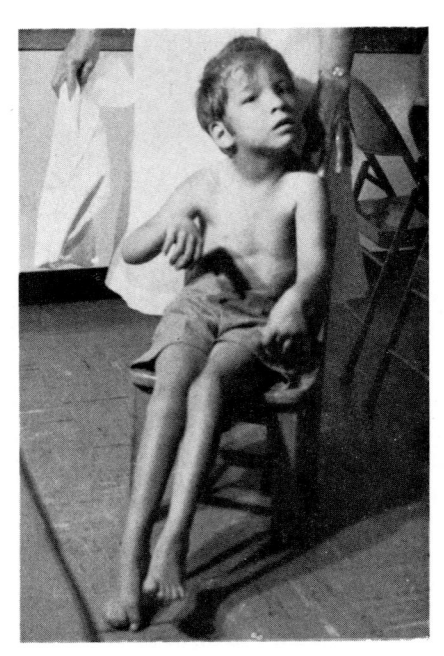

86 *Physical Therapy Services in the Developmental Disabilities*

Figure 3-23. Typical sitting posture of a child with spastic quadriplegia.

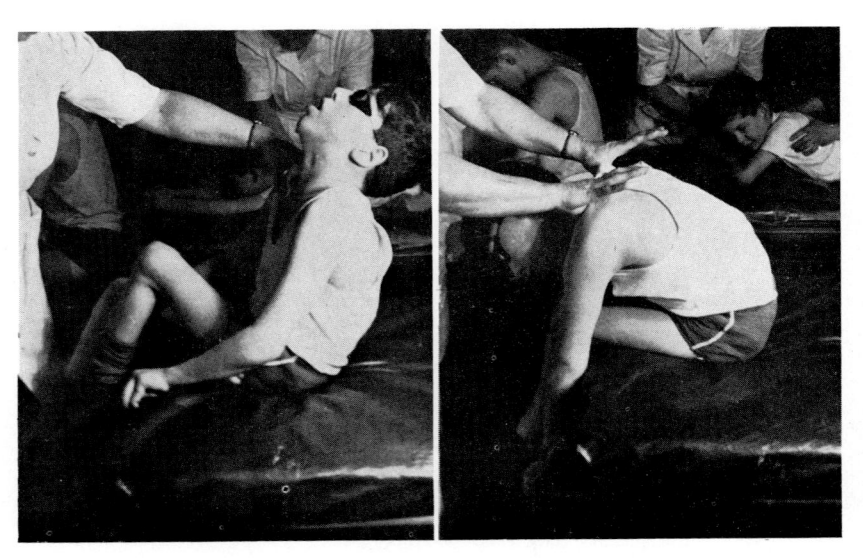

Figure 3-24. Description in text.   Figure 3-25. Description in text.

has a strong asymmetrical tonic neck reflex (which is usually stronger to the right) the child may learn to use one arm, usually the left, for grasp and release by turning his head first to one side to reach out, and then to the other to grasp the object. Hip flexion in sitting is made more difficult by the increase of extensor spasticity resulting from touch and pressure of the buttocks against the support, probably a positive supporting reaction of the trunk.

In time the child will, therefore, develop typical contractures and deformities, such as a scoliosis or kyphoscoliosis, semiflexion deformities of hips and knees, a possible subluxation or dislocation of one hip, usually the left. This dislocation is probably the result of several factors, such as the underdevelopment of the hip joints due to disuse, adductor spasticity and inward rotation of the legs, and a pelvic tilt. The latter is the result of spasticity of the side flexors of the trunk on the more flexed side, the pelvis being drawn up and tilted forward on that side, a tendency accentuated by the asymmetrical tonic neck reflex. This is probably the most important factor.

Other children may adopt an attitude of full flexion in sitting. The head is flexed forward and they will look down in order to avoid the asymmetrical tonic neck reflex as this reflex is strongest in extension. They will in this way make use of the symmetrical tonic reflex to enable them to use both hands for holding and grasping. They cannot, however, now extend the arms to reach out, and the legs and hips will tend to extend and adduct. In order to maintain sitting they will use excessive compensatory flexion of the spine and will in time develop a kyphosis and semiflexion deformities of hips and knees, with strong cocontraction of flexors and extensors of hips and knees.

The quadriplegic child with more moderate spasticity may in time acquire some of the righting and equilibrium reactions necessary for kneeling and sitting but not, however, for standing and walking. Unless the child can compensate for this lack of equilibrium by using arms and hands for support, standing and walking will be impossible. As long as these children move carefully and slowly in sitting, avoiding extreme positions, tonic reflex activity will not greatly interfere, and postural tone will not become too abnormal (Figs. 3-26 and 3-27).

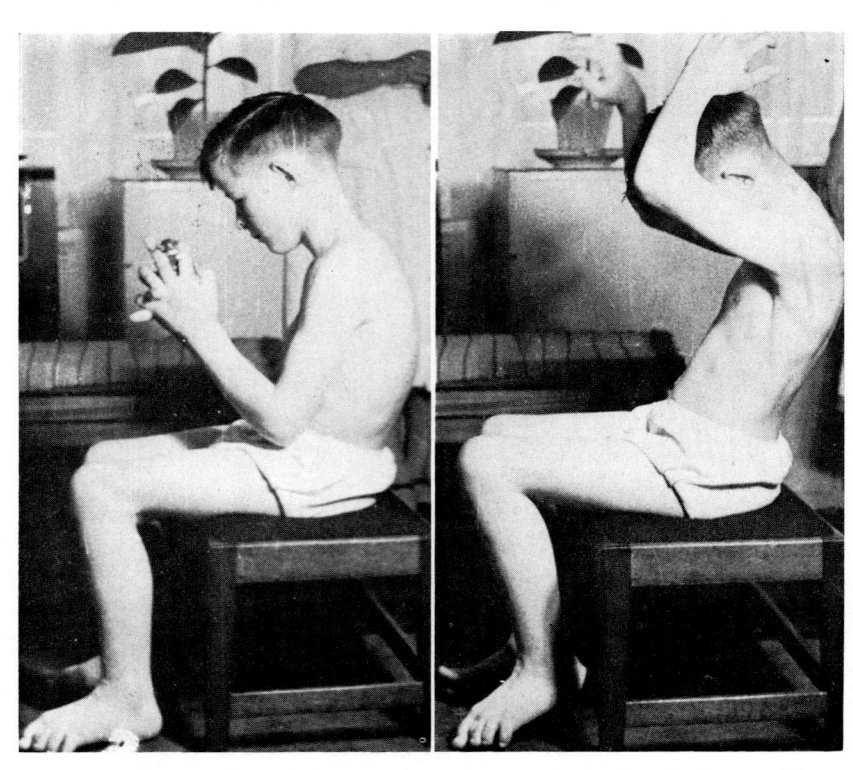

Figure 3-26. Typical sitting position.

Figure 3-27. Falling back on raising arms is prevented by flexion of head.

SPASTIC DIPLEGIA OR PARAPLEGIA. In the diplegic child the lower extremities are more severely involved than the upper ones. The condition is of a fairly symmetrical distribution. Head control and speech are usually good, although a surprising number of this type show some impairment of the coordination of the eyes.

These children may seem quite normal until they reach the age of six to eight months, since signs of spasticity may be absent or slight and the physiological predominance of flexor tone and the baby's general postural behavior may be very similar to those of a normal baby of his age. He will develop normal head-righting and, if the arms are unaffected, normal protective reactions (propping reactions) of the arms. Any abnormality may appear only when the normal process of extension reaches the lower trunk and hips. If the arms and head are involved to some extent, the appearance of head-righting and the propping reactions of the arms will be delayed and they will remain incompletely developed. Head-raising in prone and supine may be difficult and delayed due to flexor or extensor hypertonus respectively.

Though the arms may not show an asymmetrical tonic neck reflex, head-turning may produce tonus changes in the more involved legs. The child may kick only with the "occipital leg" while the "face leg" may be held in extension, first in a more primitive pattern of outward rotation; later on, the total pattern of extension, adduction and inward rotation may develop. In the more severe cases this total abnormal pattern may develop very early, before the age of six months.

If arms and hands are only slightly involved, or even unaffected, the child may, during the early phase of predominant flexion, still be able to turn to his side. Rolling over to prone will, however, present some difficulties. The child will learn this much later and will do so only with the help of his arms, while the legs remain stiffly extended. This is largely due to a lack of rotation and the inability to flex and bring the uppermost leg forward. Once he has achieved rolling into prone, he may learn to progress on his abdomen by a kind of swimming movement by alternating abduction-flexion and adduction-extension movement of the lower extremities. This is made possible by the fact that at this stage the early primitive movements of the legs still persist in prone, while in supine and sitting the legs are already stiffly extended.

Later on, creeping will become impossible as extension increases; with it, extensor spasticity of the legs becomes stronger. This happens usually when the baby acquires extension of the spine and hips, sufficient to support himself in prone on his forearms. He will now progress by dragging himself along the floor in this way which will produce associated reactions and an increase of extensor spasticity of the legs. The legs will, therefore, soon show the total extensor spastic pattern with extension, inward rotation, adduction of the legs, and plantiflexion of the feet.

Although the child may be able to raise his head in supine, sitting up will be impossible or difficult as the hips resist flexion and the legs will adduct and may even cross. Sitting up may, therefore, be delayed up to the age of three years or even longer. The child may, however, be able to sit with some support nearer the normal stage. In such a case, early detection may be delayed until the baby reaches the age of eight or nine months, when he should sit up but cannot do so, and shows poor balance in sitting. Sitting fairly safely is only possible by compensation for the insufficient flexion of hips and knees by bringing head and spine well forward.

If the arms can be extended, they will be used excessively for support, as the child lacks equilibrium of hips and legs. The child will, therefore, at best use one arm only for reach and grasp. He will be unwilling to raise his head or reach forward and up with both arms, as he will then tend to fall backward. In some children a persistent Moro reflex may add to their difficulties by making it impossible to put the arms down for support as a protection against falling backward.

In children who cannot use the arms for support, the strong flexion of the spine enabling them to sit at all will in time produce a structural kyphosis with flexor hypertonus of neck, chest, and abdominal muscles. The pelvis will be tilted forward. The original primary extensor spasticity of the hips and legs with a relative reciprocal inhibition of the flexors will gradually change into a secondary picture of semiflexion of hips and knees, with cocontraction of the hip, knee flexors and extensors. This is the beginning of the development of the well-known scissor posture of the lower extremities later seen in standing. It will become more distinct in standing through the added effect of the positive supporting reaction which will add sufficient extensor tone for standing.

The sitting pattern of the diplegic child with relatively free arms (Fig. 3-28) will be different since he can use his arms for support. He will use a pattern of strong flexion of the hips which helps him to abduct his legs and flex his knees. The pelvis is tilted forward (anteverted) and he sits with a stiffly extended spine. Later on, when standing up, extension of the hips will become difficult. In standing, the child will compensate for the insufficiency of hip extension by a compensatory extension of head and shoulders to assume and maintain the erect posture. This will result in a compensatory lordosis (Fig. 3-29). He tends to fall backward unless he can hold on to a support. Cocontraction of the muscles around hips and knees will develop in standing and walking, as in the other type of diplegia, with resulting scissoring of the legs.

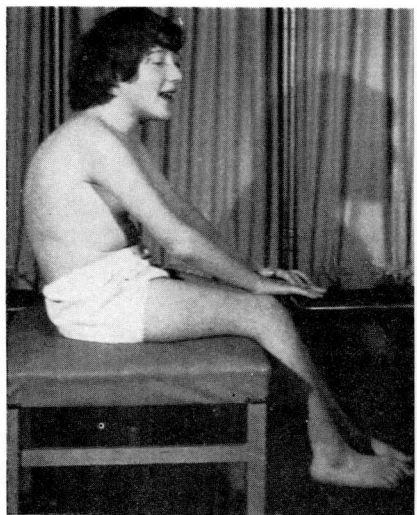

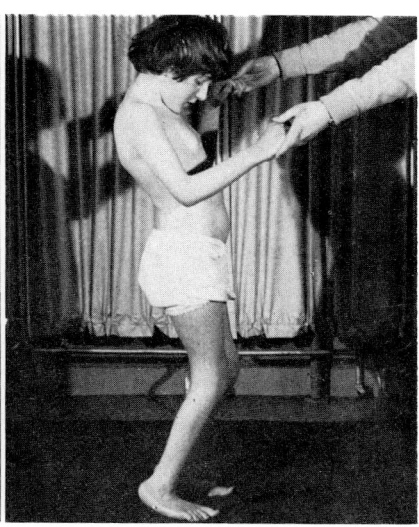

Figure 3-28. Typical sitting posture of a diplegic child.

Figure 3-29. Typical standing posture. Spastic diplegia.

Whereas the normal child achieves a fair degree of emancipation of arms and hands around 18 months, having by then acquired sufficient balance of trunk and legs, the diplegic child has to rely indefinitely on his arms for support. In early life he uses his arms for rolling over from supine to prone, and for pulling himself along the floor in prone and kneeling; later on, in standing and walking, he has to hold on to people or furniture, or has to use sticks or crutches. This involves constant and excessive use of the flexor muscles of arms and hands and of the shoulder-girdle and upper trunk which are usually involved to some extent. The child will, therefore, retain a clumsy grasp with pronation of the forearm and the primitive patterns of grasp and release belonging to earlier stages of normal child development, a time when flexor patterns predominate. Extension of wrists and fingers, abduction and opposition of thumb, and supination of the forearms and wrist will develop late and incompletely.

In standing and walking, when acquired late and possible only if arms and hands can be used, children will make excessive use of whatever righting and equilibrium reactions are present "above the waist." They will use excessive compensatory movements of head, upper trunk, and arms, as hips and legs are stiff and comparatively immobile. They lack the ability of an automatic transfer of the body weight onto the standing leg to set one leg free in order to make a step. The body weight remains on the inside of the foot. They lack balance and rotation, and in walking, seem to be falling from one leg to the other. They are unable to stand still without holding on. They seem to walk in two principal patterns, as listed below:

1. Children with strong flexion of the spine and backward tilt (retroversion) of the pelvis lean backward with their trunk in order to raise one leg and bring it forward to make a step. They then throw the body forward to transfer the weight (pigeon walk).

2. Children with a straight and erect dorsal spine and a forward tilt of the pelvis will have a compensatory lordosis of the lumbar spine, and will use alternating side flexion of the trunk from the waist in order to circumduct and bring the stiff leg forward.

Whereas a normal person walks with mobile legs and a relatively stable trunk, these children show excessive compensatory mobility of the trunk and stiff and immobile legs. They stand and walk on tiptoes, as dorsiflexion of the ankles will produce an increase of flexor tone throughout the legs. This will make standing and walking impossible, and may cause them to collapse.

The deformities which may result from the functional use of these abnormal patterns are, therefore, as follows:
1. A kyphosis of the spine.
2. A lumbar lordosis.
3. Tilting of the pelvis with insufficient extension of the hips.
4. Severe adduction of the thighs, which together with the poor development of the hip joints due to late standing may lead to a subluxation or dislocation of one or both hips.
5. The typical scissor posture of the legs.
6. An equinus or equinovalgus deformity of the feet.

SPASTIC HEMIPLEGIA. The early diagnosis of infantile spastic hemiplegia is not usually difficult because of the early asymmetry of postural and movement patterns. The affected hand will be fisted, the baby unable to open it. He will not kick with the affected leg. His head is usually turned away from the affected side. He will not pass through the symmetrical phase of normal development, starting towards the end of the sixteenth week with the disappearance of the last vestiges of an asymmetrical tonic neck response. He will not use both arms in midline, will not reach out and grasp with the affected hand, and will not support himself on the hemiplegic arm. The development in all activities which require balance of trunk and the use of both hands for support will be delayed. It will take him longer to establish balance in standing and walking. He will tend to fall towards the affected side as he lacks balance of limbs and trunk on that side, and will be unable to protect his face when falling as flexor spasticity of the arm prevents its protective extension.

The child will, therefore, in time orientate himself more and more towards the sound side. He will prefer in an emergency to fall towards that side which allows him to protect his face and head. In due course, righting and equilibrium reactions will even become hyperactive on the sound side, in order to compensate for their lack on the affected side.

At first the hemiplegic baby progresses along the floor in prone-lying, his head turned away from the affected side and dragging along the hemiplegic limbs. The affected limbs are either little used or cannot be moved at all. He does not crawl but later on will progress on his seat, pulling himself along with the sound arm and dragging the affected side behind. He will learn to sit up and stand up with the help of the sound side only, and the development of balance in standing and walking will be late. In standing he will carry his weight predominantly on the sound leg. At first the affected leg will remain abducted and relatively free of weight-bearing. At that time, the leg will appear to be weak rather than spastic, and the child will tend to collapse on it. He can usually put his heel to the ground quite easily. Because of the abduction pattern of the whole leg at this time, his foot shows eversion rather than inversion. His toes, however, are already stiff in plantiflexion and will show clawing of the toes.

As the child learns to walk, his leg and foot will gradually stiffen as he will have to take his weight, at least momentarily, on the affected leg. Extensor spasticity now gradually increases, and in many cases a pattern of inversion and plantiflexion of the ankle develops, in addition to the clawing of the toes. In walking, the child will now hyperextend his knee as he brings his weight forward over his foot without being able to flex his ankle sufficiently. He keeps his pelvis rotated backward on the affected side and his hips in some degree of flexion, as this will allow him to put his heel down. He therefore develops a pattern of walking very similar to the pattern of progression in sitting on the floor, leaving the affected side behind.

At the same time that flexor spasticity of arm and hand increases, the arm draws up in walking, and even more so in running, largely as a result of associated reactions. Associated reactions are secondary to efforts of the sound side—exclusive use of the sound hand, overactivity of the sound leg, lack of balance and the difficulty of raising the affected leg in walking. As a result, opening of the fingers of the affected hand will become more difficult and possible only with a flexed wrist. In many cases flexor contractures of elbow and wrists with pronation and ulnar deviation of the hand will develop in time.

As the child learns to carry his weight on the affected leg in standing and walking, it will become stiff in extension. The young child whose leg and foot are still mobile, has insufficient extensor tone to carry his weight, as long as his heel is on the ground, with a flexed and mobile knee. This can be observed when the child attempts to walk down some steps. He cannot do this in the normal way, stepping down with alternating legs. He uses only the affected side for stepping down while bearing his weight on the flexed sound leg. He can support his weight on the affected leg only with the help of extensor spasticity which is increased by the pressure of the ball of the foot against the ground. This means, however, that he has to walk on his toes. In time contractures of the muscles of the calf and of the long flexors of the toes may develop.

The Athetoid Child

All athetoid patients show an unsteady and fluctuating type of postural tone, but the amplitude of the fluctuations may vary widely in the individual case. These children lack sustained postural tone and cannot, therefore, maintain a stable position. There is insufficient postural fixation due to a lack of cocontraction—simultaneous contraction of agonists and antagonists to give guidance and proper support to the moving part. The grading of antagonistic activity during a movement is poor, and contraction of one group of muscles will lead to a complete relaxation by reciprocal inhibition of antagonists. The lengthening groups do not hold and, therefore, do not grade the intended movement. Because of this the movements are jerky and extreme in range with poor control of the middle ranges.

Fluctuations of muscle tone are sudden and manifest themselves in some of the involuntary movements seen in all cases of the athetoid group. In the individual case we may see the following types of involuntary movements:

1. Intermittent tonic spasms. These are predictable in pattern and are largely dependent on a change in the position of the head; that is, they are due to the influence of the tonic labyrinthine and neck reflexes. They may fix the child temporarily in certain extreme postures of total flexion or extension (tonic labyrinthine in-

fluence), or in asymmetrical postures of extension of the face limbs and flexion of the occipital limbs (asymmetrical tonic neck reflex influence). There may be a mixture of both in the individual case.

2. Mobile spasms (Walshe and Wilson 1914/15). These involve the limbs in alternating movements of flexion and extension, pronation and supination, etc. They are often rhythmic in nature. Examples are the "athetoid dance" (spinal stepping reflexes) and the pawing of the ground with one foot.

3. Fleeting localized contractions. They affect muscles or muscle groups anywhere in the body, and if they are strong and affect many muscle groups, they may produce grotesque and exaggerated postures and movements, like the grimacing of the face and the bizarre attitudes and movements of hands and fingers. Their patterns of coordination are quite unpredictable and the law of reciprocal innervation is in abeyance in this type of involuntary movement (Wilson 1925). These postures and movements defy attempts at imitation by a normal person. If these localized muscular contractions are weaker and more limited, they may show themselves only in minor localized twitches.

All these types of involuntary movement are reinforced during any attempt at volitional activity when the patient tries to coordinate a purposeful movement against the background of an unstable postural tone and in spite of the interference by tonic reflexes.

Most of the cases of the athetoid group belong to the quadriplegias in whom the head and upper parts are more involved than the lower ones. The distribution is usually very asymmetrical with one side more involved than the other. A few cases are seen among the hemiplegias who show some distal athetosis. This appears usually around or after the sixth to seventh year. More rarely one sees children with a pure hemiathetosis.

Most children of this group appear to be unstable and unpredictable in their response to stimulation. They seem to have a high threshold of stimulation with a delay of response when hypotonic. If, however, a response is obtained, it is explosive and exaggerated. They show, therefore, quick changes of extreme degree from one state to the other, both physically and emotionally. They show sudden outbursts of temper, although generally speaking, these children are often outgoing and gay. They often laugh easily and cry (after some delay) with infantile abandon.

In the athetoid quadriplegias, postural tone is usually low during the first two to three years. Their postural patterns resemble those of a premature child rather than those of a full-term baby (Fig. 3-30). Righting reactions may not develop for many years and may remain defective even in later life. Head control is absent or very poor, the baby being unable to raise his head in supine or prone-lying. In the supine position, he is unable to initiate sitting up or to turn over to prone or side-lying. The baby cannot tolerate prone-lying as he is unable to raise his head, extend his spine and hips or use his arms for support (Fig. 3-31). He cannot get up on hands and knees and is unable to crawl. He may, therefore, spend the first years of his life in supine-lying or propped-up sitting. He commonly holds his head to one side, usually the right, and cannot move it into midline or maintain it there. When pulled to sitting, the child's head lags excessively. He is unable to lift it off the support and indeed pulls it backward.

As the child grows older and starts to react more to environmental stimulation, postural tone develops and becomes stronger.

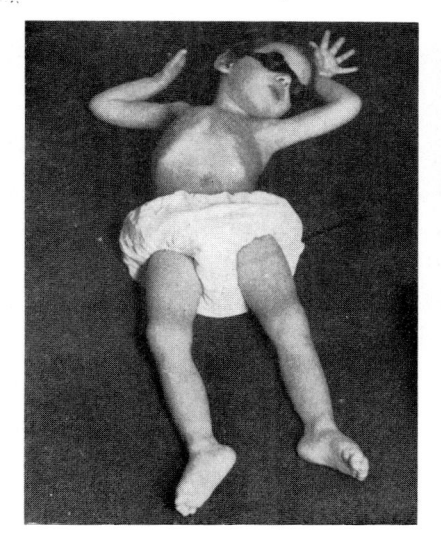

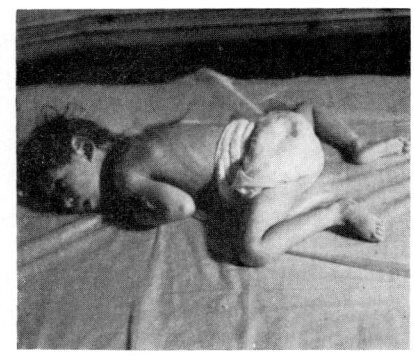

Figure 3-30 *(Left)* Athetoid quadriplegia in supine.

Figure 3-31. *(Above)*. Athetoid quadriplegia in prone.

He will now suddenly stiffen with increasing frequency and in the supine and sitting positions, throw his head backward with extension of hips and spine (Ingram 1955, Polani 1959) (Fig. 3-32).

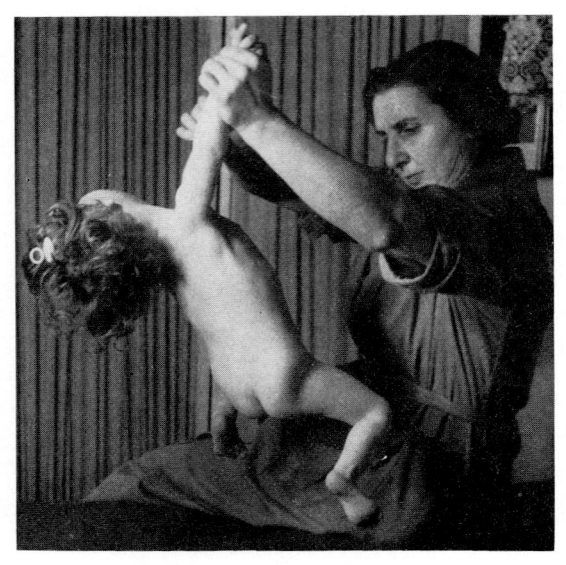

Figure 3-32. Athetoid quadriplegia. Dystonic attack.

The patterns of these intermittent extensor spasms are often the only motor patterns in the supine position of which the child makes voluntary use for moving himself backward along the floor. This he does by bending his legs and pushing his feet, which are less affected, against the floor. At this stage an asymmetrical tonic neck reflex is usually very strong and affects not only the upper limbs but the whole of the trunk. The resulting asymmetrical postural pattern may produce a scoliosis with tilting of the pelvis, which is sometimes followed by a subluxation or dislocation of one hip (usually the left).

He usually retains a primitive flexion-abduction pattern of the lower limbs unless there is additional spasticity, in which case the legs will show a typical extension-adduction pattern. The retention of the abduction-flexion pattern makes sitting on the floor possible later on, as it gives the child a wide sitting base. Sitting is also made possible through some equilibrium reactions of the less affected hips and legs. Though he may not be able to pull himself to sitting as he cannot lift his head or raise his arms, when pulled to sitting he may assist in the movement by strong active flexion of the hips.

Though unable to control his head when being pulled to sitting, once he has reached the sitting position the child may be able to hold his head up and his spine erect, but his head will be turned to one side. In sitting, he may learn to use one hand, usually the left, turning his head to the right and using the pattern of the asymmetrical tonic neck reflex for grasping. His grasp is usually weak, however, and he releases objects too easily and cannot hold on to a support. This is quite different from the tonic grasp of the spastic child, who cannot open his hands and holds on tightly to an object placed into his palm because he cannot release it.

Though the athetoid may be able to sit on the floor with extended and abducted legs, he cannot sit unsupported on a chair as this requires additional flexion of the knees. This will produce a total flexion pattern of the body resulting in the patient's falling forward and down, especially if he cannot use his arms and hands for support. If he raises his head in sitting, a total extensor pattern results and he falls backward.

If the lower limbs are not too badly affected, the child will learn to roll to his side and over to prone-lying, initiating the movements with his legs. Though he is unable to raise his head or to support himself on his arms, from the prone position he will manage to get himself to a kneeling position by pulling his legs in total flexion under his body. He can then raise his head and use his arms for support in extension, making use of the symmetrical tonic neck reflex. He can thus move into kneel-sitting, but he cannot alternately extend and flex his legs and is only able to hop along the floor in this position. Kneeling on all fours and normal crawling will be impossible.

Standing and walking will depend on the relative normality of the child's legs and on the degree of head control and equilibrium which he can develop. Usually, he cannot use his hands to hold on to a support, to pull himself up to standing, or to hold on when walking. Extensor spasms tend to make him fall backward, and both this and the asymmetrical distribution of postural tone make for insufficient support tonus. It may take him years to stand for any length of time, and many children whose lower limbs are badly involved may not stand or walk at all. When they are made to stand, the legs are in a total extension-adduction pattern and may even cross. These children stand high on their toes, their neck and shoulders are retracted, and they tend to fall backward. If they flex one leg to make a step, they may collapse in full flexion.

Other children whose lower limbs remain mobile and retain abduction, not only in sitting but also in standing, will learn to stand and even to walk. However, they use a primitive pattern of high stepping, lifting their legs too high. The abduction pattern of the lower limbs, together with the dorsiflexion and eversion of the feet will give them a sufficient walking base. They walk with hyperextended hips and knees and lean the trunk and shouldergirdle backward to avoid collapse in flexion, in this way reinforcing extensor tonus (Fig. 3-33).

Many athetoids seem to have some element of ataxia. This applies especially to the athetoid with a basically low postural tone. The ataxic element, however, is difficult to differentiate from athetosis if involuntary movements are very marked. If athetosis is slight and distal in distribution, the ataxic element may be very clear. Athetosis, with its lack of a proper grading of "reciprocal innervation" demonstrates a type of postural tone that is very similar to that seen in ataxia.

The athetoid child is not likely to develop deformities, as postural tone is generally low and he is mobile; he has, in fact, too many patterns. However, because of his hypermobility he may show a tendency towards subluxation or dislocation of the mandible, shoulder and his hip joints, and of the fingers.

The mixed cases of this group—that is, the athetoid with spasticity or the dystonic child with strong intermittent increase of postural tone—may, however, develop the following contractures or deformities:

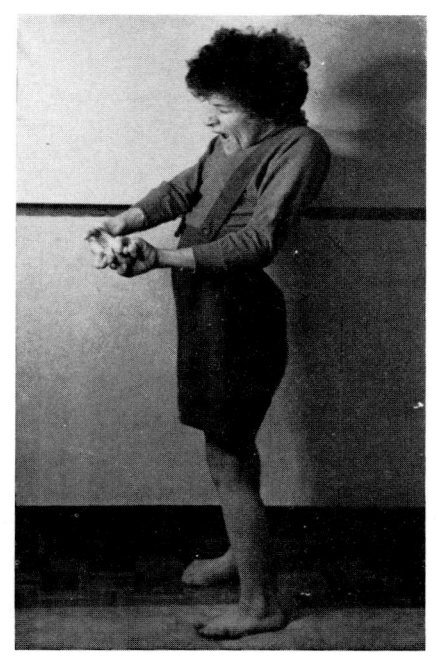

Figure 3-33. Typical standing posture of athetoid patient.

1. A scoliosis or kyphoscoliosis, often associated with deformities of the chest wall.
2. Flexor deformities of elbows and wrists, the wrists showing severe flexion with extended and "weak fingers."
3. Flexor deformities of hips and knees with equinovarus or valgus of the ankles.
4. Dislocation of one or both hips, usually the left.

DIAGNOSIS AND ASSESSMENT
Early Diagnosis

Before going into the problem of treatment, it may be important to discuss briefly the value of early diagnosis and treatment of this condition. It is now generally agreed that the early recognition of cerebral palsy is of great importance and that better and quicker results can be expected from early treatment. This has been stressed especially by Kong (1962, 1966), and also by Milani-Comparetti (1964). If treatment can be started as early as six months of age, or even earlier, the child has a better chance of improvement for the following reasons:

1. The motor behavior of babies is largely automatic. Higher centers of the central nervous system are still in the process of maturation. At this stage the brain has more plasticity than at any stage later on. Neural patterns can therefore be influenced and changed more easily. Goody and McKissock (1951) in stressing the importance of age for adjustment and learning in cases of injury to the brain state:

> Whatever the underlying anatomical basis for residual function may be, we note that the facility with which the patient can readjust himself to cerebral damage seems to be related to his age on the one hand, and to the rate of progress, if any, of the causal lesion on the other. The younger brain . . . seems more adaptable and "plastic" than the older.

2. An infant with cerebral palsy does not usually show appreciable degrees of hypertonus. Movements are not as yet interfered with by the resistance of spastic muscles, or by involuntary movements of the athetoid type. More normal movements can, therefore, be encouraged more easily at this stage, and early treatment can facilitate normal movements and prevent the development of hypertonus (Bobath and Bobath 1956, 1959, 1964, 1965, 1966).

3. If treatment is delayed, hypertonus develops sooner or later. It increases in strength, its typical patterns resulting in the well-known abnormal postures and movements of the patient. Abnormal patterns become habituated, and if the child maintains his abnormal postures for long, contractures and deformities will occur. These are never seen in the infant and young child, unless it be an associated congenital dislocation of one or both hips, and can be prevented by early treatment.

4. Cerebral palsy is a sensorimotor disorder. Movements are in response to sensory stimulation and are guided by proprioceptive information. As Goody and McKissock (1951) state:

> There is no standard brain with all its functions set and localized for

use. The brain stands ready for training. It learns, is trained, by appreciating input, sensation. It can then effect voluntarily what before has been done involuntarily.

A child's intellectual development is dependent on both environmental stimulation and the appreciation of his own body as a result of proprioceptive stimulation. During the first year of a child's life, his mental growth is dependent on an unimpeded development of his motor abilities. A child deprived of the ability to raise his head, to look around, to reach out for an object and grasp it, to bring objects to his mouth, to develop eye-hand coordination, to sit up and move around, will of necessity fall back in his mental development. If, in the more severe handicapped child, this inability to move is not overcome at an early age, mental retardation may result and may in time become indistinguishable from primary mental subnormality.

This tendency will be further strengthened and aggravated by the frequent disturbance of the normal mother-child relationship. A handicapped child will fail to emancipate himself from his mother. He will not give the mother any clues about his handling. He may not protest or adjust to the way he is handled, supported, carried, fed, etc. The mother will, therefore, often be quite ignorant on how to handle the child in the correct manner in keeping with his growing abilities. The mother will continue to treat him like a helpless baby, support him everywhere, dress and undress him, speak to him in baby language. She may handle him too quickly so that he has no time to adjust himself, and she will hinder his progress unwittingly unless specially advised and guided.

Early recognition of the more severe cases is not usually difficult. Both the retardation of normal motor development and abnormal signs of tonic reflex activity can be seen very soon. This is due to the fact that in a quadriplegic child the upper parts of the body are more involved than the lower ones. In the normal child, extension develops with head control and marches cephalocaudad. In the spastic child the abnormality (signs of a developing hypertonus and abnormal patterns) develops in the same sequence. Abnormal reflex activity will, with severe cases, interfere with the earliest signs of motor maturation such as head control, the normal development of extension against gravity in prone, and flexion against gravity in supine. Head and neck retraction in supine is soon followed by retraction of the shoulders and stiffness of the spine, a persistent and strong asymmetrical tonic reflex, the inability to raise the head in prone, and often even to turn it to one side. This will make early diagnosis fairly easy. In milder cases, however, this picture will develop more slowly and signs of abnormality may show themselves first on the more involved side only. An initial diagnosis of hemiplegia may, therefore, be made at this stage. Only in the most severe cases is spasticity strong at a very early age. However, the majority of infants do not show definite signs of spasticity and of abnormal postural reflex activity at a very early age.

In order to arrive at an early diagnosis it is important in these cases to differentiate between a general retardation of the child's motor development and early signs of a developing hypertonus and its typical patterns. Special tests are used for this purpose which provoke the abnormal patterns of hypertonus at a time when they are still latent. In other words, the child is handled in such a way as to provoke the patterns of the tonic reactions.

The tests to be described below should be used in addition to the usual techniques of history-taking and examination by the pediatrician and neurologist. None of these tests by itself is more than a pointer to a correct diagnosis. The certainty of the diagnosis is in direct proportion to the number of tests found to be positive.

Assessment

Tests in Supine

This is the position of maximal extensor hypertonus, probably as the result of the tonic labyrinthine reflex. The tests are designed to detect early signs of developing extensor hyperactivity.

TESTS FOR HEAD, NECK AND SHOULDER RETRACTION. The examiner's hand is placed behind the baby's head or shoulder and he is lifted into the sitting position. One can feel the head and neck pressing backward, or, in the more severe cases, the whole

Cerebral Palsy

spine may arch back. The arms, instead of moving forward and over the chest, are retracted at the shoulders, even after the baby has been moved well forward already (Fig. 3-34). If his head is released and allowed to drop back a little before being caught again, the baby may show a strong startle reaction, either in its early unmodified form or in its later modified form. This retraction of the head and neck explains the child's inability to raise his head actively from supine in order to initiate sitting up.

Resistance of the shoulders to forward flexion can also be tested by grasping the baby's arms at the elbows and by moving them forward and across the chest. Resistance can be felt, and when released, the arms will pull backward. This accounts for the child's inability to bring his arms forward to pull himself up to sitting, especially as he is also unable to lift his head.

The lack of head control and the retraction of head and neck can also be tested by pulling the baby up to sitting by his arms; the head will not come forward but may drop more or less back (Fig. 3-35). The baby is unable to right his head and bring it into alignment with the trunk.

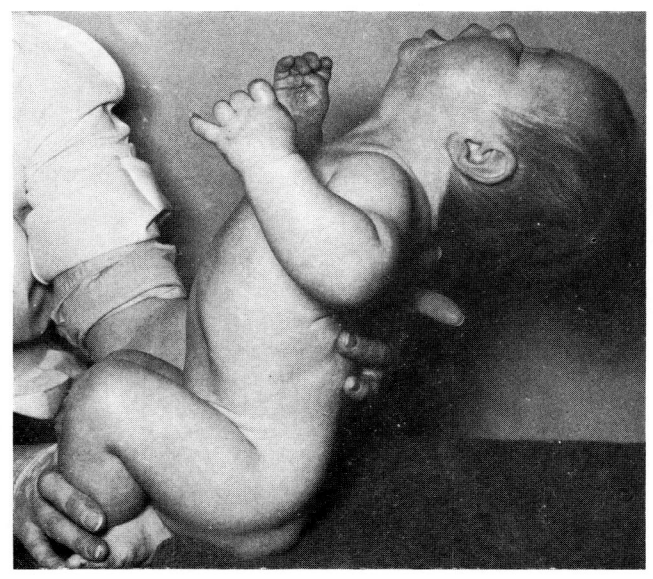

Figure 3-34. Cerebral-palsied baby. Note head and shoulder retraction.

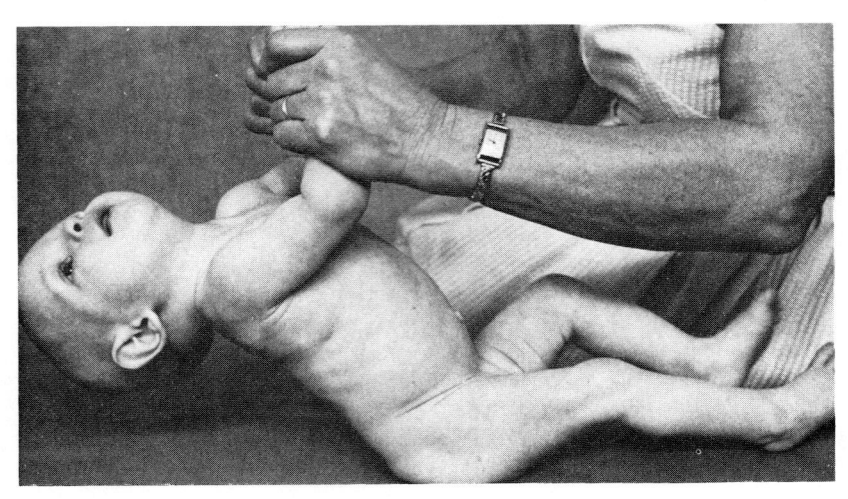

106 *Physical Therapy Services in the Developmental Disabilities*

Figure 3-35. Tonic labyrinthine influence. Note: head lag when pulled to sitting. Note lower limbs still in primitive flexion attitude.

TESTING FOR AN ASYMMETRICAL TONIC NECK REFLEX. The infant usually lies on his back with the arms in abduction and flexed at the elbows. The head is turned to one side and held for a few seconds. It is often more effective to induce the baby to turn his head actively to one side, by making him follow an object. The "face" arm may then extend spontaneously while the opposite arm may flex (Fig. 3-36). In some cases, however, the face arm

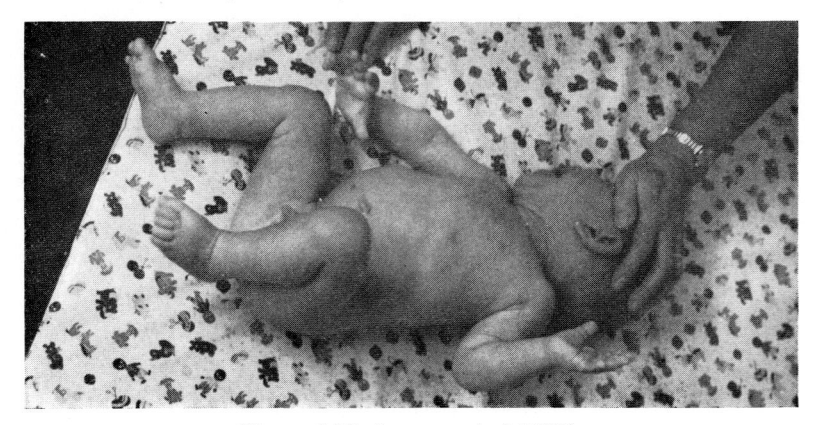

Figure 3-36. Asymmetrical TNR.

may not extend, but passive extension of this arm may now be less resisted. Passive extension of the opposite arm may, however, be more difficult. Not infrequently the influence of this reflex is more marked on one side than the other. This reflex, if of any strength, prevents the symmetrical behavior of the child—that is, the bringing together of the arms into midline. This makes it impossible for the child to play with his hands. The child cannot bring his hands to his mouth or body. He cannot control manipulation with his eyes.

TESTING FOR THE NECK-RIGHTING REACTION. If the normal child turns his head actively or passively to one side, the body should sooner or later follow and the baby will turn to his side. In cerebral palsy this reaction is prevented by the already mentioned retraction of the shoulder and of the arm.

TESTING FOR EXTENSOR AND ADDUCTOR SPASTICITY OF THE LEGS. The examiner grasps the baby's legs below the knees and moves them quickly upward to flex them against the abdomen. Resistance to this movement is noted. If the legs are quickly released, they extend immediately and may adduct and even cross. If one leg is passively flexed, the other leg may extend stiffly, rotate inward, and the foot plantiflex (a crossed extension reflex). In some children, however, both legs may flex when one is passively flexed. Adductor spasticity is usually combined with extensor spasticity. It is, therefore, best tested with the legs in extension. The examiner grasps the legs below the knees and moves them quickly apart, noting the resistance to this movement.

Tests in the Prone Position

This is the position of maximal flexor hypertonus, resulting probably from the tonic labyrinthine reflex.

A normal baby, when placed on his abdomen, will raise his head for a moment even during the first few days after birth (Prechtl 1964) and turn it to one side (Illingworth 1960). This is a protective reflex already present shortly after birth, presumably designed to keep the airways free. A child with cerebral palsy may not do this but remains face downward on the support (Fig. 3-37). It is for this reason that children with cerebral palsy whose

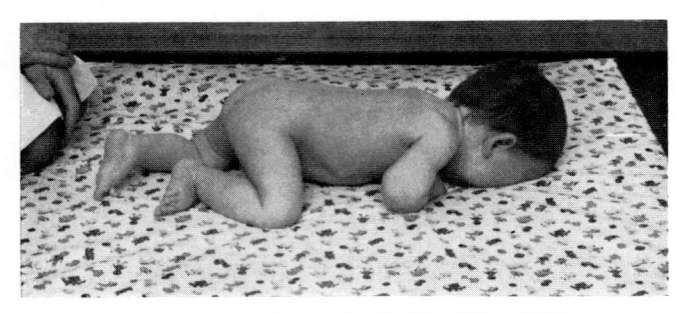

Figure 3-37. Flexion attitude. Head in midline.

head and upper parts are involved cannot tolerate the prone position. This is a valuable early anamnestic and diagnostic symptom, at a time when few other symptoms may be present.

In the prone position, the baby's arms usually show flexion and adduction and the hands are caught under his chest. If the examiner grasps the baby's hands and extends them upward to lie by the side of the head, this movement is resisted; when released, the arms will return to their flexed position.

If the examiner's hand is placed under the child's chin and the head is raised, some cases will give resistance to this movement. The head will press down or at least will feel heavier than its weight. From four months onward the normal baby will extend his arms in a propping reaction. When the child with a quadriplegia is raised by the shoulders, the arms will be pulled up in flexion (Fig. 3-38). He is unable to take his body weight on extended arms. The hips may flex also in a total flexion movement involving hips, knees, and ankles.

In more severe cases, flexor hyperactivity in prone may be so marked that the hips cannot be extended and the child cannot be placed on his abdomen. However, if the hips can be extended, this will produce the total spastic extension-adduction picture of the lower extremities in spite of the fact that spine, trunk, neck, and arms remain flexed.

If the examiner lifts the baby off the support, holding the pelvis around the iliac crests, the previously flexed legs may extend more or less strongly and resist passive flexion (influence of the symmetrical tonic neck reflex). In less severe cases the legs may flex but only slowly and after considerable delay (Fig. 3-39).

Extensor spasticity of the legs can also be detected by flexion of the knees while holding the pelvis down to the support. This must be done with the legs in adduction as any potential extensor spasticity is then more marked. Resistance to flexion is then encountered. If the hips are released, resistance will be lessened but the hips flex as well as the knees.

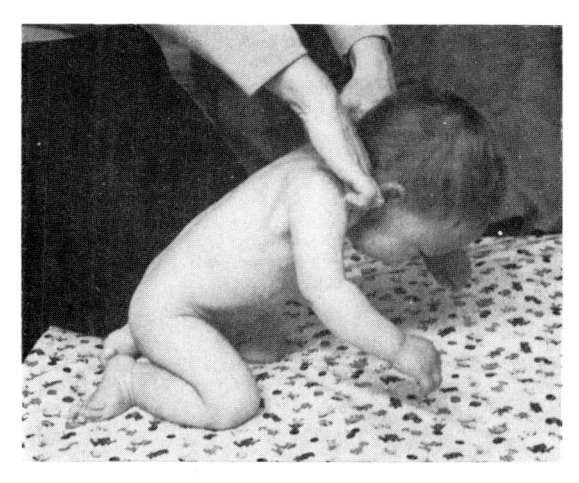

Figure 3-38. Flexion attitude. Arms tend to pull up in flexion.

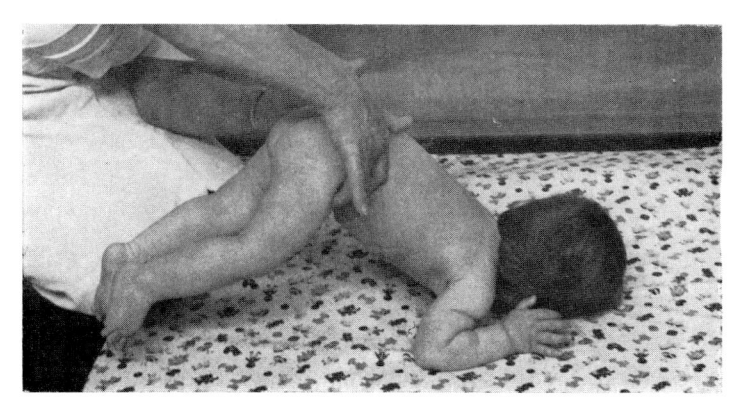

Figure 3-39. Lifted by pelvis, legs extend (see text).

110   *Physical Therapy Services in the Developmental Disabilities*

Tests in the Upright Position

If the child is lifted into the upright position, held under the axillae, and slowly lowered feet first towards a support, the legs may extend and the feet point downward (Fig. 3-40). In some more severe cases, the legs may adduct and even cross. On touching the support, the child may carry his body weight and stand on tiptoes, the legs rigidly extended and crossed (positive supporting reaction) (Fig. 3-41). Some children with more moderate spasticity may show reflex stepping, but cross their legs with every step.

The placing reaction of the legs may be absent in the more severe cases of extensor spasticity or be present only in the less involved side.

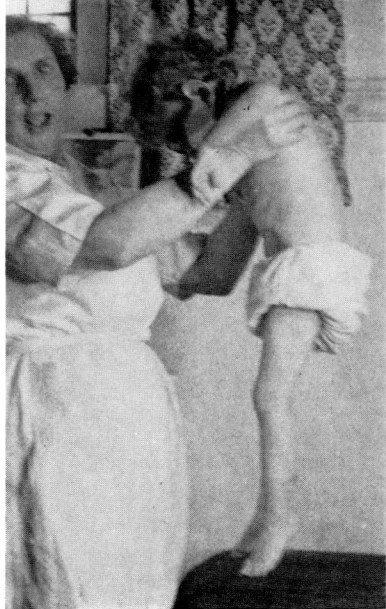

Figure 3-40. See text.

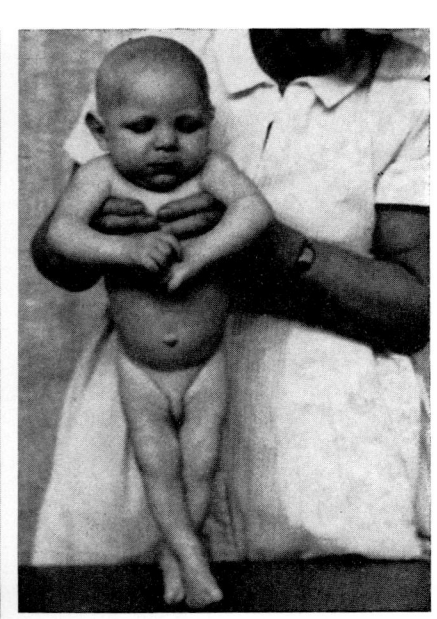

Figure 3-41. Spastic quadriplegia. Typical primary standing posture. (Severe case)

Test for the Landau Reaction

The examiner holds the child in ventral suspension in the air, and supports him under the lower chest wall. A normal baby, from the age of six months onward will raise his head and extend his spine and hips. (This reaction will normally disappear around the end of the second year.) In children with cerebral palsy of the quadriplegic type, it is usually absent; the child will neither be able to raise his head nor to extend spine and hips. He will either show a total flexor picture due probably to the tonic labyrinthine reflex, or only the knees may extend. If however, extensor spasticity of the legs is marked, the knees and ankles may extend, probably as a result of the asymmetrical tonic neck reflex Fig. 3-42). In the diplegic child, the head may be well raised but the child cannot extend the lower trunk and hips.

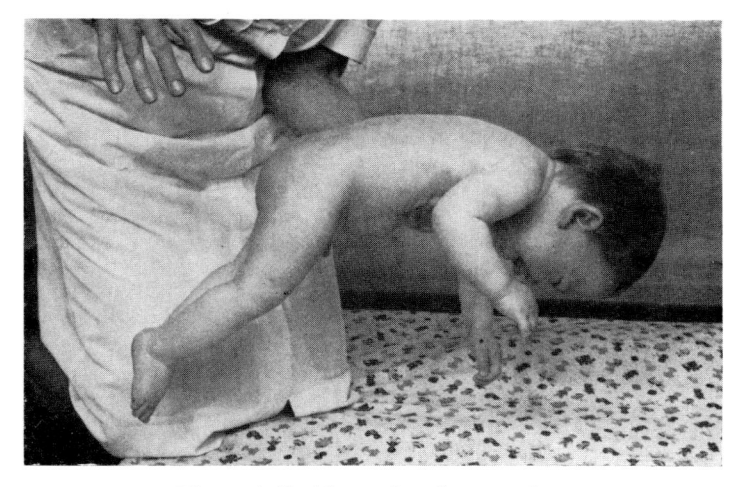

Figure 3-42. Absent Landau reaction.

Testing for the Protective Extension of the Arms

This reaction, also called "propping," "parachute," or "precipitation" reaction, has been described originally by Schaltenbrand (1927) and called by him *"Sprungbereitschaft."* From the Landau test position the child is tilted downward head first towards a support. A normal child from about six months onward will extend his arms and hands to reach out for the support. This reaction can also be tested with the baby in a sitting position. The normal baby will be able to support himself on extended arms forward at about six months, sideways at eight months, and backward between the tenth to twelfth month. In the quadriplegic child, flexor spasticity will prevent this reaction (Fig. 3-43). In the diplegic child this reaction may be delayed or interfered with, depending upon the degree of coinvolvement of the upper limbs.

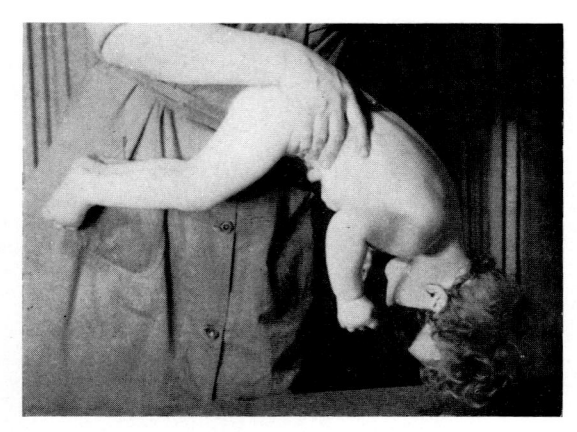

Figure 3-43. Cerebral-palsied child. Absence of head-righting and parachute reaction of arms.

The results of the examination can be summarized in Chart 3-II.

CHART 3-II
TESTS FOR CEREBRAL PALSY IN INFANCY
(SHORT-FORM CHART)

NAME_____ AGE_____
DIAGNOSIS_____ DATE OF TEST_____
TESTED FOR:
Supine
   1. Retraction of head and neck_____
   2. Retraction of shoulders_____
   3. Asymmetrical tonic neck reflex
      (a) arms_____
      (b) legs_____

Cerebral Palsy

   4. Extensor spasm of legs_____
   5. Adductor spasm of legs
      (a) in flexion_____
      (b) in extension_____

Prone
   1. Absence of protective side-turning of head_____
   2. Flexor spasm of neck_____
   3. Flexor spasm of arms_____
   4. Extensor spasm of legs_____
   5. Flexor spasm of legs_____

Sitting
   1. Protective extension of arms
      (a) forward_____
      (b) sideways_____
      (c) backward_____
   2. Head-righting trunk moved
      (a) backward_____
      (b) sideways_____
      (c) forward_____
   3. Trunk balance with use of hands_____

Landau reflex
   1. Absent_____
   2. Incomplete_____
   3. Delayed_____

Moro reflex
   1. 1st stage_____
   2. 2nd stage_____
   3. Absent_____

Upright
   1. Extensor spasm of legs_____
   2. Weight-bearing_____
   3. Balance_____

Summary

It has been argued throughout that hypertonus in all its forms is the result of a lesion to the brain and is not a muscular phenomenon. It results from the release of an abnormal postural reflex mechanism which produces hypertonus in well-defined and typical patterns. These prevent or interfere to a varying extent with normal postural control and the performance of normal movement and skills. This view has proven to be of great value in the assessment of a child's functional deficit, in the diagnosis and early recognition of this condition, and in the development of a rational approach to treatment.

PART 2

THE NEURODEVELOPMENTAL APPROACH TO TREATMENT

THEORETICAL CONSIDERATIONS

THE PROBLEM OF TREATMENT of patients with lesions of the upper motor neuron is seen as one of a disorder of coordination of muscle function in posture and movement. Every case of cerebral palsy shows a mixture of primitive and abnormal motor function, regardless of the child's intelligence. The retention of primitive patterns of motor behavior does not, therefore, necessarily indicate mental retardation.

The problem of treatment is not one of strengthening or relaxing individual muscle groups, but one of improving the coordination in posture and movement and of obtaining a more normal postural tone.

All treatment involves handling the child. Treatment, by handling, aims at influencing postural tone which can be reduced, increased, and steadied. The coordination of agonists, antagonists, and synergists can be properly regulated. Abnormal patterns can be inhibited and automatic, and active, normal responses to handling as well as willed movements can be facilitated.

Why is it necessary to handle the child? What can the child gain from being handled that he cannot learn from performing exercises at request? A normal child can do very little for himself for about the first eight or ten months. He is totally dependent at first and gradually develops postural control and the basic patterns of movement in response to being handled by his mother. He is picked up, put down, carried, fed, washed, dressed and undressed. His mother instinctively supports him when and where needed; she adjusts his posture when she feels it to be necessary.

Cerebral Palsy

There is a natural interplay between mother and child in the way the mother handles and supports him. Gradually, she withdraws her support in step with the baby's growing abilities to put himself right, to get himself out of uncomfortable positions, to right and control his head, and to hold on to his mother for support. The mother gradually withdraws her support as her child learns to move with increasing independence.

A great deal of this handling continues for at least the first three years or even longer—a period during which the child acquires all the basic patterns of many higher skills by first helping and cooperating before doing them alone. Later on, he will use the same patterns in an increasing number of combinations, changing and elaborating them for more complex functional activities. In children with cerebral palsy this relationship of mother and child, so essential to the child's development, is often grossly disturbed; therefore, in treatment and management of the child, parent counseling on how to manage her child is one of the most important factors of successful treatment. This point will be taken up again later.

The learning of movements, like any other process of learning, takes place with the help and guidance of sensory messages. A child does not learn a movement but rather, the "sensations of movements." He gradually develops the basic sensorimotor patterns which are then elaborated for future functional skills. From birth onward, we are activated by powerful afferents from the outside world, especially through our distance receptors, eyes and ears, and from our proprioceptors. Movements, initiated by the exteroceptors, are guided throughout their course by the proprioceptors. The intact and mature central nervous system has a great ability to absorb a large quantity of the afferent inflow and to react to it in a unitary and well-integrated manner, in keeping with the demands of the environment.

The central nervous system of a child with cerebral palsy cannot deal effectively with the afferent inflow. Here the input is "short-circuited" (shunted) into the synaptic chains of a few widespread and typical patterns of primitive and abnormal reflex activity. The child's responses consist, therefore, largely of a few total synergies of earliest childhood and the abnormal patterns of tonic reflexes.

Since Hughlings Jackson, we have come to look upon hypertonus as a release phenomenon, a positive sign of abnormal function of the central nervous system released from higher inhibition. What is released, however, are the abnormal patterns of hypertonus, an expression of a released abnormal postural reflex mechanism. In time the abnormal sensorimotor patterns of the hypertonic state will become firmly established in the child's nervous system. They are all the child feels and knows, and all he will use for all purposive activity. The proprioceptive system of the child can mediate only the sensations of abnormal postures and movements. The child will experience only the sensations of undue weight of the limbs, of excessive effort when trying to initiate and control a movement.

Cerebral palsy must, therefore, be considered a sensorimotor disorder rather than a pure motor disorder, and this regardless of any associated sensory or perceptory handicap. Treatment is, therefore, a sensorimotor habilitation and aims at preventing the sensory input from being channeled into the patterns of abnormal reflex activity *(inhibition)* and redirecting it into the channels of higher integrated patterns of normal motor activity *(facilitation)*.

The concept of shunting as described by Magnus (1924, 1926) may perhaps serve to explain the effect of treatment.

Sherrington (1939) found that one and the same stimulus applied to the same place may, in spinal animals, produce directly opposite reflex responses. For instance, the pinching of the toes of the extended leg of a spinal frog produced a total flexion movement of the leg, the flexor withdrawal reflex. Pinching of the toes of the fully flexed leg had the opposite effect of total extension. Sherrington called this phenomenon "reflex reversal."

Magnus (1926) made similar observations, when examining a cat. The cat was placed in side-lying on a table with the tail hanging over the edge. On pinching the heel of one leg, the tail moved upward. After placing the cat on its other side with the tail hanging down again, pinching of the same heel resulted again in an upward movement of the tail.

In seeking for a possible explanation of these observations, Magnus found it in the law of Von Uexkuell, a German biologist who had studied the response of lower animals to stimulation. This law states that in simple reflex responses and the reactions of lower animals, the response to stimulation was predictable. The afferent inflow favors the contraction of the elongated muscle groups whereas the shortened antagonists were in a state of central inhibition and were relaxed. In this narrower form, the law only applies to simple reflex responses and primitive reactions of lower animals. However, on the basis of these observations, Magnus (1924, 1926) formulated the general law of shunting as follows: At any moment of a movement the central nervous system mirrors faithfully the state of the body musculature. The state of contraction and relaxation of the body musculature determines the distribution of excitatory and inhibitory processes within the central nervous system and, with it, the subsequent outflow of excitation to the periphery. It is, therefore, the periphery—the proprioceptive system—which guides and patterns the central nervous system response.

Accepting this law, it is clear that it offers a means of influencing the central nervous system from the periphery, through the sensory side. By changing the abnormal postural patterns of a child with cerebral palsy, we can prevent the outflow of excitation from causing undesirable muscular activity (that is, away from the patterns of abnormal postural reflex activity). At the same time we can redirect the sensory inflow into synaptic chains of more normal motor activity. This then is the theoretical basis for a treatment approach which, by handling the child in specific ways, aims at the inhibition of abnormal postural reflex activity and the facilitation of normal higher-integrated automatic responses.

PRINCIPLES OF TREATMENT

An essential part of the treatment is the use of "reflex-inhibiting patterns" which serve the purpose of changing the abnormal postural patterns of the child by (1) counteracting the most dominant patterns of tonic reflex activity in any one position—supine, prone, kneeling, sitting, standing and so on, and (2) modifying the initial abnormal postural patterns and introducing the greatest possible variety of normal postural responses, all of them different from the original abnormal patterns.

By breaking up and modifying the abnormal postural patterns (the direct expression of abnormal tonic reflex activity), the latter are gradually weakened and their established shunts are constantly interrupted at many points. The excitatory outflow is thus redirected into potential motor activities previously blocked by the dominant tonic reflex activity. As has been stressed, abnormal postural reflex activity and the various types of hypertonus are coexistent. In the absence of tonic reflex activity by successful inhibition, postural tone becomes more normal. As tonic reflex activity abates, the child learns to control it.

Thus, reflex-inhibiting patterns aim at stopping abnormal postural reflex activity and producing more normal qualities of postural tone. However, the permanent inhibition of tonic reflex activity can only be obtained by activating motor function of higher organization—the inherent patterns of righting and equilibrium reactions.

It is the nature of postural tone to give way to movement. This applies both to normal and increased postural tone. Spasticity will decrease and postural tone keep fairly low as long as movement is in progress. This is generally appreciated and made use of in treatment, for instance, by Fay (1954) who used spinal and "amphibian" movement reflexes to reduce spasticity. But the only guarantee of a permanently reduced and steady postural tone is the reactivation of the higher integrated postural reactions, righting and equilibrium reactions, and the firm establishment of their synaptic connections.

This reactivation is obtained by the use of "facilitation." It consists of techniques which obtain spontaneous movement responses from the child by special techniques of handling, immediately when tone is reduced and controlled in reflex-inhibiting patterns. These movement responses are then firmly established by repetition (Bobath and Bobath 1959, 1962, 1964).

The possible explanation of the effect of facilitation may be found in the work of Ritchie Russell (1958). He states that neurophysiological studies have shown that synaptic transmission along a certain chain can be greatly facilitated by previous activity along this connection. There is, therefore, evidence of a neuronal mechanism which favors repetition, and this is true for every level of the central nervous system. He continues:

> It is equally evident, however, that this complicated neuronal activity is extremely sensitive to outside (afferent) influences. Apparently the neuronal pool can be alerted to make responses which take priority over spontaneous activity, so that if a certain response has in the past followed a given experience, there is every likelihood that this response will be repeated in the future to the same stimulus, until it acquires a remarkable degree of constancy and automaticity.

We may add that this is especially so if the newly facilitated responses belong to phylogenetically inherent and established patterns, like those of the righting and equilibrium reactions. Once established, the new response is very resistant to forgetting, not because of a hypothetical memory center, but because of the firmly established chains of synaptic connections.

As applied to the treatment, this means that the permanent carry-over of treatment depends on the extent to which the higher reactions can be facilitated and their synaptic bonds firmly established.

These higher reactions modify and keep in check the abnormal tonic and spinal reflexes. They keep postural tone steady and low. Once the higher postural reactions are firmly established, treatment can progress to the laying down of patterns of normal skills. With this approach to treatment of any particular child, the extent to which higher integrated motor responses can be evoked in treatment depends largely on the potentialities of the child's damaged brain.

In the individual case, inhibition of abnormal reflex activity and facilitation of movement may follow each other, may be used alternately, or may be used simultaneously. In whichever way inhibition and facilitation are combined, the child must be given a chance to move actively. The reflex-inhibiting postures, as used originally, controlled and fixed the whole body and tended to prevent the child from actively moving head and limbs. However, abnormal postural reflex activity originates predominantly in head, neck, and other proximal parts of the body such as the shoulder-girdle and spine. The strength and distribution of the postural tone of the extremities can, therefore, be most successfully controlled and influenced from these proximal parts, the so-called "key-points."

It is possible to effect inhibition of abnormal postural and movement patterns by changing the child's position at key-points only, and to influence and control the strength and distribution of postural tone of the limbs by using only partial reflex-inhibiting patterns. The advantage is that the child can be left free to move his limbs actively while the therapist controls certain key-points and prevents any deterioration of the movement from there. This allows for the combination of techniques of simultaneous inhibition and facilitation, and has proved to be more effective than the static reflex-inhibiting postures originally used.

When handling a child, the therapist has to be aware of the fact that active movement responses will not take place at the point or near the point at which the child is held and supported, but that the best reactions are obtained more distally from the point of control. Therefore, the key-points of control have to be chosen carefully and constantly changed and adapted to the needs of the child in order to obtain sequences of active automatic movements at the desired places.

In some of the severe cases, for instance in older children with spasticity, rigidity, or dystonic athetosis, techniques of inhibitions are still used predominantly and for a long time until postural tone has become sufficiently normal to allow for active movement responses. However, even here righting and equilibrium reactions are facilitated as soon as possible. For this purpose, from the beginning the children are moved in reflex-inhibiting patterns in the same way and direction as they are expected to move actively later on.

Movements which are apt to provoke abnormal reflex activity, and with it an increase of hypertonus, are carefully avoided, for instance, when treating a child in long-sitting with abducted and outwardly rotated legs, extended arms and flexed hips, his body should be moved sideways and forward only. Movements backward have to be avoided as they tend to increase extensor spasticity. Even in these severe cases one should always try to facilitate active motor responses, though this may at first be possible only during the initial short periods of normal postural tone.

In all other cases, especially in babies and very young children with moderate spasticity or athetosis, facilitation techniques are used simultaneously with inhibition. Babies do not usually show appreciable degrees of spasticity or athetosis and abnormal reactions can therefore be effectively prevented by obtaining the most normal movement reactions using partial reflex-inhibiting patterns. Abnormal motor patterns have not as yet become established; in fact, these babies have moved very little.

Here the development of faulty movement patterns can be prevented in many cases from the start, and normal patterns can be laid down in their developmental sequence. By facilitating righting and equilibrium reactions, entire sequences of movement, such as rolling over, sitting up, getting on hands and knees, crawling, standing up, and even walking, may be obtained. Some of the righting reactions can usually be obtained in all but the most severe cases. However, in severe cases of quadriplegia, it may be impossible to establish equilibrium reactions, especially in standing and walking.

THE PLANNING OF A TREATMENT PROGRAM

In the planning of a rational treatment program one has to take into account two factors already discussed, namely:
1. The arrest of development with a retention of primitive motor behavior.
2. The abnormal motor behavior.

Generally speaking, most therapists have so far placed the emphasis in treatment heavily, if not wholly, on the developmental aspect of the problem. Although many therapists are by now aware of the many symptoms of the neurological disorder, such as abnormal postural reflex activity with abnormal qualities and distribution of postural tone, the effect of this abnormal reflex activity on the child's motor development has not always been appreciated. This aspect has, therefore, been neglected in treatment which has been planned only to advance the child's motor behavior along developmental lines.

It is, however, necessary in the individual case to differentiate between these two factors in order to arrive at a rational treatment plan.

In every case of cerebral palsy one has to ask oneself the following questions: (1) Which aspect of a child's motor behavior, such as head control, rolling over, sitting up, standing up, standing and walking, and the use of the arms and hands, are fairly normal but have remained primitive, having stopped short of the child's chronological age? Are the various aspects of the child's arrested motor behavior closely clustered around the same stage of development or do they show a wide scatter? (2) Which of the child's motor patterns are abnormal, the result of pathological reflex activity?

These two factors produce a mixture of primitive and abnormal motor behavior with a wide scatter of the various aspects of the child's primitive patterns. Treatment must, therefore, inhibit abnormal reflex activity while advancing the child's motor behavior from its lowest level of arrest, filling in the gaps, and advancing him on a broad front. It is for this reason that it is proposed to call this treatment, hitherto known as the "Bobath approach," the "neurodevelopmental treatment."

This does not mean that one should separate the succeeding stages of development and try to perfect one activity before going on to the next stage. The normal child does not simply acquire one activity after another. There is a great deal of overlap. For instance, when he is at the stage of lifting his head in supine, he is already able to sit; while still creeping on his abdomen, he begins to sit with very little support; he moves and practices balance in sitting at a stage when he begins to pull himself up to standing. It is also important to keep in mind that some postural patterns of normal children must be avoided in treatment. The following paragraphs give examples of some postural patterns of normal children to be avoided in treatment.

When treating babies with cerebral palsy it is important to keep in mind that some of the normal motor patterns of early infancy have to be avoided as they are too similar to the abnormal motor patterns. For instance, it is quite normal for a baby of eight months in supine to arch his back, with his feet on the support, and to push his hips up, resting on head and shoulders. Though this is an important pattern to be developed in children with spastic diplegia it should be avoided or discouraged in children with athetoid quadriplegia. It is often the only activity for such children, in whom the legs are less involved than the head and trunk, and is a common way in which athetoid children progress (backward) on the floor. Its constant practice, however, will increase extensor spasms to such an extent that the head control and balance needed in sitting and standing may become impossible later on.

Another pattern to be avoided is that of kicking. The normal baby, after four months of age, kicks with lower limbs abducted and outwardly rotated, the ankles dorsiflexed. In the spastic or athetoid child however, kicking soon assumes an abnormal character with adduction, inward rotation of the legs, and plantiflexion of ankles and toes. In the child with cerebral palsy, therefore, kicking will increase extensor hypertonus of his lower limbs and, in time, will produce scissoring of the legs, toe-standing and toe-walking. For the same reason, it will also prevent sufficient hip flexion and abduction when sitting and thereby rob the child of a proper sitting base and balance.

A normal baby stops kicking altogether at eight months (Illingworth 1960), probably because at this stage he has developed a symmetrical standing pattern with abducted legs in preparation for standing and walking, abduction being essential until balance in standing has improved and walking on a narrower base has become possible. The athetoid child, however, continues to kick in a primitive as well as abnormal crossed extension pattern. In some treatment this is often encouraged as it is wrongly regarded as a "walking pattern." However, unless it is replaced with symmetrical standing before the child is made to walk, it will result in very abnormal walking if walking is achieved at all.

Another pattern to be discouraged in some children with cerebral palsy is that of support on extended arms forward when kneeling. This pattern reinforces the spastic child's tendency to flexor spasticity of shoulders and trunk with kyphosis of the dorsal spine, and the athetoid child's tendency to extension, inward rotation and adduction of the arms (decerebrate rigidity posture). Though support on the arms forward is the earliest pattern of protective extension in the normal child, in children with cerebral palsy support on extended arms sideways, or even backward, may have to be introduced first. By doing this first, flexor spasticity of the upper limbs and the pattern of adduction with inward rotation can be inhibited, before slowly and gradually encouraging the child to take his weight forward on his arms in a more normal way.

These points may best be illustrated by discussing the following case.

Name: N. D. *Age:* 3 years

Diagnosis: Spastic quadriplegia, some athetosis. Left side more involved. Relevant birth history: an only child. Full-term, birth weight —8 pounds, 9 ounces. One lung did not expand, blue asphyxia requiring oxygen.

Initial Examination: Alert and friendly child, fair head control, follows objects with eyes, reacts to noises. Understands language in keeping with his age and can say a few words. He is completely helpless; cannot roll over nor sit without support, cannot sit up, kneel, crawl, stand, or walk. He tries to use his right hand for grasp, is occasionally successful, and sometimes brings it to his face. He cannot open his left hand. Postural tone at rest is fairly good but he has, in supine, very strong extensor spasms with wide opening of his mouth and frequent tongue thrust. These spasms occur when he is excited, and makes an effort to speak or to move. He then shows also an asymmetrical tonic neck reflex to either side, but more to the left.

He was charted on a motor chart (Chart 3-III) which shows very typically the mixture of primitive and abnormal patterns. On the basis of this chart, the treatment program was sketched.

Pathological patterns to be inhibited are as follows:
1. Extensor hypertonus which is responsible for neck and shoulder retraction and the open mouth; adduction, medial rotation and crossing of lower limbs on sitting, standing and walking; medial rotation, pronation and extension of arms with clenched fists.

Cerebral Palsy

CHART 3-III
CHART OF EARLY MOTOR PATTERNS FOR CHILD

Primitive	Stage of Development	Pathology
Turns side to supine or supine to side.	2 months	Cannot turn supine to side due to extensor spasticity.
Turns prone to supine.	1 month	Does it abnormally with extensor spasm.
Excessive dorsiflexion of feet with eversion with flexed legs.	1 month	Legs are extended stiffly.
Occasionally lifts head from supine; has voluntary grasps of objects in midline.	5-6 months	Cannot lift head due to retraction; cannot bring arms forward to chest and engage hands in midline due to shoulder retraction.
Occasionally brings right hand to mouth.	2-3 months	Cannot suck fingers. Cannot bring left hand to mouth due to shoulder retraction and asymmetrical tonic neck reflex to left.
Hands clenched, tonic grasp. Arms generally flexed.	1-2 months	Pronation and extension of elbows with clenched fists.
Pulled to sitting, rights head halfway up, assists.	4-5 months	Cannot grasp and hold on to my hands. Does not right head immediately. Legs are not raised but adducted and stiff.
Sits with little support, *tends* to push backward; legs flexed and abducted.	4 months	Legs adducted and medially rotated; hips resist flexion.
Lifts head to Zone 3 in prone-lying.	3-4 months	Head control fair. When head is raised, arms extend stiffly, hands fisted; tends to fall sideways. Cannot bend elbows for support on forearms.
Landau reaction: incomplete (suspended under abdomen).	4-5 months	Head-raising is combined with stiffly adducted and medially rotated legs.
Takes part of weight standing supported. Feet everted and dorsiflexed. Rises on toes, bounces.	4-5 months	Legs adducted, medially rotated, crossing. Arms stiffly extended, adducted, pronated.
Made to walk, makes jerky uncoordinated steps.	6 months	Legs cross, extend, and turn inwards.

2. Asymmetrical tonic neck reflex patterns.

Patterns to be facilitated are as follows: (As the child's motor chart shows a scatter from one to six months, an all-around six-month level should be aimed at, before advancing the child further.)

1. Symmetrical postural patterns in supine, prone, and sitting, head in midline and hands engaging. His arms should be moved forward in supination and flexion of elbows with open hands to grasp, hold, touch his own face and body, objects and various textures.
2. He should learn to reach out with his arms—hands open—forward, upward, and sideways, and eye-hand control should be obtained. Grasp and release should be stimulated.

3. Rolling from supine to side-lying and prone.
4. Prone-lying supported first on his forearms, later on extended arms and hands. Independent head movements with a stable shoulder-girdle and trunk. Rotation between shoulder-girdle and pelvis, in order to enable him to move his arms from under his body. This rotation will also enable him to reach out with one arm while supporting his body on the other, and to creep with reciprocal movements of arms and legs.
5. Head-righting when pulled to sitting, sustained grasp in holding on should be obtained.
6. Four-foot kneeling with support and extended arms and hands. Weight transfer forward and sideways with protective extension of arms (rocking).
7. Long-sitting (that is, sitting with extended, abducted and laterally rotated legs, hips well flexed, spine extended). Support on hands forward and sideways. This is followed by side-sitting, changing from side to side.
8. Squatting and standing up with abducted, extended legs. Weight transfer sideways with mobile hips and knees. He should also learn to take his weight on semiflexed legs in various positions between squatting and standing.
9. Sequence of movement—combinations of all these positions have to be facilitated, from supine to prone, sitting up to side-sitting, kneeling, squatting and standing up.

TECHNIQUES OF TREATMENT
The Use of Reflex-Inhibiting Patterns

As has been stressed, tonic reflex patterns are most clearly seen in children with severe hypertonus. With lesser degrees of hypertonus and, therefore, more ability of movement, the child will show a greater variety of abnormal postural patterns; those due to tonic reflex activity will not be seen clearly in their pure and unmodified form, nor will they occur with regular and predictable regularity. These variations of the postural patterns and the associated modifications of the original distribution of hypertonus must be taken into account when planning treatment and working out reflex-inhibiting patterns in the individual child.

A child who has spent most of his life in sitting will often show flexor spasticity even when lying on his back, while early on he showed predominant extensor spasticity in this position. In prone, however, he still will show maximal flexor spasticity. He may, therefore, be able to lift his head in supine, using his flexor hypertonus, but not in prone. Many of these children cannot be sufficiently extended, even passively, and made to tolerate the prone position. This means that one does not necessarily see maximal extensor hypertonus in supine in all cases, but may in some cases meet with excessive flexor hypertonus.

For practical purposes, one may have to start treating this type of child with reflex-inhibiting patterns of extension in supine or side-lying first, until it becomes possible to treat him in prone-lying. On the other hand, a child who shows maximal extensor hypertonus in supine and flexor hypertonus in prone, will first be treated in prone-lying with patterns designed to counteract excessive flexor activity. One may also find children who show such excessive extensor hyperactivity being reduced to a more normal level. They may be able to lift their head well in prone, but are quite unable to do so from supine, showing at times opisthotonus in this position. They are also unable to sit without falling backward, as they press their head backward and extend hips and knees.

In these cases one may be quite unable to make the child sit up without first flexing hips and knees and abducting the legs—a partial reflex-inhibiting pattern (Fig. 3-44). It may be impossible initially to treat such a child in supine, and one will choose reflex-inhibiting patterns in side-lying (Fig. 3-45) or prone (Fig. 3-46). Other children will show arms with much flexion and threatening contractures of the elbows. Here the rotation of the head to one side may not produce a visible asymmetrical tonic neck reflex. However, it may be easier to extend the "face arm," while the other arm will show increased resistance to passive extension. The same observation can be made on the lower limbs in some children, if they are in strong flexor spasm.

In these cases, reflex-inhibiting patterns serve to counteract flexor spasticity by using symmetrical patterns of extension of the limbs with the head in midline. The easiest position to start with may be in side-lying with elevated and extended arms. When the child has become well adjusted to this position and postural tone

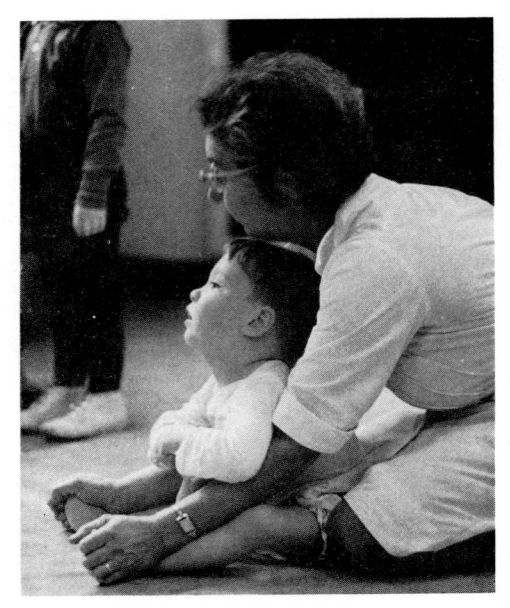

Figure 3-44. See text.

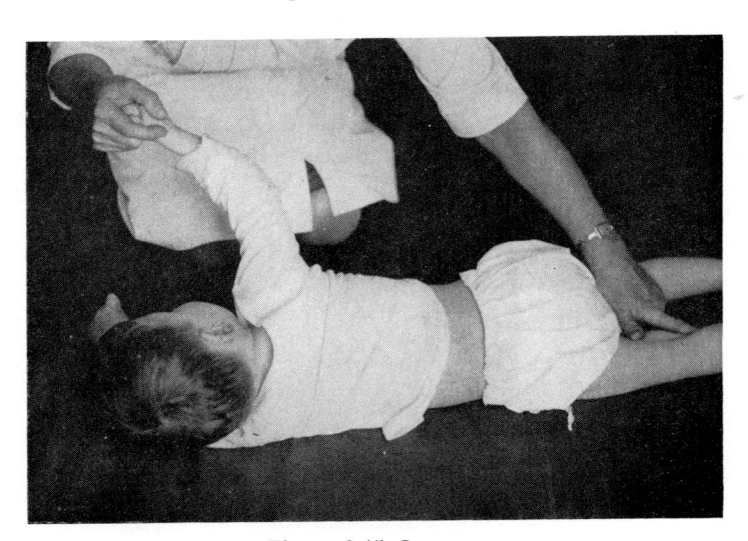

Figure 3-45. See text.

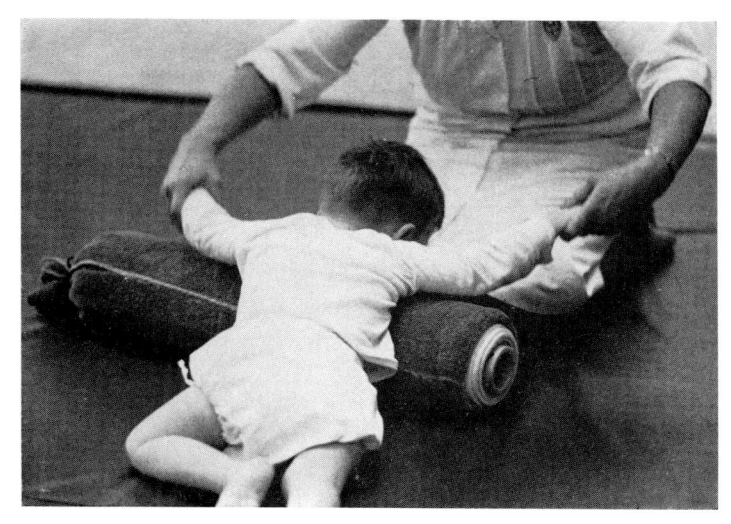

Figure 3-46. See text.

is more normal, this is followed by rotation backward of the uppermost shoulder which will bring the trunk, and later the extended hips, towards supine-lying. The patient's arms may be moved slowly from the elevated position above the head into horizontal abduction with outward rotation and extended elbows and hands. The reversed procedure may then be attempted; that is, from the side-lying position the child's pelvis may be rotated gradually forward, the hips extended and the child moved into prone-lying, his shoulders and head following (Fig. 3-47).

When trying to obtain maximal extension, it is useful to have the child's chest and shoulders supported over a roll or bolster. In prone-lying one works closely towards maximal extension of his spine and hips, especially the dorsal spine, while gradually abducting his outwardly rotated and extended arms and legs.

Rotation of the trunk between shoulder-girdle and pelvis, by moving his shoulders first backward from side-lying into supine and his hips first forward towards prone, is a useful pattern to inhibit both flexor and extensor patterns of hypertonus.

Other examples of designing reflex-inhibiting patterns are the following:

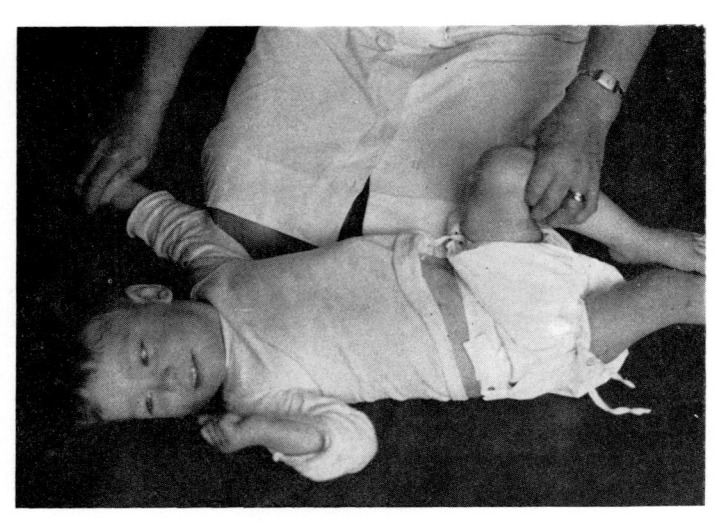

Figure 3-47. See text.

1. *Some children show postural patterns of strong flexor spasticity of trunk, shoulders, and hips, in spite of opisthotonus, and neck retraction.* They will, therefore, need patterns of extension to inhibit flexion of trunk and hips, but also inhibition of neck retraction; that is, they will need patterns of flexion of neck and head. Here the child is placed in supine on a mat, the therapist kneeling in front of him. She places his pelvis on her lap, his legs abducted and extended on either side of her. The child's head rests on the mat, his spine is extended while his neck rests on the support in such a way that the head is flexed forward. In this position the therapist can mobilize, extend spine and hips, and move his arms extended above his head, which helps to extend trunk and hips. She may also bring them into horizontal abduction to inhibit pectoral spasms and flexion of the dorsal spine.

2. *A severe case of athetoid quadriplegia, in whom there is considerable fluctuation of postural tone from hypo- to strong hypertonus, and who has strong and immediate asymmetrical tonic neck reflexes and rigid extension in supine and complete flexion in prone with no head control in any position.* In treatment one may start with a reflex pattern in supine in full flexion

with adducted and flexed legs, the arms extended, adducted and held forward, and the hands around the flexed legs. The child is, so to say, bundled up like a parcel. This will give the child a posture of symmetry and alignment of head, body, and limbs with a more stable background of postural tone for sitting. Holding him in this way in sitting but without supporting the head, the child is moved slowly sideways and backward towards supine. He is not to lose control of his head in midline and the movement must be reversed to prevent his head from falling backward. If in this position the child begins to hold on to his legs by himself and has gained head control to some extent, his legs are gradually extended and abducted, his arms placed forward or sideways for support. From there one may progress to side-sitting with support on both arms.

When analyzing the postural patterns of a child, one should look at the whole child and not at the pattern of an arm or a leg without reference to the total pattern. One should look at the way in which the postural patterns of the limbs, head, and spine are combined. In this way one can find out how one pattern affects another, whether and in what way one pattern depends on another. This is important for treatment as one can then improve the pattern of, say the limbs, by working on the patterns with which they are associated.

For instance, adductor spasticity of the legs is usually associated with flexor spasticity of the trunk, especially of the abdomen. In treatment one can reduce this adductor spasticity of the legs by extending the spine, especially the dorsal spine, in prone-lying.

Inward rotation and adduction of the lower limb is often combined with flexion and protraction of the shoulder-girdle and adduction of the arms. One can, therefore, obtain better abduction and outward rotation of the legs by treating the child with arms extended and abducted in outward rotation in supine, sitting, standing and walking.

In hemiplegias, diplegias, and spastic quadriplegias, extensor spasticity of the legs is combined with flexor spasticity of the arms and depression of the shoulder-girdle. Here one can obtain easier flexion of the legs by inhibiting depression of the shoulder-girdle and flexor spasticity of the arms. This can be done, for instance, by elevating the child's arms, lifting his shoulder-girdle, and extending the side flexors of the trunk.

It is necessary to assess a child's postural patterns in supine, prone, four-foot kneeling, kneel-standing, half-kneeling, and standing; these are more or less static positions. It is even *more* important to observe the patterns carefully while the child is moving. For instance, it is essential to assess the way in which he rolls over, sits up, gets on hands and knees, crawls, walks on his knees, stands up, sits down on a chair and gets up, walks forward, sideways, or backward, turns around, and uses his hands. In fact, the postural patterns accompanying all movements and activities the child is able to perform have to be analyzed with respect to possible abnormalities and especially with regard to the effect of abnormal postural patterns on the child's performance. Such a careful analysis is the absolute prerequisite and determines the choice of effective reflex-inhibiting patterns to counteract the abnormal patterns which interfere with or prevent normal activity. Thus, it is most important to analyze the child's postural patterns while he is moving. This is especially important in the planning of treatment of children who are only moderately or slightly affected and who can, therefore, move in many—although abnormal—ways.

One has to be careful not to reverse a total hypertonic pattern of flexion into one of total extension and vice versa. This may lead to a change from flexor to extensor spasticity and vice versa in spastic children with a great deal of cocontraction. For instance, it is wrong to place a spastic child into squatting for any length of time to inhibit the extensor spasticity of the lower limbs and toe-standing with adducted legs. This may make it impossible for the child to stand up as he becomes spastic in flexion. This will happen more easily if squatting is done with abducted legs as abduction belongs to the total flexion pattern.

It is necessary in treatment of these children to counteract both the total flexion and extension pattern of spasticity; the total patterns of either must be broken up. For instance, when trying to obtain extension of the lower limbs in supine or prone without spasticity, the legs are abducted and outward rotated, the ankles

Cerebral Palsy

dorsiflexed with hips and knees remaining extended. If in the individual child abduction increases flexor spasticity to such an extent that extension of knees and hips cannot be maintained, one may have to start by using outward rotation of the legs and dorsiflexion of the ankles only. One may have to leave abduction of the legs for the time being until extension of hips and knees can be maintained more easily. In severe cases, one may even have to leave dorsiflexion of the ankles to a later date, and start with outward rotation with some abduction only.

The following considerations must be kept in mind when using reflex-inhibiting patterns:

1. *The aim is to reduce hypertonus—spasticity, rigidity, or intermittent increases of postural tone.* This can only be obtained if the patterns are carefully chosen and graded in keeping with the child's tolerance, so that he can adjust himself to the handling. If one uses force, the child will resist and struggle and will become more hypertonic.

2. *The patterns have to be introduced gradually and not everywhere at the same time.* One begins the handling first proximally, from the head, shoulder-girdle, spine or pelvis. In this way, hypertonus and undesirable reactions of the limbs can be minimized. If necessary, changes of the abnormal limb patterns can then be effected more easily and without undue resistance such as stretch reflexes of spastic muscles.

3. *Handling must not start with the place where hypertonus is strongest and most obvious.* For instance, if adductor spasticity of the legs is strong, one must not stretch the adductors. One has to find and attack the pattern of which adductor hypertonus is a part. One has to start proximally first (for instance, at spine or shoulder-girdle) or with outward rotation of the hips and obtain abduction only later when adductor resistance has been reduced in this way.

4. *The child should gain gradually his own control of abnormal postural reactions; that is, inhibition of abnormal reflex activity must increasingly be gained independently of the therapist.* In order to give a child a chance to move actively and more normally and to learn to stop his abnormal reactions, the therapist

has to withdraw her support, to hold the child less firmly and change her points of support since the child can only learn to control and move parts that are not being held. Whenever spastic resistance is absent, even for a moment or two only, the child must be left alone to control his postures and to move. However, help has to be given immediately when hypertonus increases again before this gains momentum and the child loses control completely. In this way the child will learn the difference between the sensations of abnormal and normal motor patterns. Athetoid children have to learn to stop "spasms" at request if they occur while the child is in a controlled reflex-inhibiting pattern.

5. *It is important to give a child a great variety of postural patterns and to use similar combinations of patterns in different positions in space at certain stages of treatment.* One should not, therefore, concentrate on any one position during a treatment session, or over a period of time. If one aims, for instance, at patterns of extension in preparation for standing, one should treat the child with reflex-inhibiting patterns in side-lying, prone, supine, and if possible, standing. At the same time, patterns preparing for sitting should be included in the treatment program, e.g. side-sitting, long-sitting, supine with flexed and abducted legs, or standing with abducted legs, the child leaning forward at the hips, his hands on a low stool or on the floor.

It has to be kept clearly in mind, however, that any reflex-inhibiting pattern can be no more than a preparation for a number of movements which the child is otherwise unable to perform, or able to do only with effort, throughout a limited range and abnormal coordination. Reflex-inhibiting patterns, by inhibiting abnormal postural reflex activity, pave the way for techniques of facilitation of more normal movements and postural reactions.

Techniques of Facilitation

The techniques of facilitation of righting, equilibrium, and protective extension reactions will be described separately for clarity's sake, although normally they work together harmoniously.

Cerebral Palsy

The Facilitation of Righting Reactions

The patterns of rotation of the neck-righting and of the body-righting reaction on the body are used in treatment to facilitate rolling over from supine to prone, sitting up and lying down, getting up to kneel-standing, half-kneeling, to standing up and walking (Figs. 3-48–3-63).

The movements are initiated with the head or shoulder-girdle as key-points of control. In this way active movement responses of trunk and limbs can be obtained. They are useful techniques both with the very young children and with older ones who have fairly good head control and only moderate spasticity of trunk and upper limbs. Strong spasticity of neck and trunk will, however,

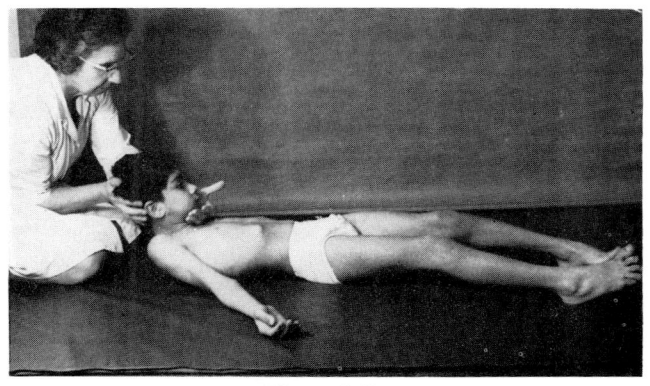

Figure 3-48.

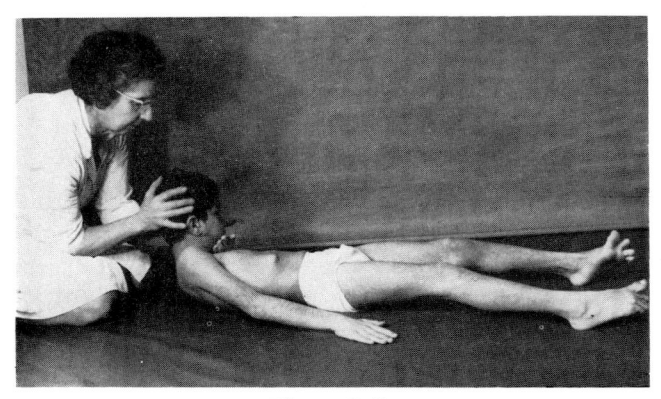

Figure 3-49.

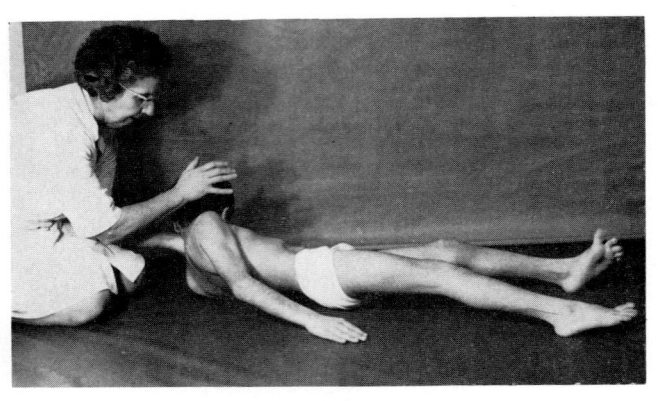

Figure 3-50.

interfere with adequate rotation of the shoulder-girdle, spine, and pelvis and thus block the desired sequence of movement at some point.

In these cases it is better to facilitate rotation from the shoulder-girdle as key-point. This has the added advantage of giving the child a chance to control and move his head actively. It has also proved more effective in controlling hypertonus of the muscles acting on the arms, trunk and neck. Furthermore, the child feels safer and more comfortable than when moved from the head.

FACILITATING MOVEMENTS FROM THE HEAD AS THE KEY-POINT. The therapist places one hand firmly under the child's chin, the other against the back of the head (Figs. 3-48–3-53). The head is then moved in a combination of either flexion forward and rotation or extension and rotation. The body should follow. In this way the patterns of rolling over from supine to prone and back again, for sitting up from prone, for getting into four-foot kneeling, and so on, are facilitated. Lateral movements of the body *in toto* must be avoided, as the main aim of this technique is to obtain rotation closely around the body axis. It is most essential not to separate flexion or extension from rotation, and to use both simultaneously. The therapist's hands should move together with the child's head and body rotation, very much like rolling a large ball between the palms of one's hands. They should

Cerebral Palsy

not remain at the child's chin and back of his head. For instance, when facilitating turning over into prone, the movement of the head is started with flexion forward and rotation to one side (Figs. 3-48–3-53). When the child is just about to turn into side-lying, a slow movement of extension of the head and lifting of the chin follows while rotation continues until the child reaches prone (Fig. 3-51). In order to return to supine the same maneuver is followed in reverse (Fig. 3-52). The change-over from flexion to extension has to be timed with great precision in order to make sure that every phase of the movement of the head coincides with

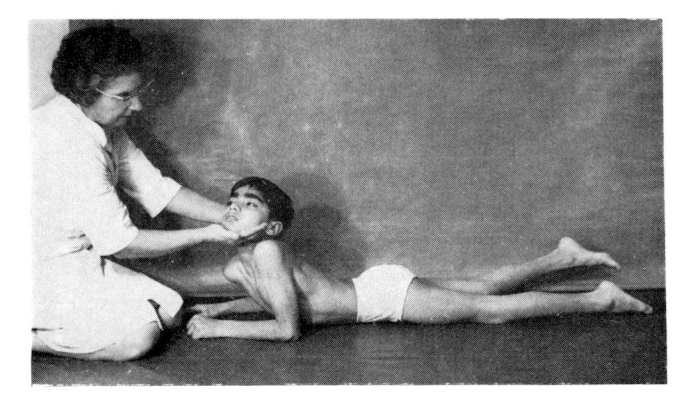

Figure 3-51.

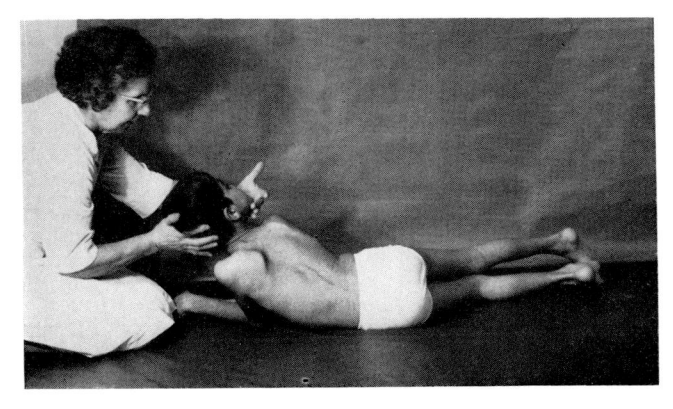

Figure 3-52.

that of the child's body. The use of force or pressure has to be carefully avoided.

FACILITATING MOVEMENTS FROM THE SHOULDER-GIRDLE AS THE KEY-POINT. The sequence of movements to be obtained are the same as those facilitated from head and neck. The hands of the therapist are placed underneath the child's axillae. The fingers are spread out in such a way as to be able to control both the shoulder blades and the upper arms (Fig. 3-53). In this way, by

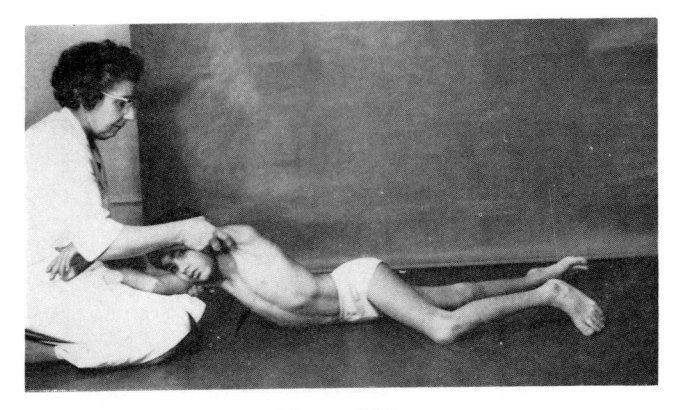

Figure 3-53.

controlling the whole shoulder-girdle, the therapist can not only facilitate movement responses of head, trunk, arms, and legs, but she can at the same time counteract any flexor or extensor hypertonus which may interfere with the intended sequence of movement at any particular stage. If, however, there is little danger of such interference by abnormal reactions and little need therefore for inhibition, the therapist may place her hands over the child's shoulders in such a way as to cover the collar bones, shoulder blades, and the head of the humerus. This makes it possible to exert pressure of graded strength and direction as the movement proceeds, and has a steadying influence on the movement. The former "grip" will serve predominantly to mobilize and lift the shoulder-girdle while the latter "grip" will result in an alignment of trunk and arms and thus tend to give increased stability. This is especially useful in the athetoid child who lacks postural stability.

MOVEMENTS TO BE OBTAINED BY FACILITATION FROM THE HEAD, NECK, AND SHOULDER-GIRDLE IN SUPINE, TO FACILITATE TURNING OVER. The following are noted:

1. Turning over to either side. The child's head is flexed forward and at the same time rotated towards one side. The child's body follows his head and he turns to his side (Figs. 3-48–3-50).

2. Turning over from supine to prone and back again. This is done by the combination of flexion of the head with rotation towards side-lying, described above, and then continued with rotation while gradually extending the child's head and spine as the body follows into prone-lying (Figs. 3-51–3-52).

Turning back to supine is done in the reverse order, thus starting with extension and rotation of the child's head and, from side-lying, continuing with rotation and flexion of his head.

IN PRONE, TO FACILITATE RECIPROCAL MOVEMENTS OF LEGS, PROGRESSION, AND SITTING UP. The methods are as follows:

1. Reciprocal movements of legs (amphibian reaction). In order to obtain this reaction the child's head is lifted by support under his chin, and simultaneously rotated to one side, thus extending and rotating his spine. He is expected to bend and abduct the legs of the side to which his face has been turned (Fig. 3-54). If rotation of the spine is blocked by flexor hypertonus of his trunk, shoulder-girdle, and arms, this normal reaction will not occur. In this case the movement is facilitated by lifting and rotating the child's shoulder-girdle while holding his arms extended above his head. The reaction will not occur unless the child's spine is well extended and his shoulders lifted well up while rotating his body. However, if his legs are very spastic and stiffly extended, his shoulder-girdle should not be lifted too high (Fig. 3-53).

2. Progression in prone-lying (Fig. 3-54). The same technique as described above is used but combined with traction on the child's head or shoulder-girdle, quickly followed by rotation of head or shoulders to the opposite side. This will lead to recip-

140 *Physical Therapy Services in the Developmental Disabilities*

rocal movements of his legs as well as a forward movement in the normal creeping pattern (Fig. 3-53).

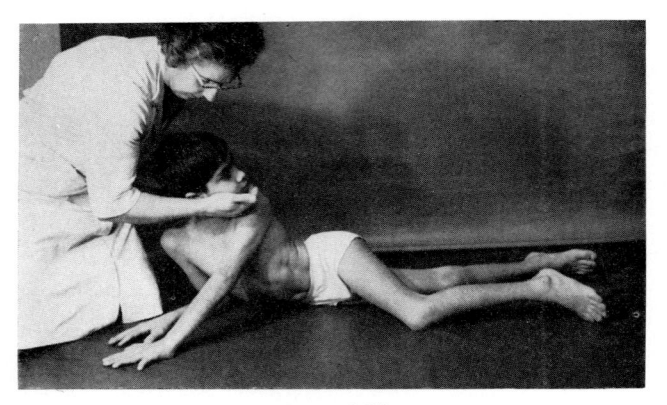

Figure 3-54.

3. Sitting up. If possible, sitting up is facilitated from the head, the child's arms being left free to move and to be used for support. If, however, there is too much flexor spasticity of his arms, the movement should be done from the shoulder-girdle. The child's head, or shoulder-girdle, is lifted and rotated to one side (Fig. 3-54). Just before his body, in following this movement, reaches the side-lying position, forward pressure is exerted against his head, shoulder, or both, thus gradually flexing the child's spine and hips while continuing with the rotation of his spine. In this way he is made to sit up (Fig. 3-55). The movement can be stopped when the child has reached the side-sitting position (Fig. 3-56), or can be continued. The same technique in reverse, starting with combined flexion and rotation and gradual extension of his spine, is used to get the child back from sitting to prone-lying.

IN SITTING, TO FACILITATE SIDE-SITTING AND KNEEL-SITTING (Figs. 3-55 and 3-56). To facilitate side- and kneel-sitting the therapist stands behind the sitting child. His head is rotated to one side, while his body is kept well forward and his hips flexed. The child's hips and legs follow the movement of his head and he moves into side-sitting. If retraction of his shoulders prevents ro-

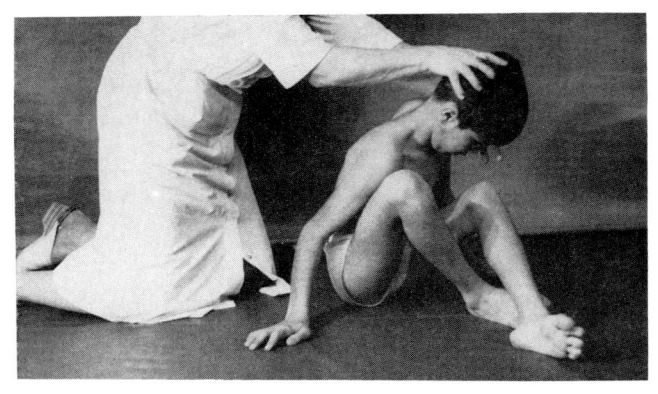

Figure 3-55.

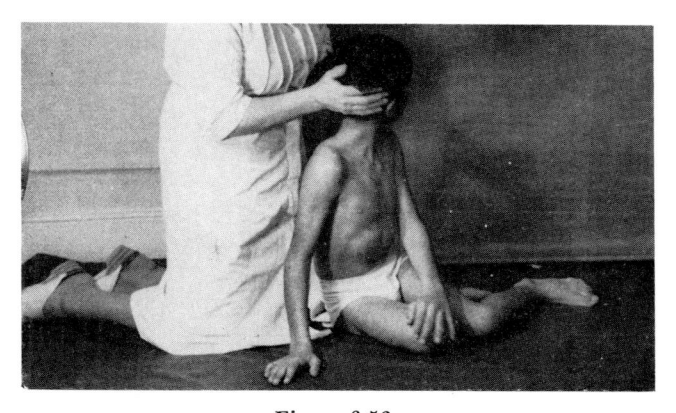

Figure 3-56.

tation forward of the trunk, facilitation will have to be done by rotating the child's shoulder-girdle and, with it, his spine and pelvis in order to obtain the desired movement of his legs to side-sitting.

The therapist moves in front of the child while continuing the rotation of his head or shoulder-girdle in order to get him onto his knees (Fig. 3-57).

Similar techniques combining rotation of head or shoulder-girdle with either flexion or extension of the spine and well-timed traction, are used to get the child from kneeling to crawling

(Figs. 3-57 and 3-58), to kneel-standing (Figs. 3-59 and 3-60), half-kneeling (Fig. 3-61), and standing up (Figs. 3-62 and 3-63).

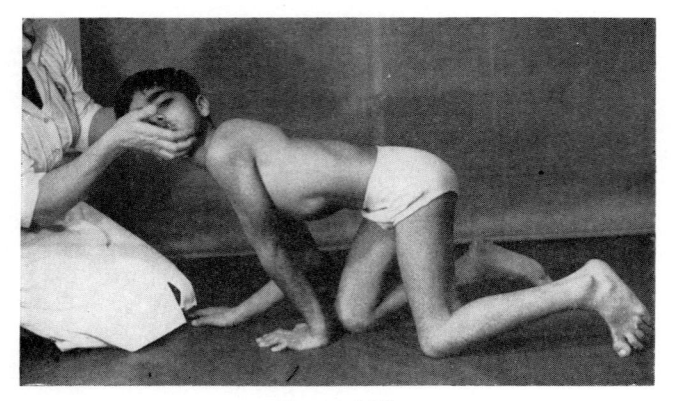

Figure 3-57.

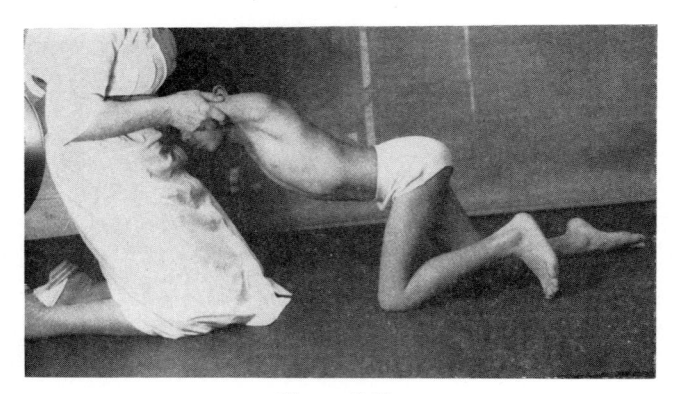

Figure 3-58.

The most important common factor in all these techniques is that of rotation as closely as possible around the child's body axis. To obtain this, lateral movements of the child's body as a whole should be avoided as much as possible.

FACILITATION OF HEAD-RIGHTING. Head-righting and control are obtained by using the patterns of the labyrinthine-righting reaction, of the body-righting reaction on head, as well as optical-righting reactions.

Cerebral Palsy 143

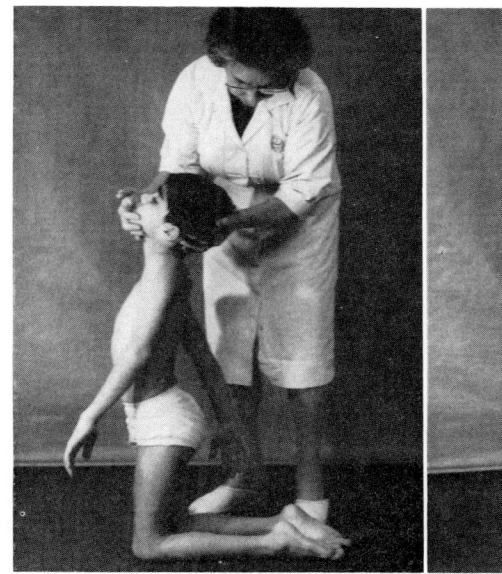

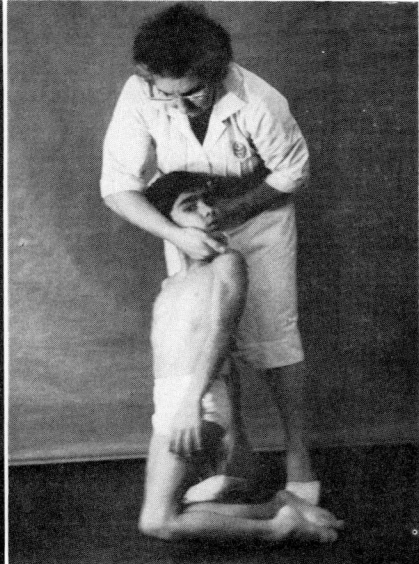

Figure 3-59.   Figure 3-60.

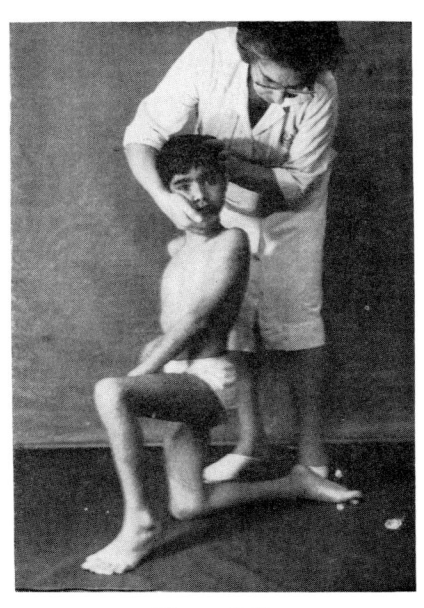

Figure 3-61.

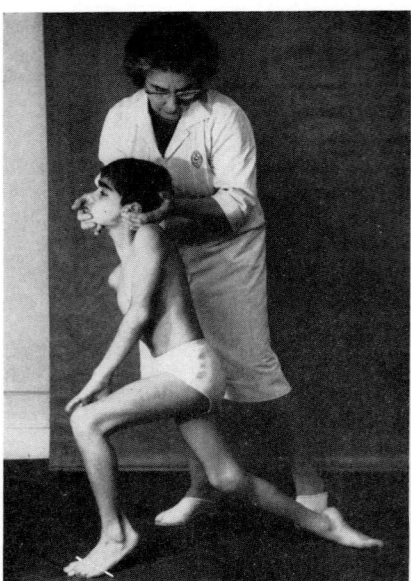

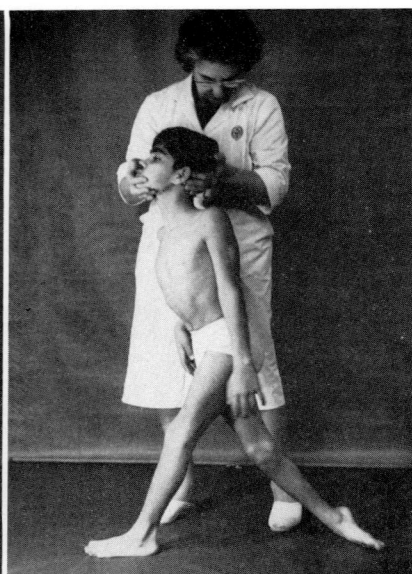

Figure 3-62.   Figure 3-63.

The child's body is moved, held and controlled from various key-points, while his head is left free to maintain or adjust its normal position in space and in relation to the trunk. In prone-lying, for instance, the shoulder-girdle is lifted and spine and hips extended, so that the child has to lift his head and hold it up (Figs. 3-64 and 3-65). From sitting he is lowered to supine and lifted up again; he has to learn to control his head position, maintaining it in alignment with the body during the movements (Fig. 3-66). This is made easier by moving his body backward either diagonally or with some rotation. Movements are first done slowly but are gradually speeded up.

ADJUSTMENT OF HEAD POSITION TO MOVEMENTS OF THE CHILD'S BODY AND HEAD IN SPACE. In *supine,* to facilitate head-raising, the therapist places the child in a position of full flexion. His legs are flexed to his abdomen and adducted and his arms are placed across his chest or around his knees, with his forearms in supination. His shoulder-girdle is then brought forward and raised

Cerebral Palsy 145

slightly off the support, while pressure is given against his upper arms to stabilize his shoulder-girdle in flexion. The child is expected to lift his head. (Fig. 3-66).

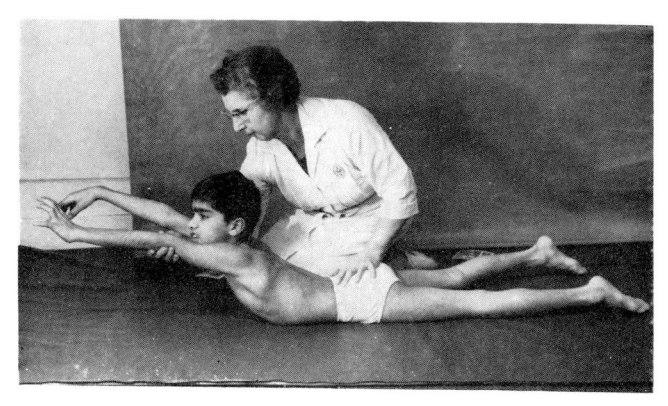

Figure 3-64.

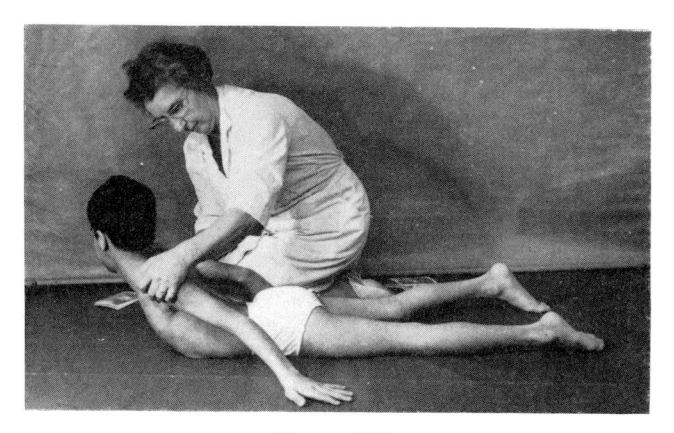

Figure 3-65.

In *prone,* head-raising is facilitated in the following ways:
1. The therapist is by the child's side. He should be fully extended with his arms above his head (Fig. 3-64). The therapist places her arm across the child's chest underneath his axillae and extends his spine by raising his chest off the support. The child's

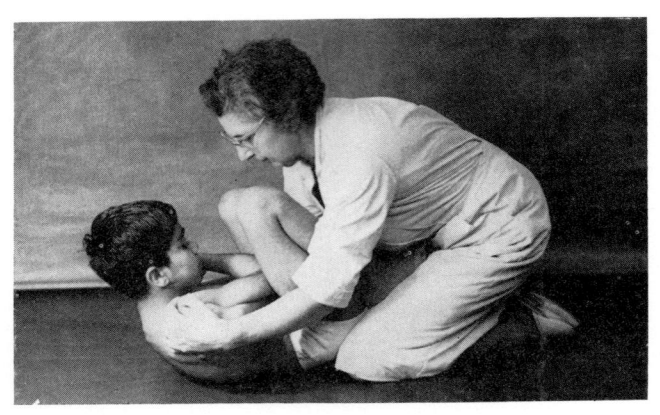

Figure 3-66.

chin may at first rest on her arm, but when sufficient inhibition of flexor spasticity has been achieved, this support is taken away by holding his arm more distally, so that he holds his head up by himself.

2. The therapist is behind the child. His arms are placed by his sides in extension and outward rotation, palms on the support. The therapist then lifts the child's shoulder-girdle up and backward, either straight or with some rotation. The child may then lift his head (Fig. 3-65).

3. A small child is held in the inverted position by his feet or knees and moved about gently. When his spine and hips extend he is gently lowered to the ground to prone-lying, chest first, then hips and, finally the legs, so as to maintain full extension. This total extension makes head-raising possible.

In *sitting,* head-righting is facilitated as follows:

1. A young child sits astride the therapist's lap facing her. His arms are extended at his elbows and adducted so that his wrists or hands can be held together by one of the therapist's hands, leaving her other hand free. He is then moved slowly backward, first with some lateral or diagonal movements of his body and later on straight backward, but only as far as he can control his head and prevent it from falling backward. At the point where the child is in danger of losing head control, the movement is reversed and

the therapist may support his head for a moment with her free hand. Gradually the range of movement backward is increased. Later on, the movement is arrested at the point where the child's head threatens to drop back, and the therapist waits for him to bring his head forward again, either moving the child not at all or just slightly forward. With an older child the same can be done, but with the child sitting on a stool or plinth (Fig. 3-67).

2. The child sits astride the therapist's lap facing forward. The therapist places her hands around his pelvis to stabilize his hips.

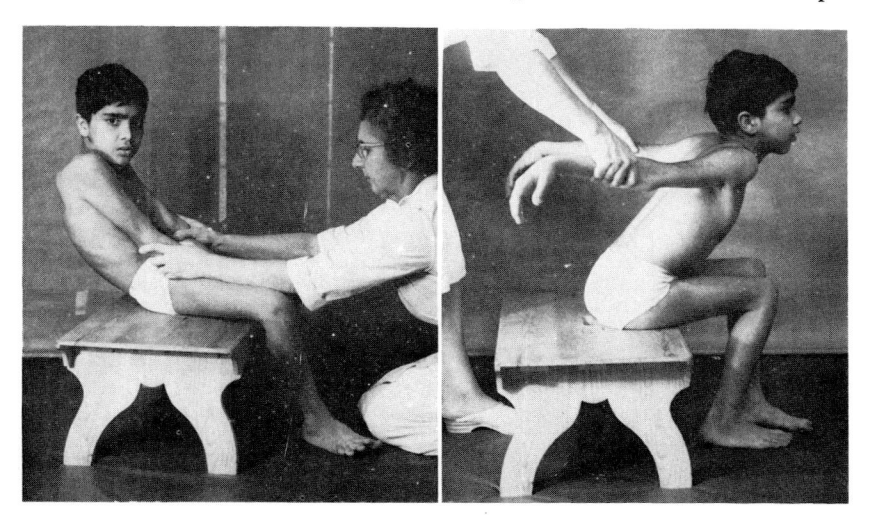

Figure 3-67.

Figure 3-68. Alternate technique of head righting.

He is made to lean forward slowly with his head and trunk, but only as far as he keeps his head upright and in the normal position. This may, at first, be combined with lateral or diagonal movements as it makes head control easier than moving straight forward. Although at first the therapist moves the child up again at the point where he starts to lose head control, he is later on expected to right his head and to get back to the original sitting posture by himself. If the child has difficulty in coming up by himself, it is advisable to put one hand under his chest and to lift him up a little, in order to find out whether there is any undue pressure downward due to a flexor spasticity. In this case, the child's chest has to be lifted from underneath by the therapist, but only to the point where no downward pressure can be felt. Pressure downward from under his chin should also be tested and the child helped to overcome this difficulty of initiating head-raising from a fully flexed position.

3. With the child still astride the therapist's lap, facing forward, his arms can be taken backward in extension and outward rotation, while his body is slowly lowered forward and downward. The combined extension of shoulders and spine helps to counteract flexor spasticity and downward pressure of his arms, head, and chest, and usually makes head- and body-righting easier. The same can be done with an older child sitting on a stool or plinth (Fig. 3-68).

4. The child sits on a plinth or stool, the therapist standing in front of him between his abducted legs. His arms are extended in outward rotation and brought forward, and his hands are held together by one of the therapist's hands; the child is then moved slowly backward in combination with lateral or diagonal movements to begin with, as it is more difficult for him to right his head when going straight backward (Figs. 3-67 and 3-68). Whenever he is on the point of losing head control, he should be moved up again (it is not necessary to get him right up to sitting again). The techniques used are similar to those described in (1). If there is much retraction of the child's shoulder-girdle due to extensor spasticity, in spite of his arms being adducted and placed forward, his hands may have to be left free and his shoulders controlled from his elbows. If necessary, his shoulders may have to be held forward by the therapist.

5. When sitting on the floor, a small child can be treated in a similar way, as described above, by making him hold on to his feet; if he cannot hold on by himself, the therapist should put each of her hands over each hand and foot of the child to hold them together. If there is adductor spasticity of the legs, the child's arms should be inside his abducted legs; however, with athetoids (who have no adductor spasticity when their legs are flexed), better alignment of head and body can be obtained with the child's arms along his legs on the outside.

Cerebral Palsy

6. In side-sitting on the floor,* the child is held by his extended left arm when side-sitting to the right or vice versa to the left. When sitting on the right, he is gently lowered toward the ground to the side of his unsupported right arm, and he is expected to right his head laterally toward the opposite side of the movement. He should not drop his head, and he must not be moved further downward than where he can control his head position. If he loses head control, it is advisable to test for pressure downward of his neck by moving him passively head up and sideways at the point of loss of head control (Fig. 3-69). If there is pressure

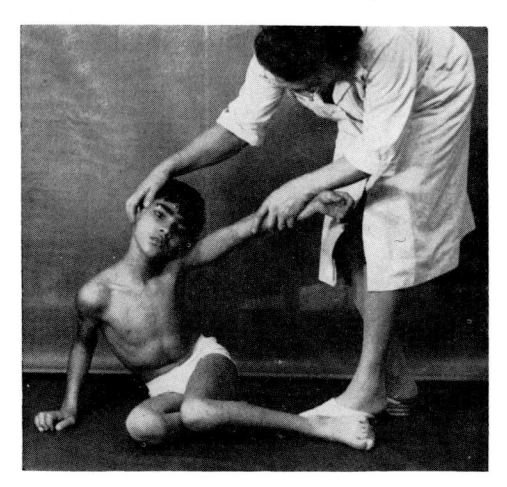

Figure 3-69.

downward, this should be inhibited before continuing with facilitation techniques. Gradually the child should learn to control his head position throughout the whole range of the movement downward to side-lying, his head touching the support only after his shoulder has reached the ground. He should also be able to lift his head at once when pulled up from side-sitting by one arm (Fig. 3-70).

In *kneel-sitting*, head-raising is facilitated as follows:

1. The therapist is behind the child and grasps him by his

---
*Side-sitting to the right means that the knees both point to the right. Side-sitting to the left has the knees pointing to the left.

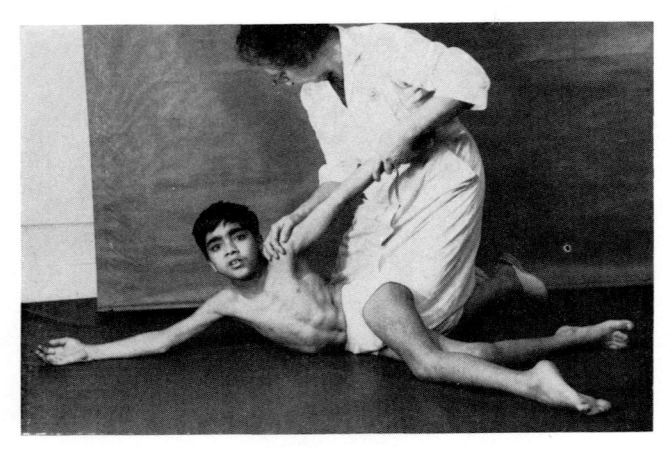

Figure 3-70.

shoulders and, pulling them backward, slowly extends his spine. He is expected to lift his head. If there is too much flexor spasticity of his shoulders and arms, this reaction will not occur. To inhibit flexor spasticity his arms are extended, abducted, and outwardly rotated, held from his elbows. The child is then moved gently forward until he lifts his head as a protection against falling on his face. This extension of his spine and shoulders may lead to a total extension involving hips and legs. To prevent this the therapist may have to stand over the child and control his hips with her knees (Fig. 3-71).

2. The therapist can also stand in front of the child. His arms are extended and lifted horizontally upward. He is then gently pulled forward and expected to lift his head. In this position he can be moved upward and downward and sideways and, by lifting one arm higher than the other, rotation can be obtained as well.

In *standing up,* head- and body-righting are facilitated as follows:

1. From the squatting position or from sitting on a low stool, the child is made to extend his legs, his heels remaining firmly on the ground. The therapist stands behind the child, her hands resting on his thighs just above his knees exerting pressure backward and downward, while he extends his knees. The therapist initially

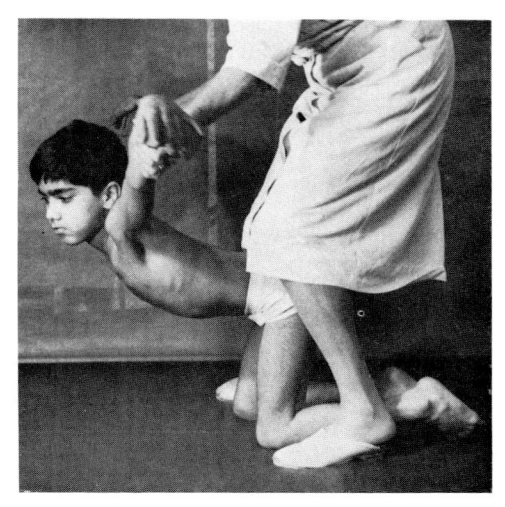

Figure 3-71.

keeps his body weight well forward, but in order to facilitate the raising of his head and body he is quickly tipped backward with his hips against the therapist, which makes it easier for him to lift his head and straighten his spine and hips. If there is a strong pressure downward of head and trunk, due to flexor spasticity, he is helped to raise his body and head throughout the first part of the movement by being lifted up with one hand under his sternum or chin (Fig. 3-72).

2. The child stands, held by the therapist at his knees from behind. The therapist's hands must cover the area both just above and below his knees to prevent flexion and, by downward pressure, to stabilize his feet which are firmly planted on the ground. He is moved gently and slowly forward, backward, and sideways, with or without rotation, and should maintain the normal position of his head (Fig. 3-73).

Facilitation of Equilibrium Reactions

This serves a twofold purpose, (1) the maintenance of balance when moving or being moved, and (2) recovery of balance when on the point of losing it.

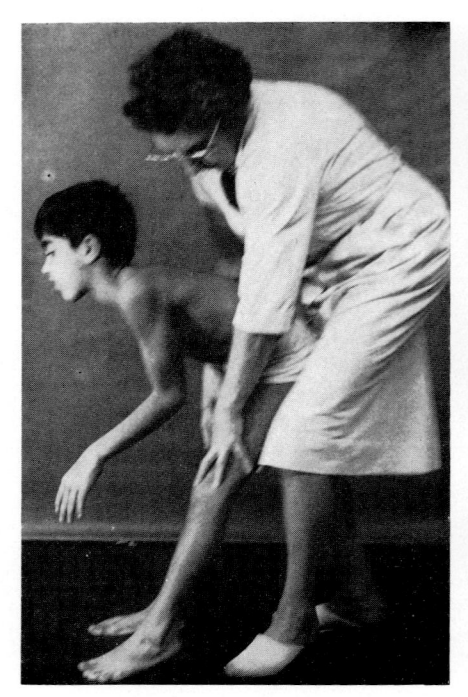

152 *Physical Therapy Services in the Developmental Disabilities*

Figure 3-72. 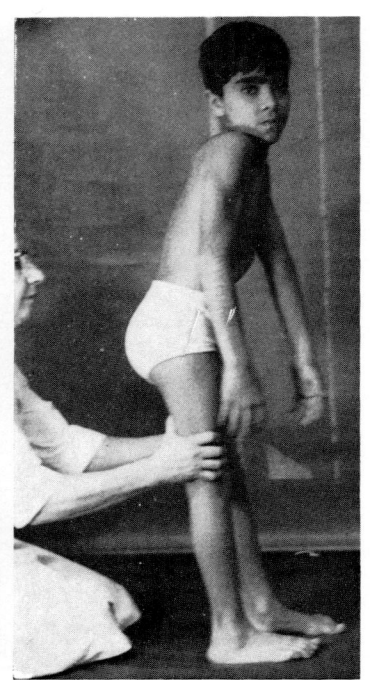   Figure 3-73.

Many children with cerebral palsy may be able to maintain a position but dare not move freely because of a lack of patterns necessary for recovering lost or almost-lost balance. In standing, for instance, one may find that if a child is supported lightly from behind under the armpits and is suddenly made to lean backward and held there, he may not be able to get his weight forward again over his feet, although some children may be able to take a few steps backward to save themselves from falling.

Equilibrium reactions are facilitated by displacing the child's center of gravity. This is at first done gently, speed and range being increased gradually. This can be done by placing the child on a movable platform such as a tilting board or by moving the child against an immovable support.

The advantages of a tilting board are that the therapist can control effectively speed, range, and rhythm of the movements of the board. The child can move freely without any interference and has free scope for any activity. In fact, he can move the board by himself. However, the disadvantages are that the therapist has insufficient control over the child and cannot prevent abnormal reactions effectively. In all but the slightest cases it is better, therefore, to practice equilibrium reactions by moving the child. The therapist has better control, can guide the child's reactions from various key-points, preventing abnormal reactions and facilitating normal ones; that is, she can effectively combine inhibition with facilitation. Furthermore, by restricting exaggerated compensatory equilibrium reactions of lesser affected parts, she can facilitate, strengthen and guide reactions of the more involved parts. This is of great importance in the treatment of children who can compensate, by exaggerated reactions of the less involved parts, for the lack of insufficiency of equilibrium reactions of the more affected parts.

In a diplegic child, for instance, one has to obtain equilibrium reactions of trunk and legs. It is, therefore, essential to prevent the child from using his arms and hands for balance. On the other hand, some athetoids with less affected lower limbs will maintain their balance in standing largely by excessive activity of hips, legs, and feet. Here, head-righting and balance of trunk and arms have to be obtained and excessive compensatory activity of the lower limbs restricted.

Equilibrium reactions can be practiced effectively only when the child is able to maintain a position against gravity, even if only for a short time. Before this, however, the experience of the sensorimotor patterns needed for maintaining or regaining balance in any particular position can be given to the child. Though he may have to be well supported in reflex-inhibiting patterns, he is already moved in patterns similar to those he will later on use for balance and postural control. The therapist will control the movement from key-points only to prevent abnormal reactions interfering with the movement.

In sitting, kneeling, and if possible in standing, a child's weight is transferred sideways, forward, backward, and diagonally, first with slow movements or by gently pushing him to and fro, and gradually with increasing speed and range of the movement. It is most important to take the hands away momentarily as often as possible, so that the child learns not to rely too much on the therapist for support and control. The child must, however, never be allowed to fall or to be afraid of falling. He must at first be given time to react adequately, and for this reason he may at first have to be held in a position where he is out of balance for a little while without being moved and with as little support as possible; he thus has to do something about the situation himself of necessity.

The facilitation of equilibrium reactions requires very careful handling of the child. If he feels too secure there will be no need to do anything. If he feels insecure and is afraid of falling, hypertonus will recur and prevent any normal reactions.

In general the first equilibrium reactions practiced are those in prone-lying, the child supporting himself on his forearms and later on extended arms. His weight is transferred by first pushing his shoulders gently from side to side. He is prevented from falling over at the last moment by pushing him back again to the midposition. This is repeated until he gradually takes over and learns to save himself from falling.

In sitting, four-foot kneeling, upright and half-kneeling, the maneuver is used at increasing speed and range, forward and backward, sideways and diagonally, using either the shoulder-girdle or hips as key-points of control. Again he is held at the exact point where his balance is threatened, and he is made to right himself, if necessary, with help.

As soon as a fairly normal standing posture is obtained, even if this should require some help from a key-point (shoulders, hips or knees), the child is swayed forward, backward, and sideways with or without rotation of shoulder-girdle or pelvis. He has to learn to keep his balance by compensatory movements of head, trunk, and hips when supported at his knees, or to counterbalance with hips, knees, and feet when supported from the shoulder-girdle or neck. Similar techniques are used with the child in a step position. The child, in preparation for walking, must learn to transfer his weight from one leg to the other without losing balance.

Once the first normal reaction has been obtained, much repetition of the same maneuver is needed to establish the new sensorimotor patterns, and to make the reaction quicker and more reliable. When pushing the child in any one direction, he should be prevented from falling by giving him a counterpush in the form of a light tap in the opposite direction. This "alternating tapping" not only prevents him from falling but also stimulates active automatic responses throughout body and limbs, as the child is left unsupported momentarily between the taps.

The following are some specific techniques for facilitation of equilibrium reactions in various positions.

In *supine,* the child is made to hold on to his feet or calves without falling to either side. He may be gently moved sideways and helped to right himself towards the midline when on the point of losing his balance.

In *prone,* the child supports himself on his forearms and his shoulders are gently pushed from side to side. He is prevented from falling over by being pushed back to the midline or to the opposite side (Fig. 3-74).

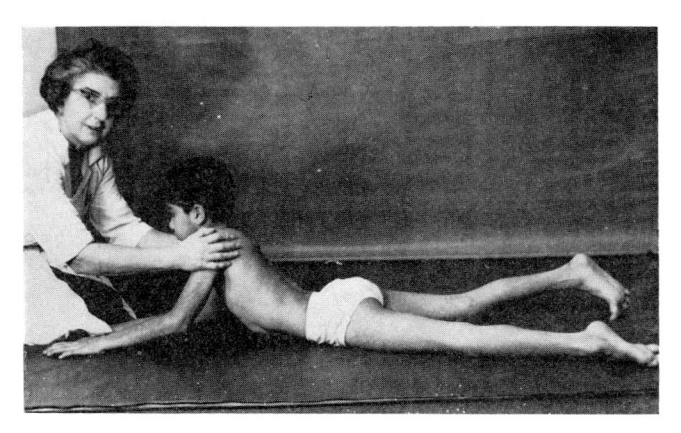

Figure 3-74.

In *sitting,* equilibrium reactions are facilitated as follows:

1. The child sits on the floor or on a stool, and the therapist, behind him, moves his body slowly to one side, holding him lightly at the sides of his chest or at his shoulders. The child should

156 *Physical Therapy Services in the Developmental Disabilities*

not use his hands for support. He is expected to right his head and to abduct and extend his arm and legs in the opposite direction to the movement of his body (Figs. 3-75 and 3-76).

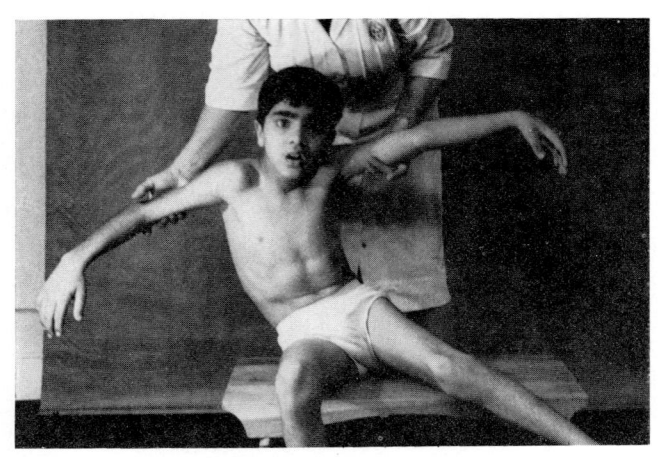

Figure 3-75.

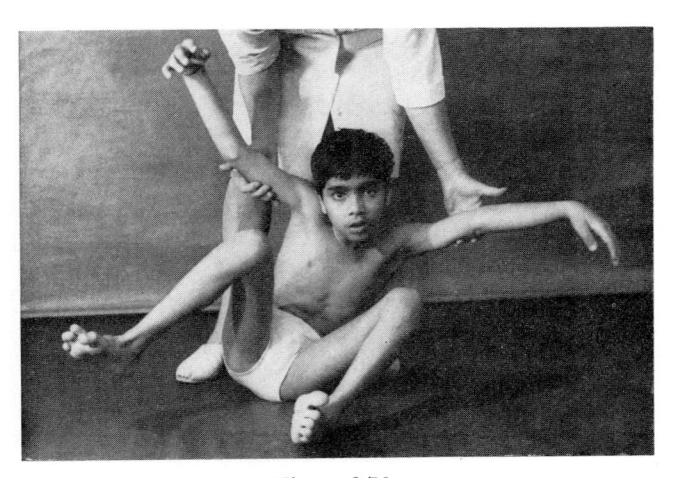

Figure 3-76.

2. The child sits on the floor. He should not use his arms for support, and he may be given a toy to hold with both hands to prevent this. The therapist then grasps his legs below his knees

Cerebral Palsy

and lifts and bends them alternately towards his body, his feet off the ground. In progressing treatment both legs are lifted and moved at the same time in the same direction. All movements should be done with his legs in abduction and outward rotation. He is expected to maintain the sitting posture and not to fall backward (Fig. 3-77 and 3-78).

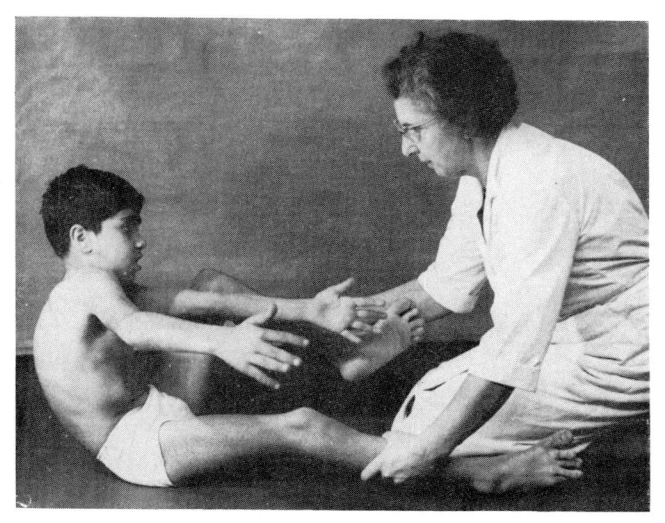

Figure 3-77.

3. The child is side-sitting without the support of his arms and hands. The therapist takes both legs by the knees and moves them slowly towards the oppoiste side. He is encouraged to remain sitting and not to fall backward or sideways (Fig. 3-79).

In *four-foot kneeling*, equilibrium reactions are facilitated as follows:

1. The child is gently pushed sideways or rocked forward and backward. He is prevented from falling over by a counterpush if he is on the point of falling. This push is given either to his shoulders or to his hips.

2. One leg or arm is lifted up and he is rocked forward and backward. The limb should only be held lightly so that he is not really supported. In order to obtain more advanced equilibrium reactions the therapist lifts one arm and one leg simultaneously—

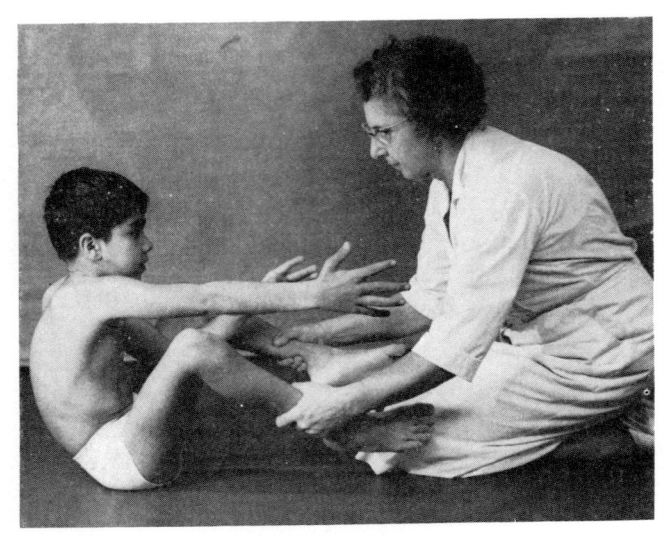

Figure 3-78.

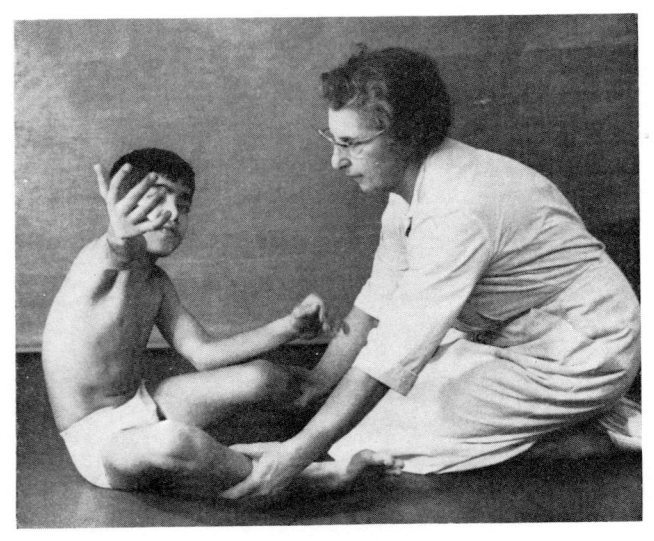

Figure 3-79.

this can be done with the limbs of the same side or of the opposite sides (Figs. 3-80 and 3-81).

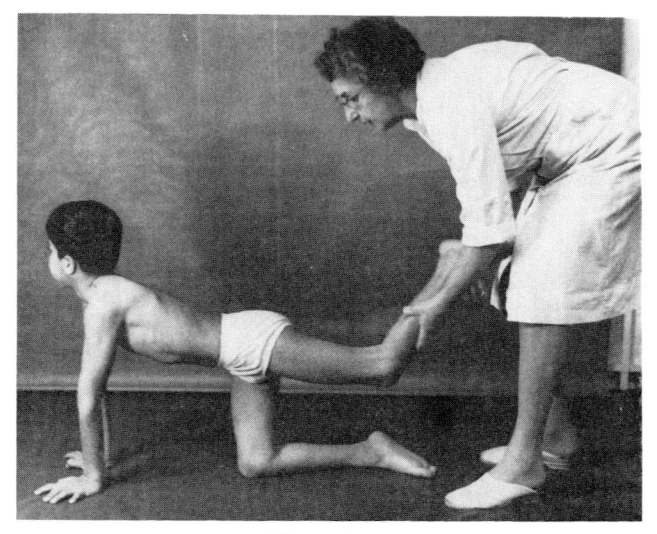

Figure 3-80.

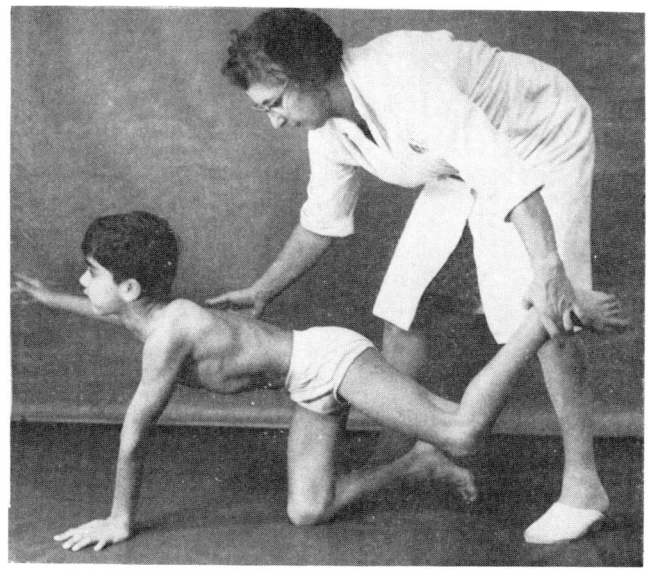

Figure 3-81.

In *kneel-standing,* equilibrium reactions are facilitated thus:

1. The child is moved from side to side, lightly held under his armpits. He is expected to abduct the weight-free leg, or lift it off the support, and to abduct and extend his arms with rotation of his shoulder-girdle. He should not put his hand to the ground (Fig. 3-82).

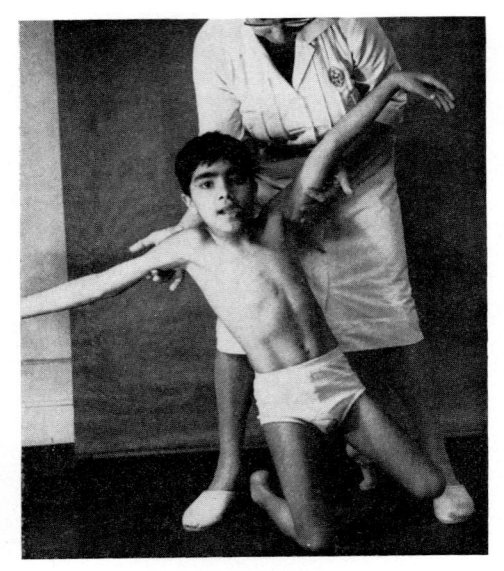

Figure 3-82.

2. The child is pushed gently backward against his lower chest wall and encouraged not to sit down. However, if he cannot maintain the upright posture and is inclined to sit down, he can be given a counterpush against his buttocks, or, if he leans too far backward, a counterpush against his back. This tapping forward and backward prevents him from falling either way and stimulates normal postural reactions of head, trunk, arms, and legs (Fig. 3-83). Alternate tapping can also be done to the sides of his hips to facilitate equilibrium reactions during weight transfer sideways.

In *half-kneeling,* the following techniques are used:

Cerebral Palsy

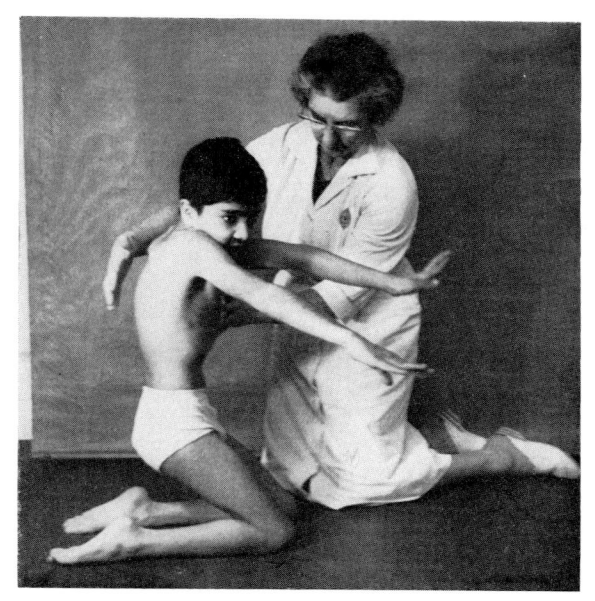

Figure 3-83.

1. The child kneels, and one leg—the left one for instance—is brought forward, with the foot firmly on the ground. Held and supported by his left knee, with some abduction and outward rotation of that leg, he is rocked forward and backward and gently moved sideways. He is expected to maintain the half-kneeling posture, and to right head and trunk. He should also balance with his arms without putting them down to the ground for support (Fig. 3-84).

2. The therapist then lifts his left leg slightly off the ground and extends his knee, bringing his foot gradually forward and down in small stages, and back again in the same way, gradually flexing his knee. The child's foot is each time lifted up and put down again (Fig. 3-85).

In *standing*, the following can be used:

1. The child stands with his legs parallel and slightly apart. He is rocked sideways held lightly by his hips or shoulder-girdle, and his weight is shifted over one leg. He is expected to abduct and extend the weight-free leg (Fig. 3-86).

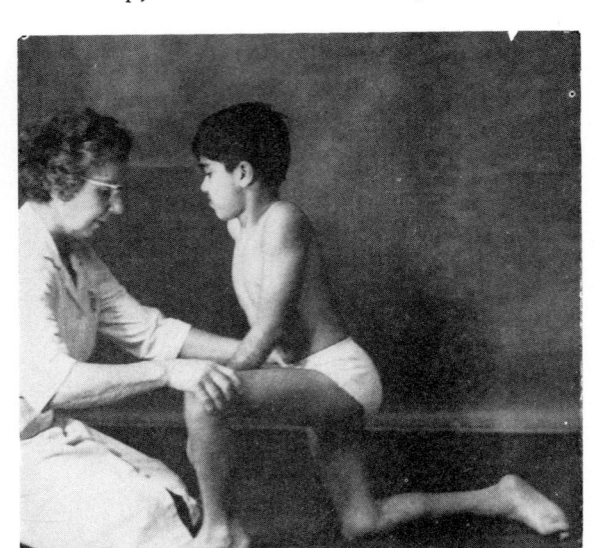

162 *Physical Therapy Services in the Developmental Disabilities*

Figure 3-84.

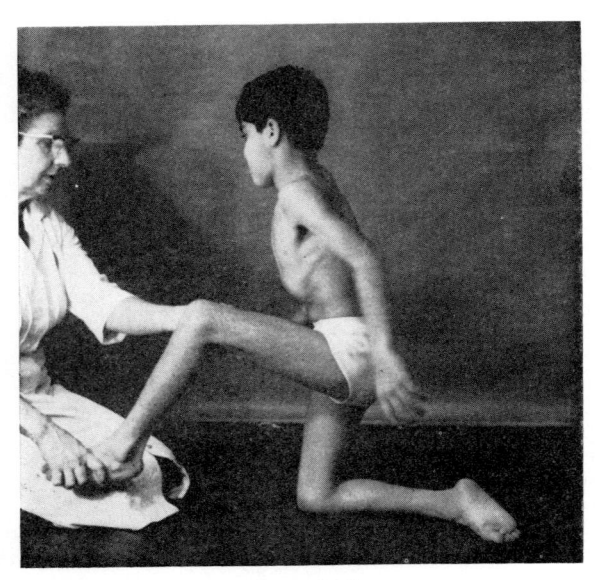

Figure 3-85.

Cerebral Palsy 163

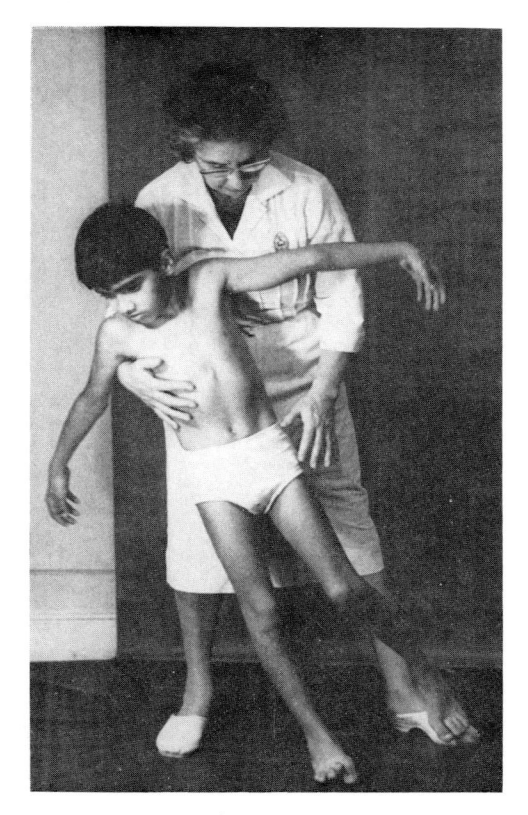

Figure 3-86.

2. The child stands in step position, one foot in front of the other, his weight distributed equally between his legs. He is then pushed gently backward and forward by alternating taps against his sternum and back. This helps him to gain control and balance during weight transfer (Fig. 3-87).

3. The child stands on one leg. The therapist, standing behind him, holds his other leg by the ankle and bends his knee to a right angle, keeping his hips extended. The child is then moved gently over his standing leg in various directions. If necessary, the therapist steadies the hip of his weight-bearing leg with her free hand (Fig. 3-88).

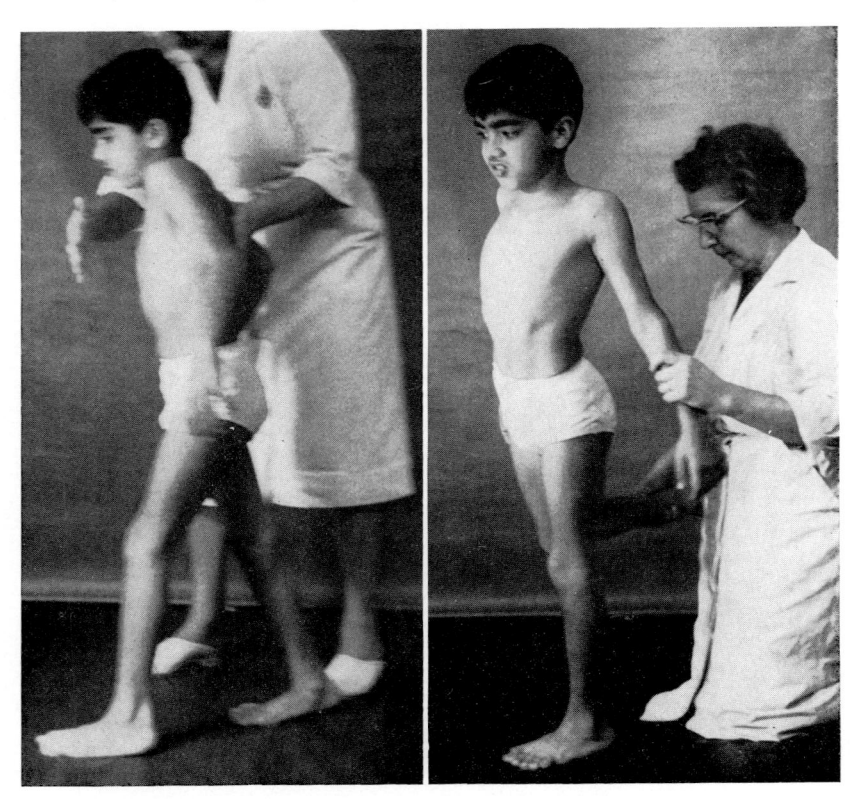

Figure 3-87.   Figure 3-88.

4. The therapist is by the child's side and lifts his leg on the same side off the ground, holding it by the forefoot with his ankle in dorsiflexion. If necessary, the child's hand opposite his weight-bearing leg is held. The therapist then gradually extends the child's knee with his leg in outward rotation, at the same time pulling his body slowly forward over the standing leg. The child is expected to react with active extension and abduction of his lifted leg, without collapsing on the standing one. This is followed by lowering his foot to the ground, heel first as in a normal large step (Fig. 3-89). (This is the "see-saw reaction," so-called by Weisz, 1938).

5. The child stands with crossed legs; both knees are turned

Cerebral Palsy 165

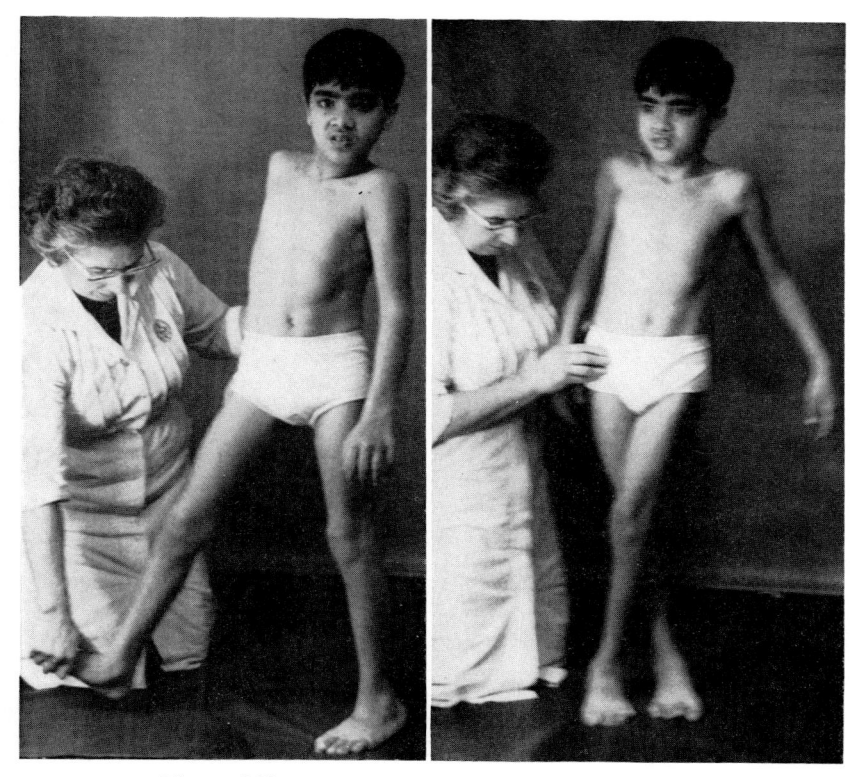

Figure 3-89.   Figure 3-90.

outward, his feet everted so that his toes are pointed toward each other. His weight is then transferred slowly backward and forward from one leg to the other. Balancing in this position makes the child put his weight on the lateral border of his feet instead of on the medial one, as usual. It also stabilizes his hips in outward rotation. Later on, the child is encouraged to walk forward and backward crossing his legs in the way described (Fig. 3-90).

6. The child stands with his feet parallel. Held by his shoulder-girdle, he is moved from side to side until he abducts his weight-free leg. When he has done so, and before he has put his foot to the ground, he is quickly pushed towards the side of his abducted leg so that he puts his foot to the ground and takes weight on his abducted leg.

166 *Physical Therapy Services in the Developmental Disabilities*

7. The child stands with his feet parallel, held lightly from behind under his armpits. He is suddenly tilted backward and told not to step backward. This movement brings weight onto his heels. He is expected to dorsiflex his ankles and toes to counteract loss of balance and falling backward (Fig. 3-91).

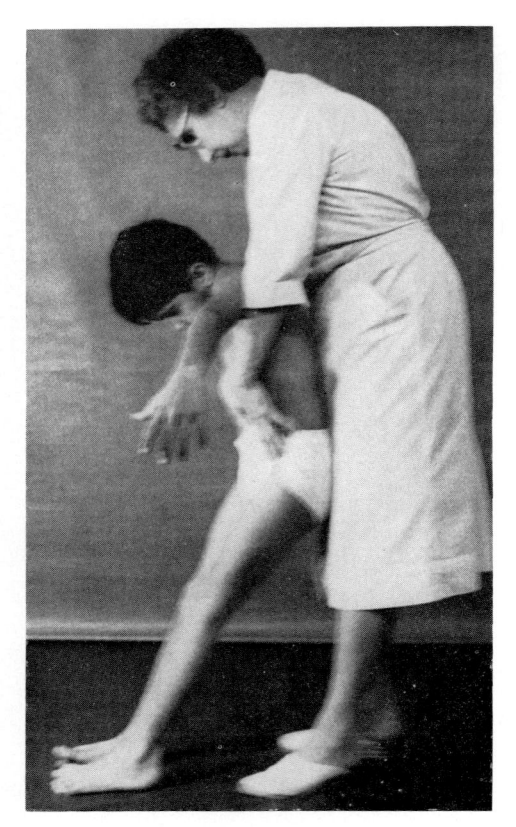

Figure 3-91.

Facilitation of Protective Extension of Arms and Hands

The facilitation techniques described below are expected to result in the child's extending his arms and hands, to support his body and to protect himself from falling on his face.

In *prone-lying*, the therapist takes the child's shoulder-girdle and pulls it backward and upward (Fig. 3-92).

Cerebral Palsy

In *sitting and side-sitting*, the following are used.

1. The child is held by one arm extended and outwardly rotated, and pushed towards the opposite side. This can be done in various directions—sideways, diagonally backward and forward (Fig. 3-93).

2. The therapist is on the side to which the child should extend his arm and take his weight when in danger of falling. She holds his elbow, wrist, and fingers extended by supporting his hand underneath his palm with one hand, while using the other hand either to keep his elbow extended if this be necessary at first, or to control his shoulder to prevent flexion and downward pressure. The child is then alternately pulled and pushed sideways, or diagonally backward and forward in quick succession, and his extended hand gradually lowered to the ground. This maneuver stimulates support tonus, and helps to keep the child's arm mobile when weight-bearing. It also allows the therapist to feel and control the child's reactions (Fig. 3-94).

In *four-foot kneeling*, the child is handled in the same way as in prone-lying. When his arms and hands extend and touch the ground he can be "bounced" up and down onto his arms and hands in order to reinforce extension and weight-bearing.

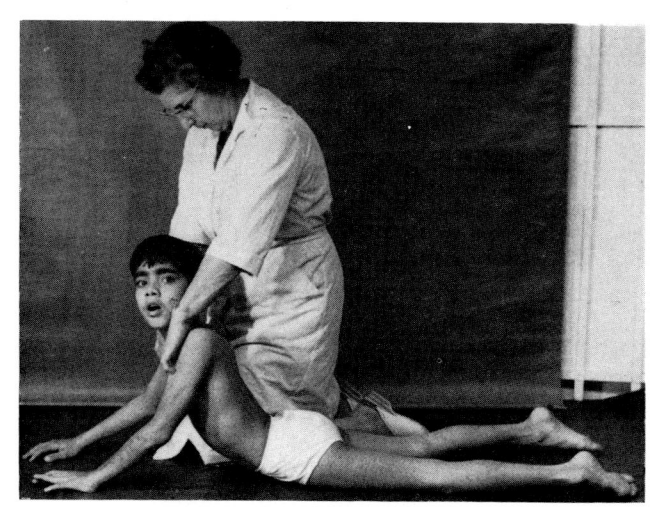

Figure 3-92.

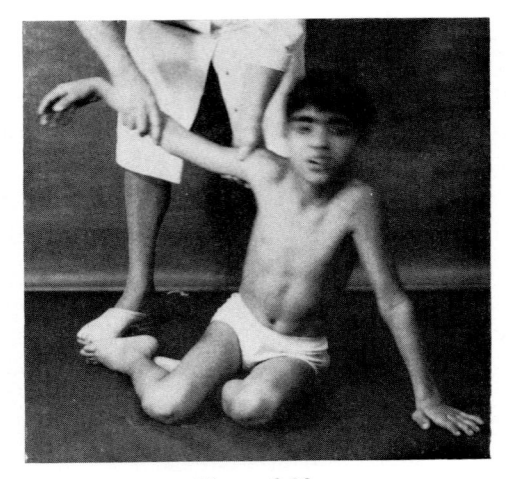

168 *Physical Therapy Services in the Developmental Disabilities*

Figure 3-93.

In *kneel-standing and standing,* these techniques are suggested:

1. The child stands on his knees. He is held by his shoulders from behind and slowly lowered forward and downward. This can also be done by holding one arm horizontally abducted in extension and outward rotation, while lowering his body, first slow-

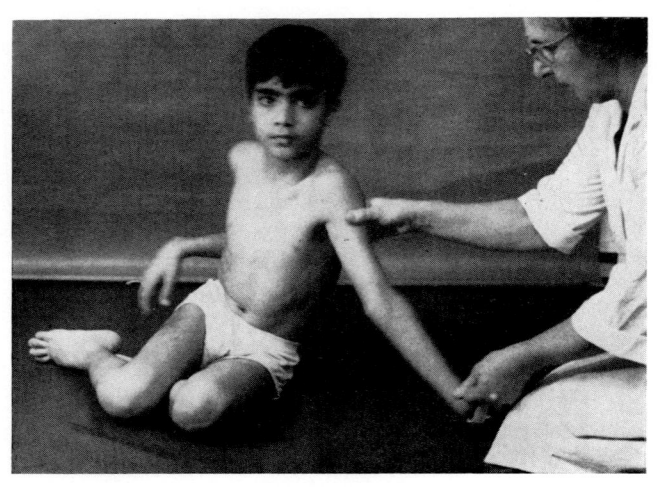

Figure 3-94.

ly and later on quickly, towards the opposite side, or diagonally or straight forward.

2. The child stands facing a table or wall forward or sideways. One arm is held as described in kneel-standing, and the child is pushed gently towards the table or wall (Fig. 3-95). He is expected to stretch out one or both arms to save himself from falling.

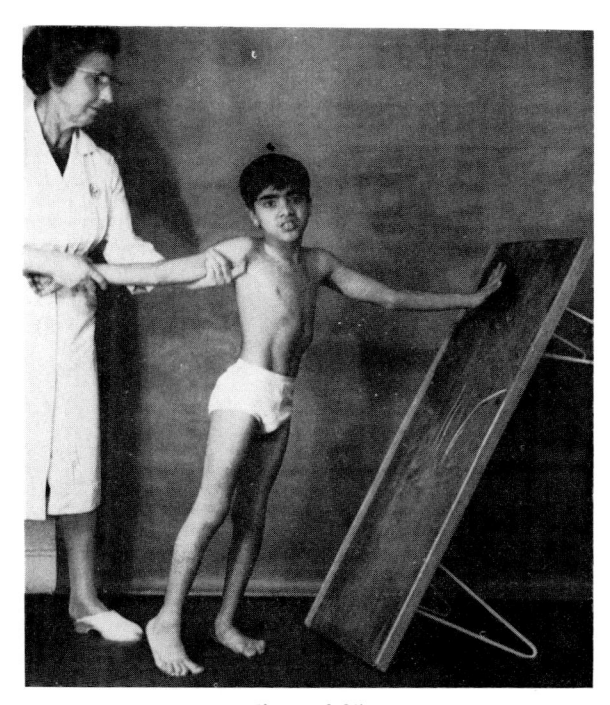

Figure 3-95.

The specific reactions to be facilitated have been described but not all of them can be used when treating the individual child. This is especially so with the facilitation of equilibrium reactions, because here one can only facilitate them when the child is able to maintain the sitting, kneeling, or standing position. A careful choice of the techniques described must, therefore, be made according to the child's needs and his ability to respond satisfactorily.

To summarize, when using techniques of facilitation the following points should be observed by the therapist:

1. Each case must first be assessed thoroughly with respect to the prevailing abnormal motor patterns and the presence of any of the normal automatic postural reactions.

2. The therapist should know beforehand what type of motor reaction she is trying to obtain and what the normal response should be.

3. She must know what technique to use in order to obtain the desired response. This depends very much on the key-point chosen and on the speed and range of the handling.

4. She must stimulate adequately, sufficiently strong enough to obtain a response but not too strongly, for if she does so, abnormal reflex activity may recur and interfere with and block the desired response. If the child is held too securely, he will feel too comfortable, and will not react but simply relax. On the other hand, the child must know that he will not fall or hurt himself. He should, in fact, enjoy the treatment.

5. The therapist must wait for the child's response and give him time to react. There is usually a delay at first, and much repetition of any particular technique is needed to obtain the first response. Still more practice and repetition are required to get the response promptly and reliably established. Not infrequently, a technique has to be adapted and modified to meet the specific needs of any particular child.

6. The therapist must never force a movement against resistance—that is, the movement initiated must never be continued if the child does not follow it.

7. Once normal reactions have been obtained, the therapist must aim at making them reliable (occurring automatically when they are activated), immediate (happening instantly), and adequate in range and pattern (in keeping with the strength of stimulation and the requirements of the situation).

Techniques of Proprioceptive and Tactile Stimulation

In ataxic children and some children of the athetoid group in whom hypotonia and impaired reciprocal innervation make postural control, fixation and the guidance of movements difficult, techniques are used to increase postural tone and regulate the interplay of agonists, antagonists and synergists. They are also used in addition to techniques of inhibition and facilitation in some spastic and athetoid children in whom postural tone is too low in the absence of abnormal reflex activity and who then seem to be "weak." The rationale of these techniques of proprioceptive and tactile simulation is probably similar to that underlying the techniques of "maximal resistance" and "rhythmical stabilization" used by Kabat (1959, 1948) and Knott (1952). These are recruiting and summation by carefully applied and repetitive tactile and proprioceptive stimulation.

The techniques are used when the following are present:

1. There is apparent or real weakness of muscle groups after hypertonus (spasticity) or intermittent spasms are reduced or completely inhibited in treatment.

2. There is sensory deficit with "weakness" of muscles due to sensory input.

3. There is no actual sensory deficit but the child does not know *how* to move because of lack of previous sensorimotor experience or because of apraxia.

In applying these techniques it is essential to avoid causing a return of spasticity or spasms by stimulating abnormal postural reflex activity. This can be done by the following methods:

1. Always combining the techniques with reflex-inhibiting patterns, in order to avoid widespread reactions, and to "shunt" the sensory input into desired channels and away from abnormal reflex patterns.

2. Stimulating carefully and only when postural tone is low. One has to stop immediately when it becomes abnormally high. In fact, techniques of stimulation are used in alternation with inhibitory techniques. Abnormal reactions have to be anticipated, if possible, and have to be stopped before they gain momentum.

3. Aiming at localized responses and avoiding widespread associated reactions.

The main techniques of stimulation are as follows:

1. Weight-bearing, pressure, resistance.

2. Placing and holding (both automatic and voluntary).
3. Tapping.

These techniques can and have to be used in combination or singly, dependent upon the needs of the child. They can be used alternately or simultaneously.

WEIGHT-BEARING WITH OR WITHOUT PRESSURE AND RESISTANCE. Static postures must not be used, especially not in the spastic child. Here intrinsic automatic movements of adjustment of trunk and limbs have to be obtained by constant weight transfer of fairly large ranges, sideways, forward, backward, and diagonally. This has to be done in all possible positions—in supine, prone, sitting, standing, and walking. In the athetoid and ataxic patient the same techniques are used but in a more static manner; movements of weight transfer must be done slowly and within a small range. A combination of weight-bearing, pressure and resistance can be used in all cases to obtain a sustained postural tone for the maintenance of posture against gravity and the control of involuntary movements.

PLACING. This is a term used to describe normal man's ability to arrest a movement at any stage, automatically or voluntarily. This can be demonstrated by moving a limb passively and with minimal support of its weight, and leaving it in various positions. The limb will then stay automatically for a moment. It feels light as the person controls the moving limb actively and automatically throughout the range of movement. Placing may, therefore, be defined as the automatic adaptation of muscles to changes of posture; this is part and parcel of the normal postural reflex mechanism. This normal reaction to placing is the prerequisite for the smooth control of every stage of a voluntary movement.

In holding, the patient's body and limbs are placed in various positions and he is to hold and control them unaided in a great variety of functional patterns and at various stages and ranges of a movement.

TAPPING. This is frequently used in combination with placing. It serves the following purposes:

1. To increase postural tone for the maintenance of a posture (pressure tapping) (Fig. 3-85).

2. To activate "weak" muscle groups, which cannot contract as a result of reciprocal inhibition by spastic antagonists (inhibitory tapping) (Fig. 3-86).

3. To obtain proper grading of reciprocal innervation and to stimulate balance reactions (alternating tapping) (Fig. 3-87).

4. To activate synergic patterns of muscle function by stimulating the specific group of muscles responsible for that action with a sweeping stroke in the direction of the desired movement (sweep tapping) (Fig. 3-88).

GENERAL MANAGEMENT

The Link-up of Physical Therapy With Occupational and Speech Therapy

The aim of all those concerned with the child who has cerebral palsy is to make him functionally as independent as possible and to develop the child's potentialities to the utmost. If this is to be achieved, it must be through a combined effort. In cerebral palsy, more than in any other condition, one has always to treat the whole child and no artificial division can be made among those responsible for the treatment and management. A united team must, therefore, have the same fundamental approach and the same concept of treatment in order to plan and execute an integrated and well-coordinated treatment program. This must include the management of the child in his home, in school, or in any community, such as a hospital for the mentally subnormal. In treatment, the two guiding considerations common to all therapists must be (1) the child's abnormal patterns of coordination, and (2) the child's arrested or retarded development.

For the speech therapist, of great importance is the sequence of development of oral patterns and its delay and abnormal deviation in the child with cerebral palsy. Breathing and feeding patterns and the establishment of a proper sequence of biting, chewing and swallowing are important precursors of phonation, beginning with vowels, then consonants, through babbling towards articulation and speech development proper. The necessity of close collaboration of physiotherapy with speech therapy is borne out by the well-known fact that children with cerebral palsy who have good head control do not usually have any speech defect. There seems to be a close relationship between the acquisition of head, trunk, and arm control and oral development.

There is also a well-known close relationship between head control and dribbling. Thus, the speech therapist, in attending to the development of articulation and speech, must see first to the forerunners of formal speech. She has to take into account factors common to physiotherapy and her own special aims. She must realize that if she goes directly for articulation, speech, and the enlargement of vocabulary, neglecting the basic principles of the common approach, she may achieve this aim to some extent. She will, however, do so by counteracting any possible progress the child may make in general physiotherapy.

For the occupational therapist the development of grasp and release, eye-hand coordination, handedness, perception, and self-help are the most important aspects of treatment. This again will overlap with developmental factors, such as head, trunk, and arm control, and the emancipation of arms and hands from the necessity of maintaining balance and support. She will have to work closely with the physiotherapist to set the child's arms free for manipulation of his own body and surrounding space.

Perceptual and spatial orientation training is not only the task of the occupational therapist but is the aspect common to all concerned with the child. This aim is furthered by the close handling of the child by the physiotherapist, by the establishment of correct oral behavior by the speech therapist, and by the occupational therapist's direct concern for the child's manipulation of his own body and objects. Obviously the occupational therapist will use special techniques of sensory and perceptory training in addition, such as the handling of objects, play with sand and materials, and other special techniques of perceptory training. Moreover, she is an important connecting link between the treatment center and the home, advising and guiding parents, teachers, and nurses.

For all those concerned with the child, it is important to appreciate that in normal child development certain abilities appear simultaneously or closely together. For instance, certain patterns appearing at some stage will give the child head and trunk control which are important both for speech and manipulation. Head control, for instance, influences feeding, phonation, and articulation as well as manipulation. The development of symmetry of motor behavior—beginning around the fourth month with the disappearance of the last vestiges of an asymmetrical tonic neck reflex response—goes together with better head control and hand-eye coordination. It enables the child to bring his hands together. Rotation within the body axis—appearing from the sixth or seventh month—enables the child to use one hand for support while reaching out with the other. Progression in any manner, whether first by rolling over, then by creeping and crawling, and later in sitting and walking, will give the child the chance to explore his environment and to relate his own body to surrounding space.

The Importance of Play

The normal child plays with his hands and his body. Mouthing of his hands and of objects serves to develop his body percept and at the same time prepare the child for self-help. By playing with his lips and tongue he prepares for vocalizing and speech. Play therapy is an important adjunct of physical, occupational and speech therapy. It is an important way of coordinating treatment with the management of the child at home or in a nursery or hospital. The normal child babbles, makes sounds, and later speaks while playing. He is never silent, talking to himself when he plays. Movement stimulates vocalizing and vice versa.

A normal child needs many ways of playing. He also needs activity to no apparent purpose, moving, vocalizing, exploring, and thus finding out by trial and error the motor patterns which he will later on need for complex and purposive skills. Before he is able to feed himself, to dress and undress, wash and bathe himself, he must have control of his head, trunk, and limbs, and balance in all positions. He acquires these abilities first by cooperating when being handled by his mother or nurse. The child with cerebral palsy must go through these same preparatory steps. Play therapy, alone or in groups, in the setting of a hospital or training center,

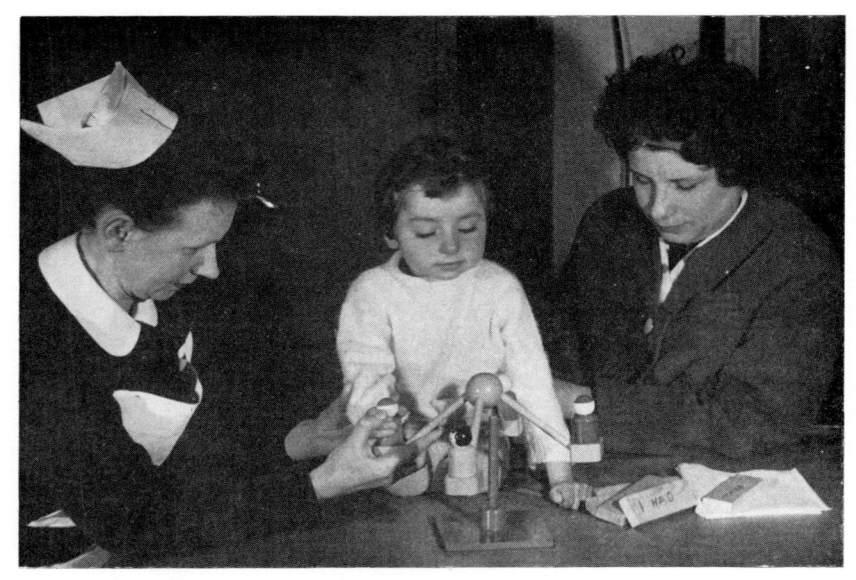

176 *Physical Therapy Services in the Developmental Disabilities*

Figure 3-96. Harperbury Hospital. Play therapy.

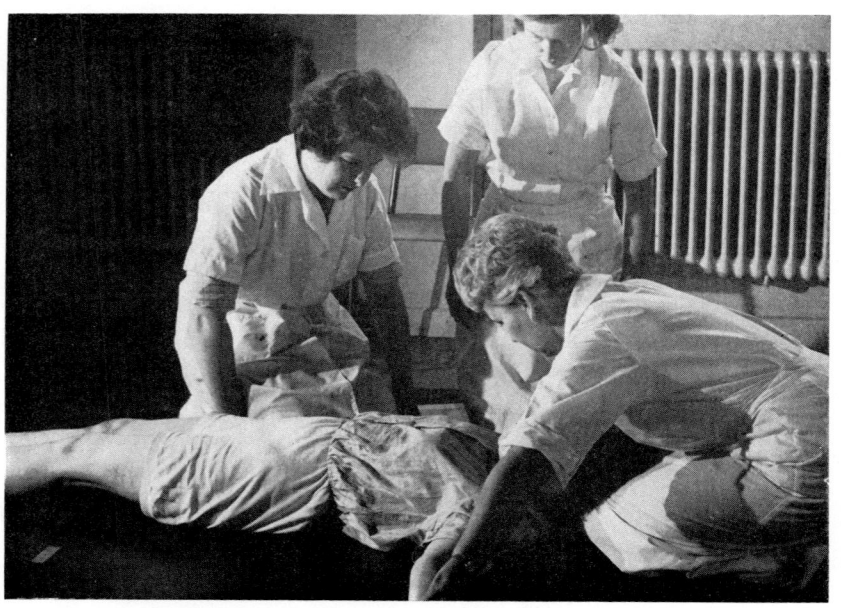

Figure 3-97. Harperbury Hospital. Instruction of therapists.

in school or nursery, can give the child this possibility if everybody concerned with the child works to that end and if parents, teachers, and nurses are properly advised and guided by the therapists. (Fig. 3-96, 3-97, 3-98).

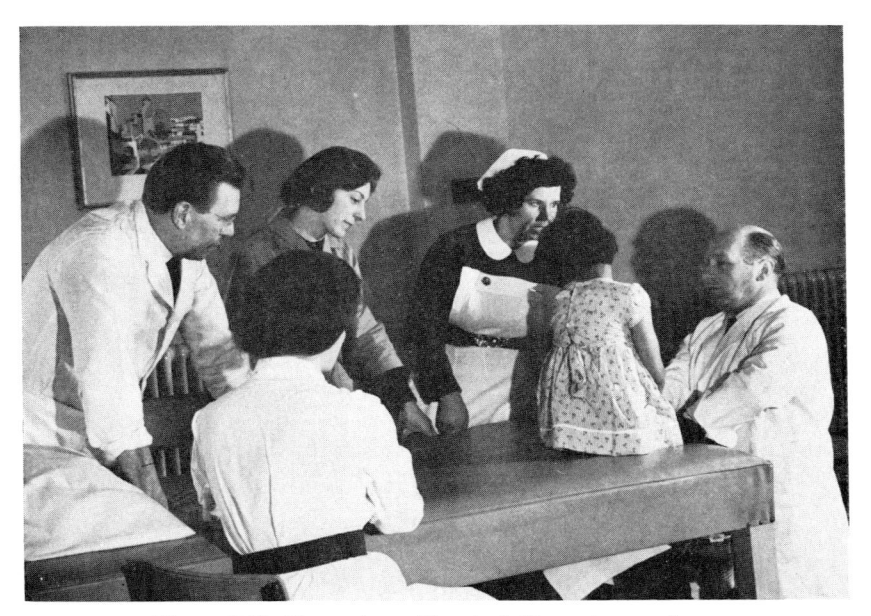

Figure 3-98. Harperbury Hospital. Nurse instructions.

The Management of the Child Outside Treatment Sessions

The management of the child at home or in a nursery or hospital for the mentally subnormal is a most essential aspect of the total treatment program. Even if a child spends a whole morning all through the week in the treatment center, he will still be most of the time in his home or in a hospital ward. This aspect is even more important if a child attends an outpatient center twice or three times a week only.

By its very definition cerebral palsy is a condition existing from earliest childhood, at a time when the child's brain is still immature and when he is totally dependent. He develops his physical and mental abilities through close contact with his mother. In the child with cerebral palsy with normal or subnormal intelligence, this mother-child relationship is severely disturbed. Without guidance by the therapist, the mother will often be helpless and unable to guide the child to develop to the utmost his physical and mental potential. With the best will in the world, the mother may prove to be a hindrance rather than a help to the child.

This early period is a time during which the mother is particularly in need of advice and guidance (Finnie 1968). A great deal of trouble and anxiety can be avoided, if at this stage the mother is made an active member of a treatment program. She must be advised on how to handle the child, what positions to avoid, how to carry, feed, dress and bathe him. Most important, the disturbed interplay of mother and child must be restored with full appreciation of the child's disabilities. She must learn again to experiment, to give help where it is needed but only to the extent that the child's expanding abilities require. All this must be done in a way which will support treatment rather than counteract it.

She must be taught to speak to the child in terms appropriate to his age, rather than in baby language. As the child is often more or less immobile, things of interest should be brought to him. He should not be nursed in a cot or propped up in a chair or divan, but should be on a mat on the floor for at least part of the day. His mother should play with his body and limbs, should bring his hands in contact with his mouth, lips, tongue, and feet, and let him play with his hands together. The child should be stimulated, and experiences in keeping with his age should be brought to him. Later on, in play form, he should handle things of variety while they are being named. He should try to find things hidden in a sand pit, and name them before he sees them. It is a good thing to let him mix with other children of his age or perhaps slightly younger. All this may help to keep the child's mentality in step with his true potential.

In a hospital for the mentally subnormal the children should be able to form special bonds with a small but constant circle of nurses who must be specially advised by the therapists in the daily handling of the children and trained on the same lines as the mother. Constancy of nursing care of a small group of children by any one particular nurse is desirable. The cot system of nursing should be abandoned. If placed on a mat on the floor, the child will be able to move harmlessly within his potential ability. Usually, the worst possible position for the cerebral-palsied is on his back. Maximal extensor hypertonus makes these children utterly helpless in this position. Most children are far better off if nursed in prone-lying, if necessary with the upper chest over a bolster to keep the head free.

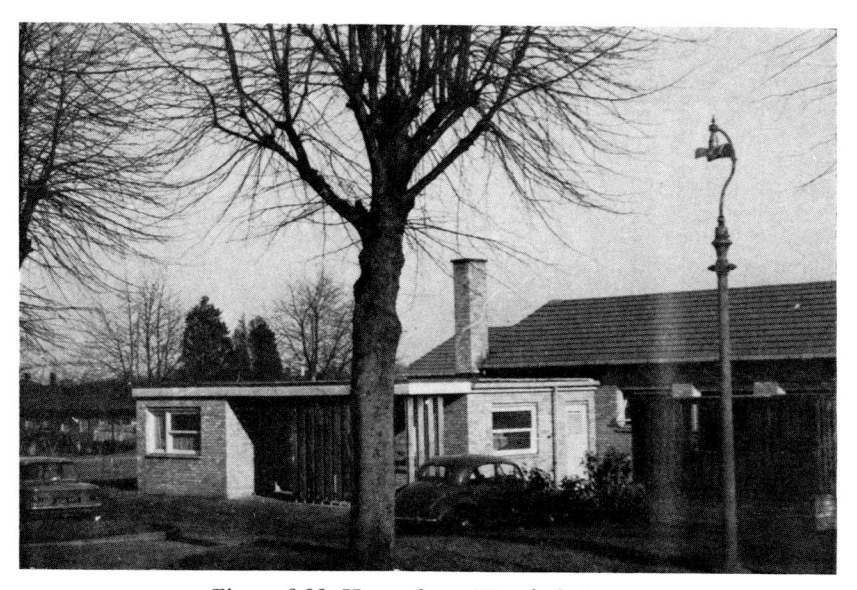

Figure 3-99. Harperbury Hospital. C.P.U.

The speech therapist and occupational therapist should advise the nurses, and be present at mealtimes, supervising the feeding habits of the children. The day should be organized, the children occupied; their minds must not be allowed to get dulled.

Mothers and nurses should persist in training these children in bladder and bowel control. This can be achieved in many more children than has been done, even in children with more severe degrees of mental subnormality. It will, however, take very much longer than with normal children.

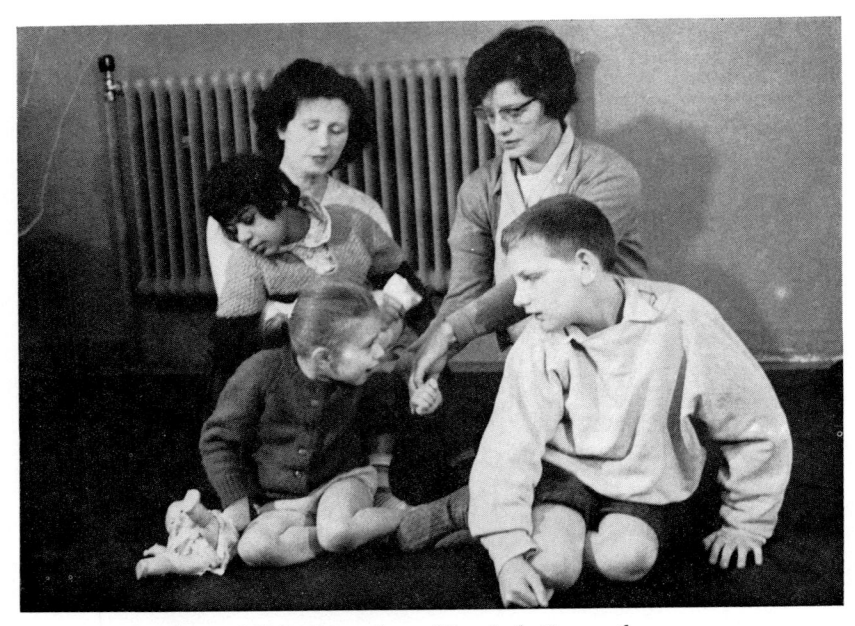

Figure 3-100. Harperbury Hospital. Group therapy.

Wards should not be too large and should cater for about 20 children at most. They should be well-staffed and allow for individual attention to the needs of the individual child. Contact with the outside world, outings, shopping excursions, etc., will tell the child more than picture books. It would be desirable to allow at least some of these children to meet normal children of their age—if necessary their mental age—if the discrepancy be not too great. This has proved of great value in enlarging a child's vocabulary and language facility. Commitment to a hospital for the mentally subnormal must not mean the end of the road, but should mean the beginning of an active program of treatment and management aimed at improving the child's physical condition and maintaining his mentality and personality to the utmost of his potentiality.

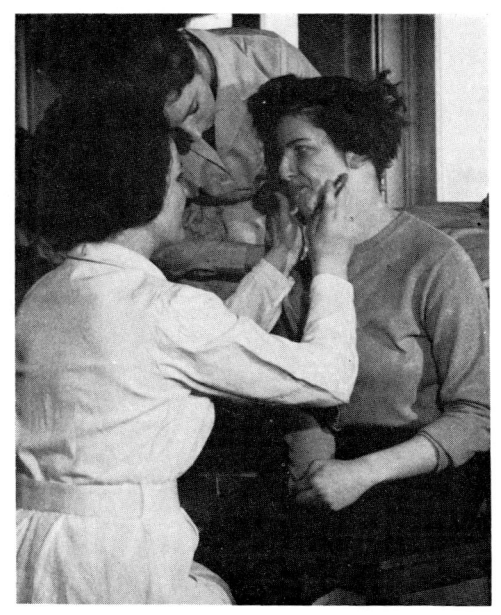

Figure 3-101. Harperbury Hospital. Cosmetic session.

BIBLIOGRAPHY

Abercrombie, M.L.J.: Perception and eye movements; some speculations on disorders in cerebral palsy. *Cerb Palsy Bull,* 2:142-148, 1960.

Abercrombie, M.L.J.: Eye movements, perception and learning. In Smith, V.H. (Ed.): *Visual Disorders in Cerebral Palsy.* London, Heinemann, 1963, pp. 52-58.

Abercrombie, M.L.J.: *Perceptual Visuomotor Disorders in Cerebral Palsy.* The Spastics Society, Medical Education Unit. London, Heinemann, 1964.

André-Thomas, Chesni, Y., and Saint-Ann Dargassies, S.: *The Neurological Examination of the Infant.* Little Club Clinics in Developmental Medicine No. 1. The Spastics Society. London, Heinemann, 1960.

André-Thomas, Chesni, Y., and Saint-Ann Dargassies, S.: *Etudes Neurologiques sur le Noveau-Ne et le jeuns Nourrisson.* Paris, Masson and Cie, 1952.

Asher, P., and Schonell, F.E.: A survey of 400 cases of cerebral palsy in childhood. *Arch Dis Child,* 25:360, 1950.

Bender, L.: A visual motor gestalt test and its clinical use. *Amer Orthopsych Ass Res Monog No. 3*, New York, 1938.

Bobath, B. *Abnormal Postural Reflex Activity Caused by Brain Lesions*. London, Heinemann, 1965.

Bobath, K.: *The Motor Deficit in Patients with Cerebral Palsy*. The Spastics Society, Medical Education and Information Unit. London, Heinemann, 1966.

Bobath, K.: The Prevention of Mental Retardation in Patients with Cerebral Palsy. Paper read at the 5th International Congress of Child Psych. Scheveningen, 1962.

Bobath, K.: The neuropathology of cerebral palsy and its importance in treatment and diagnosis. *Cereb Palsy Bull, 1*:8, pp. 13-33, 1959.

Bobath, B., and Bobath, K.: The facilitation of normal postural reactions and movements in the treatment of cerebral palsy. *Physiotherapy*, August, 1964a.

Bobath, B., and Bobath, K.: Grundgedanken zur Behandlung der Zerebralen Kinderlaehmung. Beitr Orthop Trauma, Heft 3, pp. 1-28, 1964b.

Bobath, B., and Bobath, K.: An analysis of the development of standing and walking patterns in patients with cerebral palsy. *Physiotherapy*, June, 1962.

Bobath, B., and Bobath, K.: The diagnosis of cerebral palsy in infancy. *Arch Dis Child, 31*:159, 1956.

Bobath, B., and Finnie, N.: Reeducation of movement patterns for everyday life in the treatment of cerebral palsy. *Occup Therapy*, pp. 21-23, June, 1958.

Brandt, S., and Westergaard-Nielsen, V.: Etiological factors in cerebral palsy and their correlation with various clinical entities. *Danish Med Bull. 5*:47, 1958.

Buehler, Ch.: Kleinkindertests. Leipzig, p. 110, 1932.

Buehler, Ch.: Inventar der Verhaltungsweisen des ersten Lebensjahres, Jena, 1927.

Clarke, A.M., and Clarke, A.D.B.: *Mental Deficiency; the Changing Outlook*. London, Methuen, 1958, pp. 236-239.

Doll, E.A.: The psychological significance of cerebral birth lesions. *Amer J Psychol, 45*:444-452, 1933.

Dunsdon, M.I.: *The Educability of Cerebral Palsied Children*. London, Newnes, 1952.

Fay, T.: The use of pathological and unlocking reflexes in the rehabilitation of spastics. *Amer J Phys Med, 33*:347-352, 1954.

Finnie, Nancie: *Handling the Young Cerebral Palsied Child at Home*. London, Heinemann, 1968.

Fisch, L.: Deafness in cerebral palsied school children. *Lancet, 2*:370, 1955.

Floyer, E.B.: *A Psychological Study of a City's Cerebral Palsied Children*. Brit. Counc. Welf. Spastics. Manchester, 1955.

Fulton, J.F.: *Physiology of the Nervous System.* New York, Oxford U. P., 1951, pp 105-134.

Gesell, A., and Amatruda, G.S.: *Developmental Diagnosis.* 2nd ed. London, Harper, 1947.

Goldstein, K.: *Language and Language Disturbances.* New York, Grune, 1948.

Goldstein, K.: *The Organism.* New York, American Book Co., 1939.

Goody, W., and McKissock, W.: *Lancet, 1:*481, 1951.

Guibor, G.P.: Some eye defects seen in cerebral palsy with some statistics. *Amer J Phys Med, 32:*342, 1953.

Illingworth, R.S.: *The Development of the Infant and Young Child, Normal and Abnormal.* London, E. and S. Livingstone, 1960.

Illingworth, R.S.: *Recent Advances in Cerebral Palsy.* London, Churchill, 1958.

Ingram, T.T.S.: *Pediatric Aspects of Cerebral Palsy.* Edinburgh, E. and S. Livingstone, 1964.

Ingram, T.T.S.: A study of cerebral palsy in the childhood population of Edinburgh. *Arch Dis Child, 30:*85, 1955a.

Ingram, T.T.S.: The early manifestations and course of diplegia in childhood. *Arch Dis Child, 30:*244, 1955b.

Jackson, J. Hughlings: *Selected Writings of John Hughlings Jackson.* Taylor, James (Ed.). London, Staples Press, 1958, Vol. 2, p. 29.

Jones, Blundell A.: Dislocation of the hip in asymmetrical spasticity of the thigh adductors. *Cereb Palsy Bull, 3:*190, 1961.

Kabat, H., and Knott, M.: Principles of neuromuscular reeducation. *Phys Ther Rev, 28:*107, 1948.

Kabat, H.: Athetosis: Neuromuscular dysfunction and treatment. *Arch Phys Med, 40:*7, 1959.

Kirman, B.H.: Epilepsy and cerebral palsy. *Arch Dis Child, 31:*1-7, 1956.

Knott, M.: Specialized neuromuscular technics in treatment of cerebral palsy. *Phys Ther Rev, 32:*73, 1952.

Kong, E.: Die Fruehdiagnose der zerebralen Laehmung. In Rossi, E. (Ed.): *Diagnose & Therapy zerebraler Laehmungen in Kindesalter.* Karger, Basel, 1962.

Kong, E.: Very early treatment of cerebral palsy. *Develop Med Child Neurol, 8:*198-202, 1966.

Little Club, The: Memorandum on terminology and classification of cerebral palsy. *Cereb Palsy Bull, 1:*27, 1959.

Luria, A.R., and Yudowich, F.: *Speech and the Development of Mental Processes in the Child.* London, Staples Press, 1959.

MacKeith, R.: The primary walking response and its facilitation by passive extension of the head. *Acta Paediat Lat, 17:*710, 1964.

Magnus, R.: Some results of studies in the physiology of posture. *Lancet, 2:* 531-535, 585, 1926.

Magnus, R.: *Koerperstellung*. Berlin, Springer, 1924.

Magoun, H.W., and Rhines: *Spasticity. The Stretch Reflex and Extrapyramidal Systems*. Springfield, Thomas, 1947.

McGraw, M.: *The Neuromuscular Maturation of the Human Infant*. New York, Columbia, 1943.

Mein, R.: Use of the Peabody Picture Vocabulary Test with severely subnormal patients. *Amer J Ment Defic, 67:*2, September, 1962.

Mein, R.: A study of the oral vocabularies of severely subnormal patients. *J Ment Defic Res, 5:*1, June, 1961.

Mein, R., and O'Connor, N.: A study of oral vocabularies of severely subnormal patients. *J Ment Defic Res, 4:*2, 130-143, 1960.

Milani-Comparetti, A.: Spasticity versus patterned postural and motor behavior of spastics. *Europa Medicophysica, 1:*3, September, 1965a.

Milani-Comparetti, A.: La Natura del Diffeto Motorio Nella Paralisi cerebrale infantile. *Infanzia Anormale Fasc 64,* Luglio, Agosto, 1965b.

Milani-Comparetti, A.: Lo Sviluppo Motorio Infantile Normale e Patologico. *Infanzia Anormale 57,* Marzo-Aprile, pp 207-288, 1964.

Paine, R.S.: Neurologic examination of infants and children, *Pediat Clin N Amer, 17:*3, August, 1960.

Paine, R.S.: The evolution of infantile postural reflexes in the presence of chronic brain syndromes. *Develop Med Child Neurol, 6:*4, 1964.

Peiper, A.: *Die Eigenart der Kindlichen Hirntaetigkeit*. VEB. Leipzig, Georg Thieme, 1961.

Phelps, W.M.: Bracing for cerebral palsy. *Crippled Child, 27:*10, February, 1950.

Phelps, W.M.: New Jersey Cerebral Palsy Survey. Sth Med. Rec. 1955.

Polani, P.E.: The natural history of choreo-athetoid cerebral palsy. Guy Hosp Rep, *32:*1959.

Prechtl, H., and Beintema, D.: The Neurological Examination of the Fullterm Newborn Infant. Little Club Clinics in Developmental Medicine, No. 12. The Spastics Society, London, Heinemann, 1964.

Purdon, Martin: Verbal communication, 1961.

Rademaker, G.G.J.: *Reactions Labyrinthiques et Equilibre*. Paris, Masson and Cie, 1935.

Rademaker, G.G.J.: *Das Stehen*. Berlin, Springer, 1931.

Riddoch, G., and Buzzard, E.F.: Reflex movements and postural reactions in quadriplegia and hemiplegia with special reference to those of the upper limb. *Brain, 44:*397, 1921.

Rushforth, G.: Spasticity and rigidity. An experimental study and review. *J Neurol Neurosurg Psychiat, 23:*99, 1960.

Rushforth, G.: Muscle tone and muscle spindle in clinical neurology. In Williams, D. (Ed.): *Modern Trends in Neurology*. No. 3. London, Butterworths, 1962.

Russell, Ritchie W.: The physiology of memory. *Proc Roy Soc Med Sect Neurol, 51*:9, January, 1958.

Schaltenbrand, G.: The development of human motility and motor disturbances. *Arch Neurol Psych, 18:* 1927.

Schaltenbrand, G.: Ueber die Entwicklung des menschlichen Aufstehens und dessen Stoerungen bei Nervenkrankheiten. *Deutsch Z Nervenheilk, 89*:82, 1926.

Schaltenbrand, G.: Normale Bewgungs-und Lagereaktionen bei Kindern. *Deutsch Z Nervenheilk, 87*:23, 1925.

Schilder, P.: *Brain and Personality*. New York, 1931.

Schonell, F.E.: *Educating Spastic Children*. Edinburgh, Boyd and Oliver, 1956.

Shapiro, A., and Bobath, K.: The Relationship of Intelligence to Cerebral Palsy. II Congress of Child Psychiatry, Rome. Assissi, Tipografia Porziuncola, 1963.

Sharrard, W.J.W.: Danger of dislocation of the hip in asymmetrical spasticity of the thigh adductors. *Cereb Palsy Bull, 3*:72, 1961.

Sherrington, C.S.: *Selected Writings*. Brown, Denny (Ed.). London, Harnish Hamilton, 1939.

Sherrington, C.S.: *The Integrative Action of the Nervous System*. New York, Cambridge U. P., 1947.

Sherrington, C.S.: On reciprocal innervation of antagonistic muscles. *Proc Roy Soc, 337*-349, 1907.

Sherrington, C.S.: Reflex inhibitions as a factor in the co-ordination of movements and posture. *Quart J Exp Physiol, 6*:251, 1913.

Tardieu, G.: Danger of dislocation of the hip in asymmetrical spasticity of the thigh adductors. *Cereb Palsy Bull, 3*:71, 1961.

Tizard, J.P.M.: The future of infantile hemiplegics. *Proc Roy Soc Med, 46:* 637, 1953.

Vassella, F., and Karlsson, B.: Asymmetric tonic neck reflex. *Develop Med Child Neurol, 4*:363, 1962.

Walshe, F.M.R.: On certain tonic or postural reflexes in hemiplegia with special reference to the so-called associated movements. *Brain, 46*:2, 1923.

Walshe, F.M.R., and Wilson, S.A.K.: The phenomenon of tonic innervation and its relation to motor apraxia. *Brain, 37*:199, 1914/15.

Weisz, St.: Studies in equilibrium reactions. *J Nerv Ment Dis, 88*:153, 1938.

Wilson, S.A.K.: The croonian lectures on some disorders of motility and muscle tone with special reference to the corpus striatum. *Lancet, 2*:169, 1925.

Woods, G.E.: *Cerebral Palsy in Childhood*. Bristol, John Wright and Sons, Ltd., 1957.

Yannet, H.: The etiology of congenital cerebral palsy. *J Paediat, 24*:38, 1944.

Zador, J.: *Les Reactions d'Equilibre*. chez l'Homme. Paris, Masson, 1938.

Zapella, E.M., and Foley, J.: The placing and supporting reaction in cerebral palsy. *J Ment Defic Res, 8*:17, 1964.

Chapter Four

A SENSORIMOTOR APPROACH TO TREATMENT

Shirley A. Stockmeyer

BASIC CONCEPTS
The Contribution of Physical Therapy Treatment to the Total Development of the Child

The treatment and care of the multiply handicapped child should be directed toward the development of his full potential in all three areas of learning—motor, cognitive, and affective. It is a long-range goal that the child be able to respond appropriately and effectively in his movements, his intellectual functions, and in his attitudes and feelings. Although physical therapists might be primarily concerned with the motor aspects of behavior, seldom does learning take place in one domain at a time. Schilder (1964) points out that "In every stage of development, the motor reactions are in close connection with general psychic attitudes. It is well to bear this in mind even if one talks about the grasp reflex and the Moro reflex."

Many responses which are fully manifest in the early stages of development have a protective or avoidance role to play in the behavior of the organism. Growth does not take place unless the individual can progress from a stage of protective avoidance or withdrawal to a stage of extending toward the environment and exploring it during continued contact. Intellectual, emotional, and motor development can take place only if there is basic stability which modifies reactions to danger. The combination of responsiveness plus stability enables the child to "risk" himself in new experiences, to try new "postures," to learn their limitations and uses, and to make them a part of his expanding resources.

This concept applies to the total functioning of the child. A deficit in just one form of behavior may influence all other forms. It is quite possible that the child who needs motor stability is also psychologically in need of stability, and that the sensory influences used to change one area of response may influence the other area. Consider the child who is sluggish in his general motor performance and has difficulty initiating movement: his need for controlled and purposeful arousal may be demonstrated in his physical and mental functions. His lack of movement-generated impulses may compound problems of diminished central facilitation.

The therapeutic situation is structured to provide for the learning of motor skills, but should also be planned to assist in the development of other aspects of behavior, especially in the affective area. How regretful it is to see a child who has gained some elementary motor ability through treatment but who has also learned to dislike the therapeutic situation as well as his own physical being because he has never experienced movement which is both effective and easy. The therapist must know how to structure the treatment sessions so that there is positive reinforcement of specifically desirable behavior. This planning involves care and judgement in the selection of therapeutic tasks to insure some successes which are spontaneous and pleasing to the child.

Duality of Sensorimotor Functions as a Basis for a Therapeutic Approach

The progress of the child toward higher levels of maturity in motor control may be brought about by the blending and interaction of two fundamental reaction systems. The sensorimotor mechanisms which provide the organism with a means of changing position and executing movements free of weight-bearing represent one system, and the sensorimotor mechanisms which enable him to maintain contact and body posture are involved in the second system. Working together, first in weight-bearing activities and then in non-weight-bearing activities, these two systems bring the individual to a level of fine manipulative and articulative skills. Experimental evidence for a new concept of motor control with two systems, one for axial and proximal limb musculature, the other for distal musculature, has been presented by Kuypers (1963). These systems are not the same as those of the classical pyramidal and extrapyramidal divisions, a point which has been made by Buchwald (1967) in her comparison and discussion of the concepts of motor systems.

Of the two reaction systems with which this treatment approach is concerned, one system can be described as the dynamic or phasic component which gives the individual the mobility necessary to move in the environment or to act upon the environment. Mobility responses are characterized by quick initiation, full range of movement, and heightened speed. The other system is the static or tonic component which contributes the stability necessary to maintain position or prevent overreaction. It is essential to the understanding of the role of these two systems in treatment to think of stabilization as being regulatory or controlling in nature in addition to providing a means of maintaining position or posture.

Just as there are dual functions related to response, there are dual functions related to stimuli. The degree to which a receptor adapts to a stimulus is a determinant of its involvement in tonic or phasic reflexes (Eldred 1967a). For each sensory modality which might be used therapeutically to bring about a phasic or tonic response, two different qualities of stimuli, one of a continuous or maintained nature, the other of an intermittent or changing nature, can be described. The maintained stimulus would be used with slowly adapting receptors related to tonic motor functions. The single or changing stimulus would be used with the rapidly adapting receptors related to phasic functions.

The Influence of Sensory Factors in Total Development

The nature of the responses of the child and how they develop depend on many factors including the manner in which his nervous system reacts to incoming stimuli in a given situation. It is necessary to consider therapeutic procedures as a part of these environmental stimuli, since the child is stimulated by handling and positioning and provides self-generated sensory input as he moves in response to treatment.

All the avenues by which therapeutic procedures can exert an influence are through sensory channels. Treatment to bring about change in motor ability has a motor activity as its goal but must ultimately be concerned with the normalcy of the sensory feedback from that motor activity as well as the sensory influence of specific therapeutic procedures. In regard to sensory input, there are a number of points of importance to the therapist who is attempting to bring about a change in response. The therapist must know that the environment, the attention to the task, and the state of the central nervous system can influence the transmission of sensory impulses. He must understand the role which various motor responses can play in the regulation of sensory input. He must be able to recognize the possible nature of the feedback from a specific response and judge whether this feedback could facilitate a desirable subsequent response. Finally, the therapist must consider his own role in treatment to be something more than one in which he applies a procedure.

Influences on the Transmission of Sensory Impulses

Of the information generated in the sensory receptors, only part reaches the higher levels of the central nervous system. Livingston (1959) has reviewed pertinent research on the subject of control exerted by the central nervous system on sensory receptors and sensory transmission. He notes that a reduction or inhibition of sensory information can result from tonic central nervous system influence on points as remote as peripheral receptors.

The influence of the environment and of the patient's attention on sensory input are of particular importance to the therapist because they can be manipulated in the treatment situation. Livingston (1959) points out that ". . . activity along sensory pathways appears to be modifiable to some extent according to an animal's environmental experience and according to its overtly expressed direction of attention, the interference with sensory transmission appears to be regulatory and to constitute a goal-seeking physiological mechanism." Two questions arise which are related to treatment. In central nervous system disorders, is there a change in the regulatory tonic inhibition of sensory transmission so that sensory input has too great an influence or a reduced influence on centers which effect responses? Can therapeutic measures provide enough of the appropriate type of stimuli and direct attention and effort away from or toward the activity in such a manner as to alter the influence of sensory input? Working hypotheses derived from these questions need to be developed for use in the treatment situation.

The Role of Certain Motor Responses in the Regulation of Sensory Input

The muscles around the eyes, mouth and nose, the tensor muscles of the ear, the flexor muscles of the hands, and the physiological flexors of the feet play a distinct role in the regulation of sensory input. The distance receptors, the eyes, ears, and nose (olfactory bulb), and the specific receptors in the distal parts of the extremities, are the sensory "explorers" of the environment. Also, it is conceivable to think of the taste buds as being the distance receptors for the digestive system. The sensory input to these receptors following the initial stimulus can be regulated to some extent by motor activities.

Peiper (1963) has described this motor-sensory relationship in the infant. "The sensory reactions, from which the facial expressions have developed, originally decrease or improve the perceptive ability of the sensory organs of the face by narrowing the openings of the sensory organs through the circular muscles or by enlarging them through the radiating muscles." Peiper (1963) describes what he calls the "spreading reaction," a phenomena in which a reaction may spread from a stimulated to a nonstimulated organ so that the hands and possibly the feet, acting as sensory organs, may be involved in a receptive or defensive response.

Peiper also notes that the reception of a sensory organ may be changed by a non-specific as well as a specific stimulus. With many brain-damaged children we are dealing with the problem of an immature central nervous system, arrested or delayed in development because of the influence of damaged areas. It may be fruitful in developing principles for management and treatment to consider that some of these children have not progressed in the modification of their receptive and defensive responses nor in the integration and inhibition of "spreading reactions."

The Nature of Feedback from a Specific Response

Any active somatic motor response will generate sensory input which can further affect the motor mechanism involved. Some forms of feedback are involved in servomechanisms in which they supply the information necessary for adjustments in different dimensions of the motor response. Stimuli generated by movement do not always facilitate the active muscles, but rather may facilitate the antagonists. There are at least three factors which determine the influence of feedback from active movement—namely, the classification of the muscle, the duration of the contraction, and the degree of resistance, stretch or joint approximation involved. Rood (1962) has described the stimulus-response relationship in active motor functions and has developed exercise principles based in part on this relationship.

Since the Rood treatment approach is largely based on the use of physiological mechanisms, muscles are classified according to the physiological sensorimotor system, tonic or phasic, to which they belong. Comparing the anatomical and physiological classifications, the tonic muscle group includes deep extensor muscles acting on one joint, limb adductors and external rotators, and shoulder-girdle adductors and downward rotators. The phasic group includes all physiological flexors, internal rotators, limb adductors, shoulder-girdle abductors and upward rotators, and superficial extensors crossing more than one joint. The physiological classification is based on such characteristics as speed of contraction time, receptor concentration and feedback influence, and primary level of central activation.

It appears that motor neurons of phasic muscles are usually facilitated and their antagonists inhibited by resistance as well as stretch applied to the agonist. If resistance to a phasic muscle is very heavy but brief it may leave the muscle inhibited. Possibly through the influence of their Golgi tendon organs, phasic muscle motor neurons can be inhibited in a nonresisted contraction of that muscle, necessitating continued supraspinal facilitation in the form of increased voluntary effort if the contraction is to continue. Motor neurons of tonic muscles are thought to be facilitated and their antagonists inhibited by moderate resistance and stretch applied to the tonic muscle. When high levels of resistance are given to tonic muscles it appears that antagonistic flexors are facilitated for cocontraction. Stretch of tonic muscles well into the range seems to be inhibitory to these tonic muscles and facilitatory to antagonistic flexors. The flexor facilitation which occurs with greater resistance or stretch to tonic extensors may be a result of the influence of secondary afferent receptors of the muscle spindle which are part of a multisynaptic flexion reflex regardless of the muscle in which they lie.

The Role of the Therapist in Using Sensory Input Therapeutically

The relationship between therapist and patient is a continuous cycle. The interaction occurs rapidly enough to require that the therapist be able to monitor and interpret what he senses about the patient's response, act upon the patient with that information, and at the same time be receiving more sensory information about the patient from his own visual, tactile and proprioceptive mechanisms (Fig. 4-1).

The therapist must learn a motor strategy which enables him to act upon and interact with the patient with the use of selected types of sensory information. The development of such a strategy can be accomplished only if there is an integration of the sensorimotor and cognitive skills of the therapist.

GENERAL TREATMENT PROCEDURES

Several guiding ideas are proposed to aid in determining the treatment program of the child with a central nervous system deficit. Since part of the problem lies in an immaturity of the sensorimotor mechanism, it is essential that the order in which treatment activities are carried out be consistent with the se-

A Sensorimotor Approach to Treatment

THERAPIST

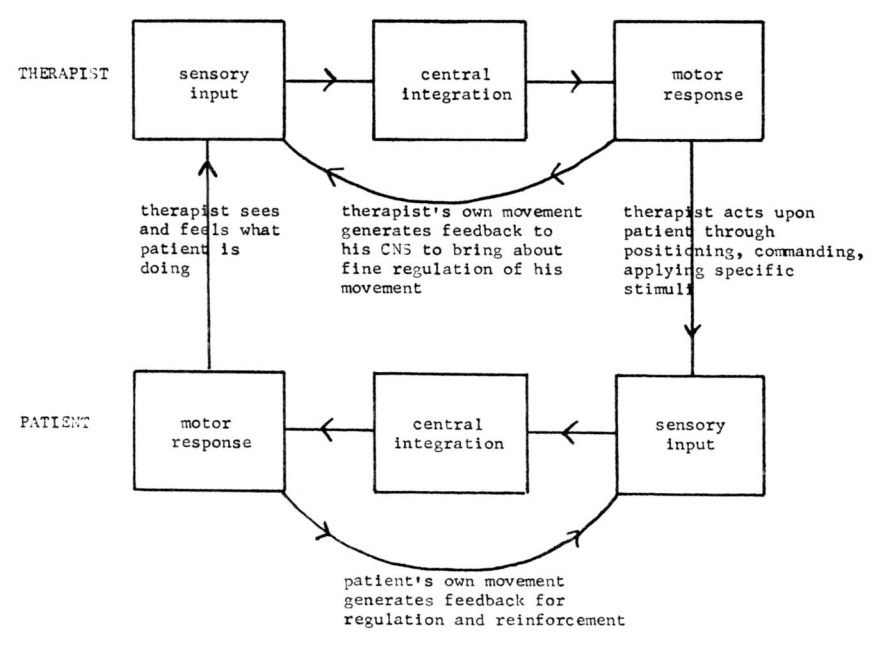

sensory input → central integration → motor response

- therapist sees and feels what patient is doing
- therapist's own movement generates feedback to his CNS to bring about fine regulation of his movement
- therapist acts upon patient through positioning, commanding, applying specific stimuli

PATIENT

motor response ← central integration ← sensory input

patient's own movement generates feedback for regulation and reinforcement

Figure 4-1. The relationship between the sensorimotor processes of the patient and of the therapist.

quence for acquiring and integrating mobility and stability functions (Table 4-I). In addition to immaturity there is a central defect which may suppress functions of areas primarily unaffected. This problem calls for measures which will reflexly facilitate dormant functions or those with the potential to emerge. Various forms of sensory stimulation, selected on the basis of the relationship between receptor discharge and reflex response, serve the purpose of reflex activation. Generally speaking, maintained stimuli given to excite the static or slowly adapting component of receptors are used to facilitate tonic actions for the purpose of achieving stability; single or changing patterns of stimuli given to excite the dynamic or rapidly adapting component of the receptors are used to facilitate actions for the purpose of increasing mobility.

Avoidance-withdrawal responses as (Fig. 4-2, 4-3) indicated

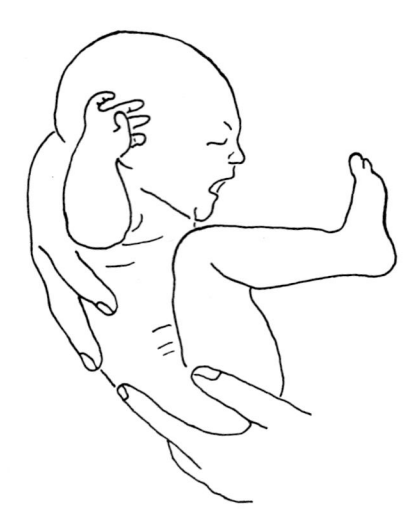

194 *Physical Therapy Services in the Developmental Disabilities*

Figure 4-2. The newborn: withdrawal responses in the upper and lower extremities.

must be modified so that changing or intermittent stimuli bring about controlled movement for more precise action. Protective responses would normally remain prepotent over controlled movement only when danger was real or the threat unexpected. The development of coinnervation, maintained contact of the distal part of the body with supporting surfaces, and progression toward unilateral weightbearing will modify avoidance-withdrawal responses.

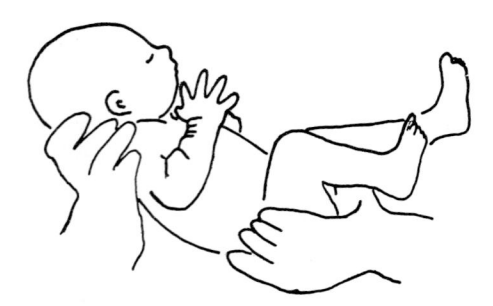

Figure 4-3. The newborn: avoidance reaction of the hand; the fingers extend and spread.

A Sensorimotor Approach to Treatment

Traction responses or strongly predominant flexor tone (Fig. 4-4, 4-5) must be modified if weight-bearing activities are to be accomplished. Initially, this modification will occur when tonic

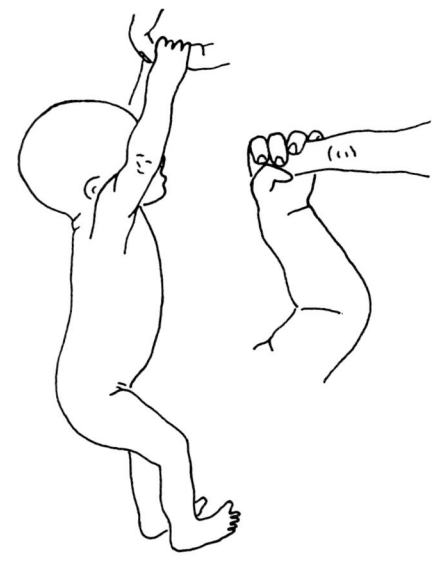

Figure 4-4. The newborn: the traction response.

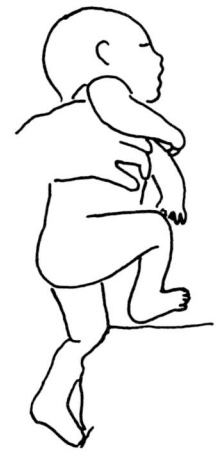

Figure 4-5. The newborn: the placing response with full range of flexion.

postural extensor patterns develop their full potential. In the presence of abnormal flexor stretch sensitivity, it may be necessary to inhibit flexor responses in order to activate extensors. Later, flexor action would be reactivated when coinnervation has developed.

Movements which alternate quickly from one extreme of the range to the other result from lack of regulation of range, speed, and direction normally provided by three-dimensional stabilization. The stepping response of the newborn which has been well illustrated by André-Thomas and Autgaerden (1966) is an example of this type of movement. Twitchell (1965) describes the stepping in terms of "overflexion," "overextension," and "overadduction." The stabilizing elements which regulate excessive range are not well developed until after stages of unilateral weight-bearing. The proprioceptive feedback from heavy resistance and stretch of tonic extensor muscles is essential for the development of stability.

Growth or progress in gaining control may be thought of as a process of modification through balance of extremes. This modification would lead to more precise and appropriate responses but at the same time to greater variety rather than narrowing of the number of responses. If the extremes of behavior were characterized by mobility and stability, the modified form would be described as the ability to maintain basic control of behavior while responding to and acting upon changing environments. More specifically, if motor behavior were described in the same terms, maturity in motor activities would be described as control of basic posture despite a changing environment or the ability to change position with precise control in order to manipulate a part of the set environment.

These points are made in order to establish the concept that the ultimate goal of a therapeutic program is to achieve blending of mobility and stability so that movements are purposeful and precise rather than being extreme and labile or the opposite, rigidly unchanging. Evaluation procedures attempt to identify the absence or excessive dominance of either mobility or stability. Treatment attempts to restore the balance between these fundamental components.

The Development of Mobilizing Responses and Their Role in Coordinating Movement

Mobility is a basic functional characteristic of any movement. It can be described simply as that characteristic which enables the organism to change position. In locomotor activities mobility is manifest as the limbs advance in space. In manipulative functions or any fine skill it is present in the form of rapidly alternating movement and in the great ease of overcoming inertia. Phasic reciprocal movements of non-weight-bearing limbs have the greatest mobility.

The responses of the newborn are characterized by mobility. The withdrawal, avoiding or defensive action patterns are rapidly initiated and usually move the individual as far from the stimulus as possible or prevent him from sustaining contact. Such reactions are elicited by exteroceptive stimuli. Distal parts of the body with high concentration of rapidly adapting receptors are involved in these reflex responses. The receptors are possibly the same ones involved in discriminating functions after there is modification of their influence. Stimuli which activate phasic responses are quick and changing. The Moro reflex, a phasic vestibular reflex, is elicited by a sudden movement of the head (Peiper 1963). Phasic reflexes frequently demonstrate a secondary component which is the reverse movement of the initial response, a phenomena which may be related to Sherrington's "successive induction" (1906).

The protective type patterns are essential for the survival of the individual but must be modified if advanced motor functions are to take place. Twitchell (1965), in describing development of voluntary prehension, indicates that avoiding responses and grasp reactions balance each other out. Nociceptive responses are not repeatedly elicited as a therapeutic measure because of the difficulty in controlling them. However, in selected instances they may be used to initiate movement where no other sensory avenue is open. In addition to the protective or nociceptive responses of the newborn there are three advanced levels of mobility development.

198   *Physical Therapy Services in the Developmental Disabilities*

Movement into an Oriented Position

The labyrinthine-righting reflex, the optical-righting reflex, and the body-righting reflex acting on the head bring the head into a position with the vertex up and the mouth horizontal. Then through the chain reflexes, the rest of the body is brought to a position where equilibrium can be maintained (Peiper 1963). So many functions are built upon the ability to right the head in relation to gravity that only small progress can be made until this is accomplished. As the head is righted the stimulus from lack of alignment between the head and neck will bring about change in the position of the body. The head-neck relationship of the normal righting reflexes contributes to the mobility

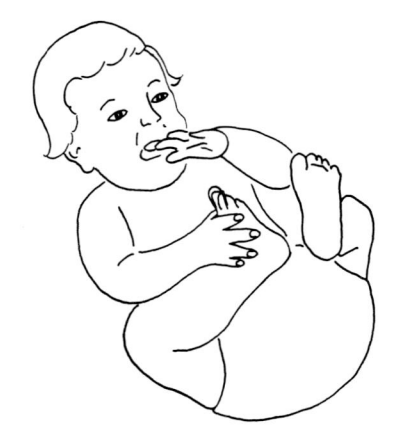

Figure 4-6. Supine: controlled flexion toward the midline with development of the supine righting reflexes.

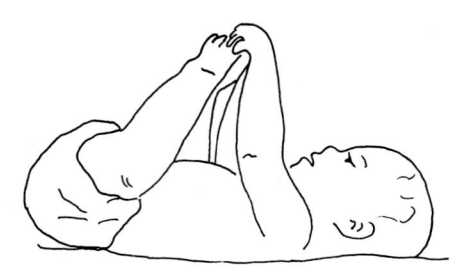

Figure 4-7: Supine: controlled flexion.

A Sensorimotor Approach to Treatment

component of movements by bringing about general change in body position.

To elicit a head righting reflex the child must be strongly subjected to gravity. For example, to obtain head orientation in a

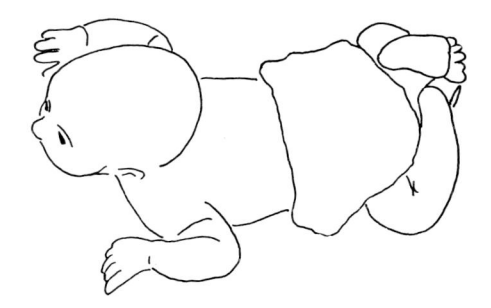

Figure 4-8. The labyrinthine-righting reflex of the head; the arms spread horizontally.

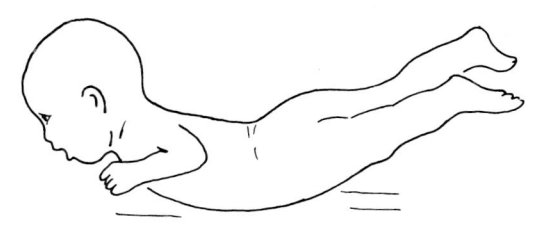

Figure 4-9. The labyrinthine-righting reflex of the head with the symmetrical chain reflex.

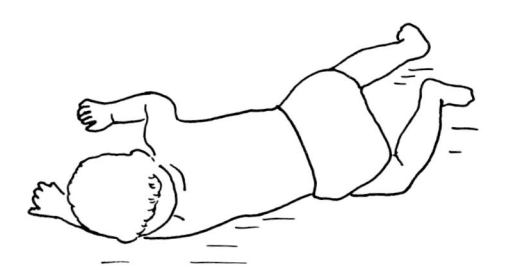

Figure 4-10. The head moves from the position of the labyrinthine-righting reflex to the position for stretch of tonic extensors, neck cocontraction resulting.

prone position along with the first associated chain reflex, suspend the child in the prone position holding him around the waist. Tilt him obliquely downward, keeping the lumbar and lower thoracic region extended. The correct response will be neck extension with a total extensor pattern following (Fig. 4-9). It is important to give a minimum amount of trunk support. This is difficult to do while keeping a secure hold on the child at the same time. Various devices can be used to assist with the movement (for example, a swing with a canvas seat across which the child lies, a narrow padded bench on rockers, or a large ball). If only the head and upper trunk response is to be evoked, the child can be tilted from a sitting position.

Righting of the head in the lateral and supine positions can be achieved with similar oblique and backward suspensions. Peiper (1963) illustrates various positions for eliciting the labyrinthine-righting reflex. If there is extreme weakness in head control or overstretch from overactive antagonists the child will be unable to initiate from the fully stretched position and must have his head supported or positioned in a moderate range while being tilted. Derotative righting occurs as a child rolls in response to head turning. In immature forms of rolling, the trunk will move as a unit. As maturity occurs neck-trunk action will be of the spiral type; this is the most likely basis for trunk rotation components of upright activities.

Movement to Recover Balance

Equilibrium responses serve to keep the center of gravity of the body over the base of support. When balance is disturbed there are two recourses. There can be shifting of parts away from the direction in which the body is falling. This shift redistributes the center of gravity because of changes in the mass. As a result there are abduction and lateral trunk flexion reactions to side-falling, movement of the extremities and head forward when pushed offbalance backward, and movement of the extremities and head backward when balance is lost forward. There can also be movement of the base of support back under the center of gravity, such as stepping movements in the direction of the fall. If redistribution of body weight or change in base of support is not successful there is quick and full-range movement into a position of support.

The first responses to balance disturbance are quickly initiated and phasic and therefore contribute to the mobility component of movement. It is extremely important that they be "captured" and sustained if the movement is to be reinforced. The therapist must maneuver the patient in and out of the point of balance so that the response is repeatedly being evoked, and the reversal of the response is not allowed to occur. Shift from a bilateral to a unilateral weight-bearing position evokes an equilibrium response in a less obvious form. The limb on which weight is borne increases its stabilizing cocontraction, and the limb which is relieved of weight-bearing and subject to slight stretch from traction increases its mobility.

Discrete Distal Movement

When proximal regions immediately adjacent to the distal parts of the body become stabilized, distal movements with tremendous ability to overcome inertia can be developed. Such movements are more discrete and varied than any of the more general body responses manifesting mobility.

The Development of Stabilizing Responses and Their Role in Coordinating Movement

There are certain postural functions which must be linked into one concept in order to see the emergence of skilled activity. Basic posture or position can be held at one point in space by the action of stabilizing muscles. Also, posture can be thought of more dynamically as the background for a movement. Postural mechanisms furnish the proximal stabilization which enables distal movement to be skilled. Rather than posture as the fundamental factor, stability might be considered even more encompassing.

When the body or part of it is strongly stabilized in all dimensions by muscle action, it will be fixed in place and prepared for weight-bearing. If a goal demands movement of a limb while weight-bearing on it, stabilizers are capable of allowing some movement although this will be understandably restricted. If movement while weight-bearing were not limited, balance would be lost, as is the case with some central deficits affecting stability. The stabilizers keep the range of movement in check so that the posture can be held. During unilateral weight-bearing, when maintenance of position is dependent on the response of the limb, the action of the stabilizers is at its maximum preventing movement almost entirely. As stabilization develops and unilateral weight-bearing is possible, the extremity on the other side of the body is free to move and reach out.

The movements of the child after he has accomplished weight-bearing are quite different from those same attempts prior to weight-bearing. The child has lost the tremulous, athetoid-like movements of the normal three-month-old. He is able to place the distal part of the extremity with more precision, and he is able, in the case of the upper extremities, to hold the arm in position while the hand manipulates. All of his accomplishments demonstrate restriction of unnecessary movement components which detract from achieving a specific goal. This restriction of control of movement appears to be the function of stabilizers. In its extreme form, which is seen in unilateral weight-bearing, stabilization prevents movement through coinnervation of synergistic and antagonistic muscles. In more modified form, stabilization allows limited and specific movement directed toward achieving a goal, or it may simply serve to protect the joints from excessive ranges during free-swinging movement. Stability develops in three stages.

THE DEVELOPMENT OF MIDLINE HOLDING. The labyrinthine-righting reflex raises the child's head to a face-vertical position. The responses which follow this reflex are, according to Peiper (1963), "chain reflexes dependent on the labyrinthine reflex of the head." Pieper points out the difficulties in determining the extent to which other tonic and righting reflexes contribute to the adjustment of the body to the head. His use of the term "chain reflexes" refers to the combination of reflexes which bring the child to the position where, in a given instance, he can maintain equilibrium.

In the supine position the trunk and neck flexors which act later in coinnervation are first activated to hold for extremity movement. It appears that the bilateral holding action of proximal flexors against the pull of gravity on the limbs follows from the development of righting reflexes. (Figs. 4-6, 4-7) Bilateral midline hand activities and related visual functions may be partly dependent on this controlled flexion for their development.

The "symmetrical reflex in the abdominal position," a term used by Peiper, is the activity which first develops extensor action in the child (Fig. 4-9). The extensors of the neck, trunk, lower extremities and proximal regions of the upper extremities are held in a shortened position against gravity. It is theorized that activity in a sustained position sets the stretch reflex at a new length (Eldred 1967b). It does not seem remote to think of the symmetrical chain reflex serving the purpose of determining the stretch sensitivity of extensor muscles. The reflexes involved in stretch responses must be functioning before the child can maintain balance as he bears weight.

Observe the normal child between the ages of two and six months of age, and notice that as he begins weight-bearing on the upper extremities as well as the lower extremities, he frequently alternates between the position of holding the extensors in the shortened range and bringing them into a stretched position ready for weight-bearing; or, he may actually put weight on the extremity. It almost seems as though he first gains a small amount of stretch sensitivity and then "tries it out" or "uses it up" and goes back for more. The key factors to keep in mind when developing this stage of stability through treatment are that the extensors must be a maintained contraction in their shortened range against resistance (usually gravity) and this response must be in the prone position.

THE TONIC EXTENSORS ARE STRETCHED AND RESISTED. The tonic extensors which have been exercised in their shortened range must be put on a stretch and given resistance in order to bring about coinnervation of muscles on all sides of the joint. The stretch to the tonic extensors does not have to be extreme stretch, but it needs to be stretch relative to the completely shortened range. The neck and trunk are stretched when the child goes from the extremely extended position to the unsupported horizontal position. (See Fig. 4-11 for the neck progression.)

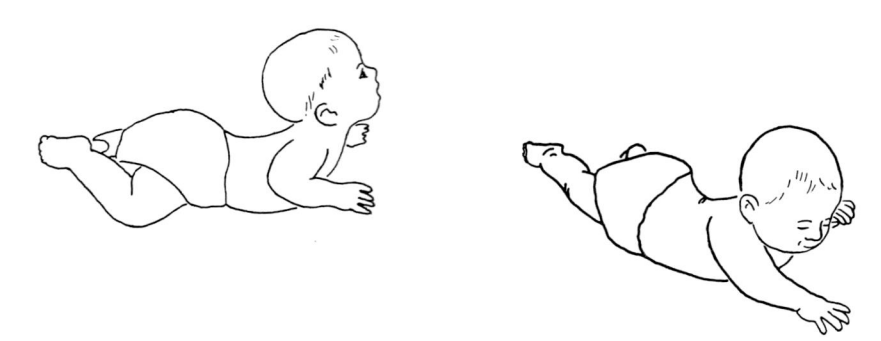

204 *Physical Therapy Services in the Developmental Disabilities*

Figure 4-11. Rolling over in response to head-turning.

For the trunk, the position achieved in creeping is the furthest point in the second stability stage. It is difficult to imagine how, with the extremities weight-bearing, the horizontal position places a stretch on trunk extensors. Rood has drawn attention to the fact that the tenth thoracic vertebra is a pivot point toward which and away from which action takes place. When the tonic extensors of the trunk work to stabilize, they pull from the pivot point toward the hips if they are below the pivot, and toward the shoulders if they are above the pivot. The action of the extensors would lift the center of the trunk upward so that the vertebral column would have moved from a point of extension, especially in the lumbar and low thoracic regions, toward a midpoint between extension and flexion. The effect of the relative stretch and the great amount of resistance to the movement is to bring about coinnervation of flexors and extensors.

One mechanism which may prove to contribute largely to coinnervation patterns is the feedback from the high-threshold receptors in the muscle spindles of tonic extensors. The greater the stretch and resistance to a tonic extensor, the more influence from these receptors in the form of flexor facilitation. The result may be that a greater postural or gravitational demand signals the balancing out of forces around a joint to restrict movement in all directions.

For the upper extremities the first coinnervation pattern

occurs when the child bears weight on his elbows (Figs. 4-12 and 4-13). The scapular adductors and downward rotators and the shoulder extensors and external rotators (which belong to the tonic extensor pattern) are stretched, and resistance is provided by the weight of the upper trunk and scapulae. Additional resistance and increased joint compression are present when the

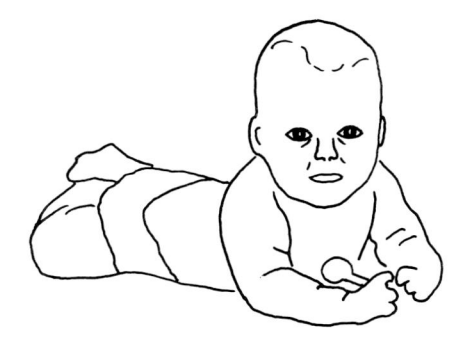

Figure 4-12. Bilateral weight-bearing on the elbows.

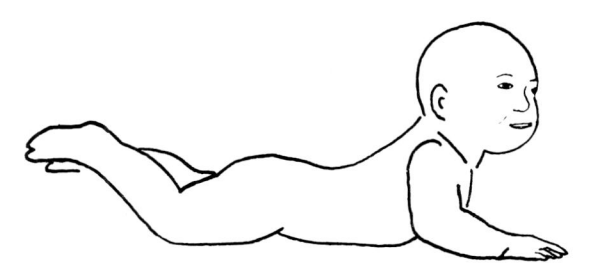

Figure 4-13. Bilateral weight-bearing on the elbows.

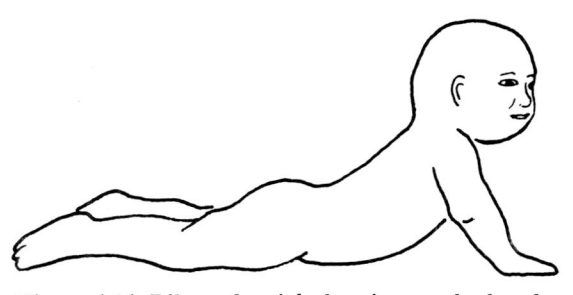

Figure 4-14. Bilateral weight-bearing on the hands.

child shifts to bearing weight on one elbow and reaches forward with the free upper extremity. Unilateral weight-bearing stimulates the receptors for high-threshold joint compression. The influence of these receptors is thought to be related to facilitation of coinnervation patterns.

The lower extremities enter the second stage of stability development when weight-bearing on the knees begins. Stability in

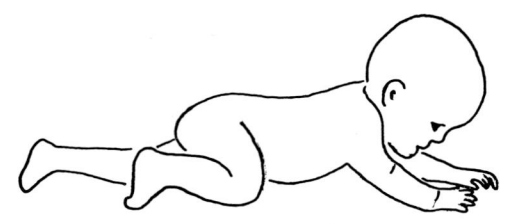

Figure 4-15. Beginning to move into the creeping position; the trunk not yet stable enough to support the pull of the extremities.

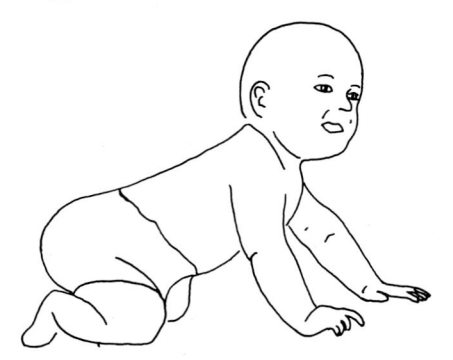

Figure 4-16. The quadruped with hips back in heel-sitting fashion; the trunk not fully horizontal.

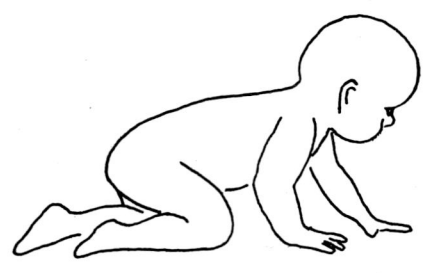

Figure 4-17. The full quadruped with trunk horizontal and stable.

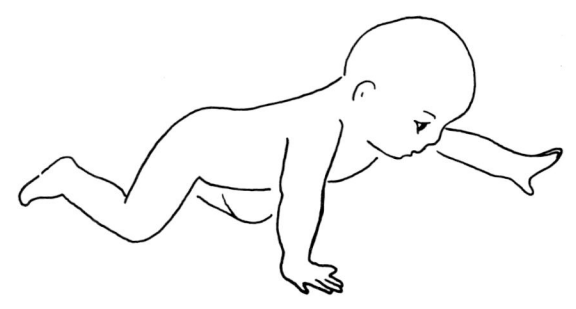

Figure 4-18. Unilateral weight-bearing for the upper extremity, full stability development; beginning skill in placement of the free extremity.

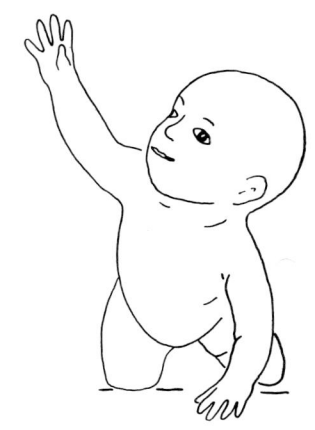

Figure 4-19. Unilateral weight-bearing for the upper extremity; the free extremity in controlled reach.

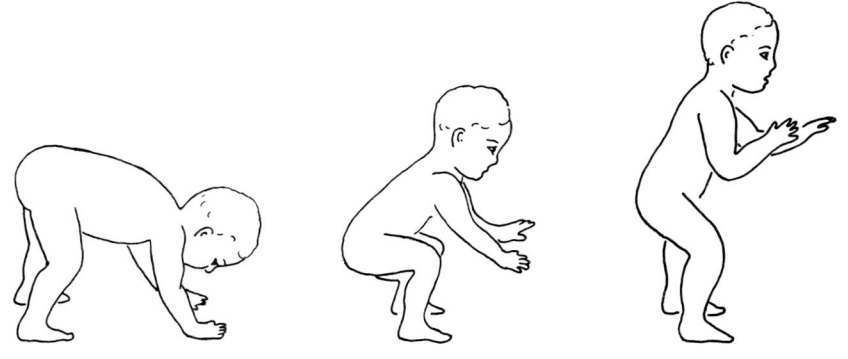

Figure 4-20. Movement from plantigrade to semisquat to standing; bilateral weight-bearing involving more than one joint.

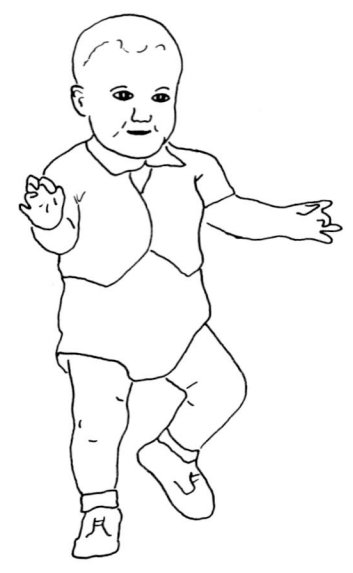

208 *Physical Therapy Services in the Developmental Disabilities*

Figure 4-21. Unilateral weight-bearing for the lower extremity; beginning skilled placement of the free extremity.

the lower extremities is closely linked to lower trunk stability, just as the upper extremities are linked to upper trunk stability. The child may assume a quadruped position in which he tends to sit back on his heels (Fig. 4-16). This position may indicate incomplete development of trunk stabilization.

STABILIZATION OF ADDITIONAL LIMB SEGMENTS. The third stage of stability development does not apply to neck and trunk development, only to the extremities. Stability is further developed when additional joints are involved in the weight-bearing process. The child advances from the position on elbows to weight-bearing on hands. He may do this without change in the lower extremity pattern (Fig. 4-14), and will eventually use the upper extremity pattern in the quadruped positions (Figs. 4-17–4-20). The lower extremities add the knee and ankle joints to the weight-bearing pattern when going from quadruped on hands and knees to quadruped on hands and feet (plantigrade standing) and then on up to erect standing (Fig. 4-20).

A Sensorimotor Approach to Treatment

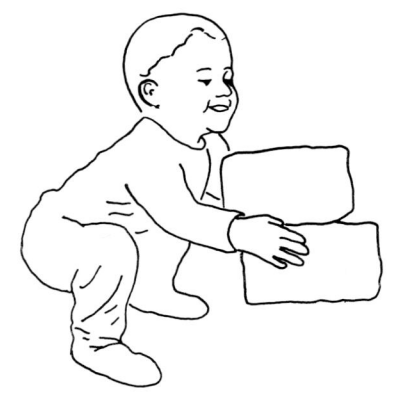

Figure 4-22. Holding the squat position; tonic holding of the distal part of the lower extremities.

The addition of other joints to the pattern places the center of gravity further from the base of support, thereby requiring more stabilization to maintain balance. More weight is superimposed on the limbs resulting in greater joint compression, and proximal muscles must work to stabilize longer levers. If the child shifts to unilateral weight-bearing, he further increases the demand for stabilization (Fig. 4-18) and elicits cocontraction in its most extreme normal form.

In addition to increased resistance, joint compression, and

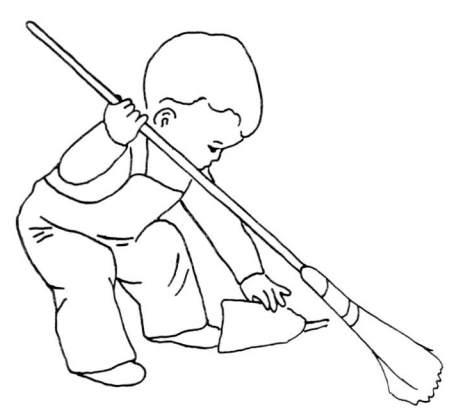

Figure 4-23. Semisquat; resistance and stretch to the tonic extensor pattern.

stretch, there is another form of sensory input which occurs at this stage which has great therapeutic importance. During bilateral and especially unilateral weight-bearing the soles of the feet and palms of the hands are in maintained contact with the supporting surface. The continuous pressure from this contact is thought to be part of the normal mechanism for modifying responses to tactile stimuli. Specific receptors found in abundance in distal parts of the body and originally involved in mobilizing responses, adapt rapidly to continuous stimuli. Following adaptation, specific receptors appear to contribute to functions of discrimination rather than causing labile movement responses away from the stimulus.

Combining Mobility and Stability Functions

In the preceding sections on mobility and stability, the dynamic and static qualities of motor functions are discussed separately although they actually are combined for a total response. Soon after beginning bilateral weight-bearing in various postures, the child may rock in place moving his body on a fixed distal point. This may be a normal type of rhythmic behavior preparatory to weight shift. It may also be found in emotionally disturbed and retarded children. Provence and Lipton (1962) propose that there are at least four forms of rocking with different origins and meanings. Where the infant does not appear to be emotionally disturbed, the rocking movement may be interpreted as a purposeful developmental activity.

Lurie (1949) notes that rhythmic patterns are common in transitional stages. A child may be able to hold a posture but not have the control to locomote in the posture. For example, he can hold the quadruped and rock in it before he can creep. He can stand and bounce and rock before he can step forward. If this rocking appears in normal children it may be serving the purpose of stimulating joint and muscle receptors to prepare for increased weight-bearing on one side and for freedom of movement on the other side. Once there is unilateral weight-bearing on one extremity the other extremity moves outward with more precision than demonstrated in previous stages. The upper extremity which reaches forward participated in the stages of stability development which have modified earlier patterns of traction and avoidance.

As movement takes place, the reciprocal contractions are regulated by coinnervation which developed during weight-bearing. If the child is stepping forward in the erect posture, the advancing extremity has gone through stability developing stages. The withdrawal and positive supporting reactions which are reciprocal have been modified with the development of coinnervation. The early steps or the first reaching in the quadruped are far from being extremely accurate. However, enough stability has developed to assure general accuracy in reciprocal actions. As more and more unilateral weight-bearing is practiced and stability is further developed, the precision of placement of the extremity will become greater.

The most advanced combination of stability and mobility occurs when all regions proximal to the fingers are stabilized so that the fingers can move selectively and rapidly. In the hand, the reciprocal action of the extensors was first seen in the avoiding reaction, while the flexors were active in traction responses. During weight-bearing on the open hand the traction response is modified. When strong ulnar grip is activated, the tonic dorsal interossei are stretched and metacarpals are stabilized. At the same time, the wrist is stabilized and thumb adductors and opponents are activated. The development of ulnar grip appears to be prerequisite to the skillful use of the hand, which requires stabilization of all metacarpals and the wrist.

From very early stages there are indications that stability and mobility not only develop concurrently but that there is an interaction between them which results in a higher level of performance than the sum of the two components. Three different types of combined action can be identified. In the weight-bearing position there can be movement and postural holding at a given joint —for example, in shifting weight on and off a weight-bearing extremity. In a non-weight-bearing action such as reaching toward a definite point with the hand or foot, phasic movement would be the mobilizing component and the stabilizing component would come from postural muscles which are providing control of regulation of the speed, range, and direction of movement. A more advanced combined action would be demonstrated by fine manipulation in which stabilizers would hold proximal regions so that distal fine skill could take place at a given point in the range of the reach.

In each case the interaction between the tonic and phasic system results in a modulated motor response. A central or peripheral source triggers off a response which must be controlled if it is to have any purpose other than protection or withdrawal. Control seems to be brought about directly by the restricting, holding effects of cocontraction or possibly in an indirect way by inhibition from the tonic system.

TREATMENT OF SPECIFIC PROBLEMS

There are a vast number of possible combinations of problems which a therapist might have to deal with in selecting treatment procedures. Therefore, it is impossible to outline a program which will be appropriate for a given child. However, a basic plan for evaluation and progression coupled with thoughts about the needs of children with specific types of problems should provide the framework for treatment selection.

The process of evaluation is threefold, as shown below:

1. Identification of unmodified patterns of the newborn such as those of avoidance or defensive responses, the Moro reflex, active traction responses, stepping responses, or proprioceptive positive supporting responses. These responses would normally be found active in the neonate (Twitchell 1965). A number of outstanding works on the neurological examination of infants are available to assist in the identification of these early patterns (Beintema 1968, Paine and Oppe 1966, Prechtl and Beintema 1964).

2. Identification of the spontaneous progress which has been made in the integration of patterns found in the newborn. Table 4-I can be used as a guide in this evaluation. The work of Paine and associates on the evaluation of postural reflexes is invaluable in the study of progression from the neonate stage (Paine 1964, Paine et al. 1964).

3. Identification of patterns released from control because of the pathological condition. Examples of such patterns are seen as maintained or obligating tonic neck reflexes and tonic labyrinthine reflexes. The spontaneous movements of the normal infant readily move him away from these responses (Peiper 1963). Vassella and Karlsson (1962) found that only 8 percent of neonates demonstrate true asymmetrical tonic neck reflexes, their criterion being the consistency with which the reflex can be elicited. By seven months of age, none of the infants in that 8 percent segment of their population demonstrated the reflex.

Planning of the treatment program grows out of the findings of the evaluation. The initial program will usually consist of two parts, first the sequence of activities which will bring the child up into at least one stage of control beyond his present level, and secondly, the selection of procedures which will facilitate or activate the responses to be gained. Many of the treatment procedures suggested are based on the work of Rood (1954, 1956, 1958, 1962, 1963). The mobility-stability model represents an interpretation of some of the concepts of Rood's approach to treatment (Stockmeyer 1967).

The Child Whose Sensorimotor Activities are Normal but Delayed in Relation to His Chronological Age

The level of motor maturation of the child can be judged by one of many tests available (Bayley 1933, Gesell and Amatruda 1947, Knobloch et al. 1966, Milani-Comparetti and Gidoni 1967, Sloan 1955, Willson 1969). It is important to ascertain if the only motor problem is one of delayed maturation. The question to ask during observation of the child's responses to motor development tests is this: Given an item which would be performed at a specific chronological age, does the child perform the activity as you would expect a child of that chronological age to do it? In other words, does he perform activities at the six-month-level with the same quality of movement you would expect of a normal six-month-old?

Sometimes a mild tremor or athetoidlike movement is not

abnormal if one considers the maturation level rather than the chronological age. On the other hand, if the child is performing an activity where normally there would be no such incoordination and he displays a deviation, we attach a different meaning to the clinical sign and would explore further for a specific deficit. It is difficult to determine if the quality of a movement is normal for the activity even though the activity achieved is below the chronological age of the child. The problem lies in finding the criteria which define the quality of normal movement in measurable terms and provide a standard to which the patient can be compared. At the present time we have only impressions to guide us. However, the work of Milani-Comparetti and Gidoni bear watching for the promise their motoscopic examination holds (1967).

The purpose of treatment for the child with delayed development is to encourage activities which become possible as maturation provides the readiness. The activities which comprise the treatment program can be drawn from different sources. Tests of motor maturation usually contain performance items which represent a sequence of activities. The progression of control as outlined in Table 4-I can be used to identify the general nature of responses which need to be activated. The therapeutic programs for children with delayed maturation are usually not definitive because of the very general nature of the motor problem. The sensory input normally generated by movement and holding are not supplemented unless specific deficits are identified.

The Child Whose Movements Are Slow, Stereotyped, and Difficult to Initiate

Even though the child's voluntarily initiated movement may be lacking the quality of mobility, he may respond quite readily to stimuli which evoke protective or early phasic responses such as withdrawal and the Moro reflex. Sustained postures of the trunk and lower extremities are not uncommon. Rood (1963) has identified such postures as a type of reversal of pattern in response to repeated stimulation. For example, in some children it can be observed that repeated stimulation of a withdrawal response in the lower extremities is followed by a period of heightened tension in the reverse extensor pattern and increased difficulty in voluntarily initiating the flexor pattern. The clinical picture is generally characterized by responses in which early reflexes persist, superficial phasic muscles hold the child in sustained positions, and tonic postural functions have not developed.

Treatment can be initiated at two points. Preferably the righting reflexes, especially in the prone position, will be strongly emphasized in the program. If the phasic holding is marked or persists in one area, the therapist may find it more effective to begin by inhibiting the holding action of superficial muscles. Eventually, treatment must progress through the stages of stability development if there is to be consolidation of the gains made in releasing superficial holding. High-threshold joint compression, moderate to heavy resistance to tonic extensors, and vibration of tonic extensors would be appropriate facilitating procedures.

The Child Who Is Hypotonic and Lacks the Reflex Basis for Movement and Posture

Evaluation may reveal that even reflexes found at birth are severely reduced in strength. It is important to distinguish between the lack of a reflex which should be present and the apparent absence of a reflex because of integration by higher level functions. Performance in three essential patterns should be evaluated. These patterns are prone extension, supine flexion, and rolling activities (Figs. 4-6–4-11) which are manifestations of the righting reflexes.

Treatment could begin with activation of the earliest reflexes; however, there are some potential dangers involved with such an initiation. Many of the responses of the newborn can be classified as protective reactions. Such reactions are often difficult to modify if they become too firmly established. Although protective responses must remain prepotent if they are to serve the organism effectively, as the child matures it should take an increasingly stronger or truly noxious stimulus to set them off. If treatment is begun with the activation of protective reflexes, the child should be advanced to the next stage as soon as a response at the lower level is elicited. It may be more advisable to begin with righting reflexes which develop neck and trunk responses and even advance to some weight-bearing activities before returning to establish protective reflex behavior.

The Child Who Lacks the Controlling Influence of Stabilizers

The more frequently seen clinical signs in children who lack stability are athetosis and hyperflexibility. One factor these two signs have in common is a lack of regulation or restriction of excessive movement. The child with athetosis will generally have difficulty with activities requiring holding, whether weight-bearing or non-weight-bearing. He does not have the ability to move with limited direction or range because of interference with feedback from tonic muscles. Observation of his movements, especially during locomotor activities, reveals that at a given joint he must move further than normal into the range to get a response to stretch. The result of this lack of stretch sensitivity is that the movements have greater range than is efficient for maintaining balance.

Balance or equilibrium is a result of rather discrete and sensitive adjustments to gravity. Receptors stimulated by minor changes in stretch, compression, pressure, and head position play a role in the activation of the tonic holding we call posture. Hyperflexibility may be seen as a clinical sign alone or accompanying athetosis. It is usually an indication that tonic stabilizers do not have enough tone or stretch sensitivity to confine movements to ranges which will preserve the integrity of joint structures.

Evaluation of the child with athetosis should include identification of unmodified neonate patterns. Many of these movement patterns involve avoidance or withdrawal responses in reaction to changing stimuli. Although flexor actions predominate in the athetoid child, movements are often from one extreme of the range to the other as seen in their "wooden soldier" type movements in supported ambulation or the use of the infant "cry pattern" for speech articulation.

The treatment sequence of major importance to these children is one which follows the three stages of stability development identified earlier in this chapter. Every effort should be made to reduce the presence of frequently changing stimuli in the child's treatment environment. Maintained stimuli alone should be selected to facilitate the holding responses needed by the athetoid child; for example, maintained contact with even but not rough supporting surfaces, sustained weight-bearing, close-fitting clothing (at least in cooler weather), firm and continuous contact in handling the child. Stimuli such as light touch or cold should be avoided.

The Hyperactive Child Whose Sensorimotor Activity Is Dominated by Tactile Avoidance Responses and a Low Threshold for Environmental Stimuli

The most obvious signs of this type of disturbance may be in the child's psychosocial behavior. These children are often spoken of as being stimulus-bound or having an impulse disturbance, and can attend to an object or task for only short periods of time. Frequently, such children do not like to be touched or restrained in any way. If they are at the creeping rather than the walking stage, they may bear weight only on the fingertips and knees, the knee being flexed so that the lower leg and foot are not in contact with the supporting surface. A mild tremor or slight ataxia may be seen.

Treatment is directed toward generalized reduction of activity and increased tolerance for maintained positions. The influence from distal parts of the extremities should be reduced by maintained contact with a supporting surface. The quadruped position with increased joint approximation given by the therapist is an important part of treatment. Neck cocontraction needs to be developed or repeatedly facilitated in order to stabilize visual and auditory input. All contacts with objects and surfaces and all handling of the child should be firm. Heavy resistance should be given to postural patterns. Cold or very rough surfaces should not contact the hands and feet. The emphasis is on a constant input, not on stimuli which are changing in their level of intensity.

TABLE 4-I
STAGES OF CONTROL
FRAMEWORK FOR PROGRESSION OF TREATMENT*

Mobility		Stability	
Stage 1 Neonate Responses, Extreme Positions, Movement with Much Range	Stage 2 Early Modification of Neonate Patterns	Stage 3 Tonic Extensors in Non–Weight-bearing Midline Holding	Stage 4 Bilateral Weight-bearing, Cocontraction
Non–Weight-bearing Movement, Phasic Responses			
Protective responses—withdrawal and avoidance (2,3) † Moro reflex Traction response (4) Stepping, placing (5)			
	Righting reflexes give rise to chain reflexes Supine flexion (6,7) Prone extension (8,9,11) Rolling (11)	Prone extension (8,9,11)	Deep atlanto-occipital extensors on a stretch cocontraction holding weight of head (11) Tonic extensors on stretch in elbow weight bearing (12,13), Bilateral weight-bearing on hands (14) Bilateral weight-bearing on hands and knees (16,17)
			Bilateral weight-bearing on hands and feet, plantigrade position (20) Bilateral weight-bearing on feet (20)
		Hold semisquat and squat (22,23)	Up to standing from squat

*Based on the Ontogenetic Motor Patterns according to Rood (1962).
†Numbers in Table 4-I indicate figures which illustrate the activity.

A Sensorimotor Approach to Treatment

Combined Mobility and Stability Weight-bearing		Combined Mobility and Stability Non–Weight-bearing Movement	
Stage 5 Movement with Bilateral Weight-bearing	Stage 6 Maintained Unilateral Weight-bearing	Stage 7 Controlled Placement of Distal Part Axial and Proximal Limb Stabilization for Distal Mobility	Stage 8 Precision of Distal Movements
On elbows rocking push backward	Weight shift to unilateral weight-bearing on one elbow with unilateral reaching Equilibrium responses		
Rocking in quadruped	Weight shift to unilateral weight-bearing on one upper extremity—the other extremity reaches forward or advances in creeping (18,19)		
	Unilateral weight-bearing on one knee—other extremity advances in creeping		
Rock back to semisquat, up to standing (20)			
Bounce in standing			
	Step in place Side step holding on	Step forward, upper extremities held forward, in readiness to catch weight (21) Step forward, upper extremities at sides	
			Heel-toe gait, base smaller, Fine manipulation by hands

BIBLIOGRAPHY

André-Thomas, and Autgaerden, S.: *Locomotion from Pre- to Post-natal Life.* Little Club Clinics in Developmental Medicine, No. 24. The Spastics Society. London, Heinemann, 1966.

Bayley, N.: Mental growth during the first three years: An experimental study of sixty-one children by repeated tests. *Genet Psychol Monogr, 14:*1-92, 1933.

Beintema, D.J.: *A Neurological Study of New Infants.* Little Club Clinics in Developmental Medicine, No. 28. The Spastics Society. London, Heinemann, 1968.

Buchwald, J.S.: A functional concept of motor control. *Amer J Phys Med, 46:*141-150, 1967.

Eldred, E.: Peripheral receptors: Their elicitation and relation to reflex patterns. *Amer J Phys Med, 46:*69-87, 1967a.

Eldred, E.: Functional implications of dynamic and static components of the spindle response to stretch. *Amer J Phys Med, 46:*129-140, 1967b.

Gesell, A., and Amatruda, C.: *Developmental Diagnosis.* New York, Paul B. Hoebner, 1947.

Knobloch, H., Pasamanick, B., and Sherard, E.S.: A developmental screening inventory for infants. *Supplement to Pediatrics, 38:*1095-1108, Part 2, 1966.

Kuypers, H.G.J.M.: The organization of the "motor system." *Int J Neurol, 4:*78-91, 1963.

Livingston, R.B.: Central control of receptors and sensory transmission systems. In Field, J., Magoun, H.W., and Hall, V.E. (Eds.): *Handbook of Physiology, Section 1: Neurophysiology.* Washington, D.C., American Physiological Society, 1959, Vol. 1, pp 741-760.

Lurie, R.S.: The role of rhythmic patterns in childhood. *Amer J Psychiat, 105:*630-660, 1949.

Milani-Comparetti, A., and Gidoni, E.A.: Routine developmental examination in normal and retarded children. *Develop Med Child Neurol, 9:*631-638, 1967.

Paine, R.S.: The evolution of infantile postural reflexes in the presence of chronic brain syndromes. *Develop Med Child Neurol, 6:*345-361, 1964.

Paine, R.S., Brazelton, T.B., Donovan, D.E., Drorbaugh, J.E., Hubbel, J.P., and Sears, E.M.: Evolution of postural reflexes in normal infants and in the presence of chronic brain syndromes. *Neurology, 14:*1036-1048, 1964.

Paine, R.S., and Oppe, T.E.: *Neurological Examination of Children.* Little Club Clinics in Developmental Medicine, Nos. 20 and 21. The Spastics Society. London, Heinemann, 1966.

Peiper, A.: *Cerebral Function in Infancy and Childhood.* New York, Consultants Bureau, 1963.

Prechtl, H., and Beintema, D.: *The Neurological Examination of the Fullterm Newborn Infant.* Little Club Clinics in Developmental Medicine, No. 12. The Spastics Society. London, Heinemann, 1964.

Provence, S., and Lipton, R.C.: *Infants in Institutions.* New York, International U. P., 1962.

Rood, M.S.: Neurophysiological reactions as a basis for physical therapy. *Phys Ther Rev, 34:*444-449, 1954.

Rood, M.S.: Neurophysiological mechanisms utilized in the treatment of neuromuscular dysfunction. *Amer J Occup Ther,* Part 2 *10:*4, pp. 220-225, 1956.

Rood, M.S.: Eleanor Clarke Slagle Lecture: Every one counts. *Amer J Occup Ther, 12:*326-329, 1958.

Rood, M.S.: The use of sensory receptors to activate, facilitate, and inhibit motor response, autonomic and somatic in developmental sequence. In Sattely, C. (Ed.): *Approaches to Treatment of Patients with Neuromuscular Dysfunction.* Study Course VI, Third International Congress, World Federation of Occupational Therapists, 26-37. Dubuque, Iowa, W. C. Brown, 1962.

Rood, M.: P.T. 511, Neurophysiology in the Treatment of Neuromuscular Dysfunction, 1960. P.T. 521, Neurophysiological Response Mechanisms in Therapy, 1963. Unpublished notes from University of Southern California.

Schilder, P.: *Contributions to Developmental Neuropsychiatry.* Bender, Lauretta (Ed.). New York, International U. P., 1964.

Sherrington, S.C.: *The Integrative Action of the Nervous System.* New Haven, Yale, 1906.

Sloan, W.: The Lincoln-Oseretsky Motor Development Scale. *Genet Psychol Monogr, 51:*183-252, 1955.

Stockmeyer, S.: An interpretation of the approach of Rood to the treatment of neuromuscular dysfunction. *Amer J Phys Med, 46:*900-956, 1967.

Twitchell, T.E.: Normal motor development. *J Amer Phys Ther Ass, 45:* 419-423, 1965.

Vassella, F., and Karlsson, B.: Asymmetric tonic neck reflex. *Develop Med Child Neurol, 4:*363-369, 1962.

Willson, M.A.: Use of a developmental inventory as a chart of progress. *J Amer Ther Ass, 49:*19-32, 1969.

SELECTED BIBLIOGRAPHY

American Association on Mental Deficiency and Mental Retardation Branch, Division of Chronic Diseases, Public Health Service, Department of Health, Education, and Welfare. Role of Physical Therapy in Mental Retardation. Proceedings of Workshop for Physical Therapists, May 9-10, 1966.

Berkson, G.: Stereotyped movements of mental defectives. V. Ward behavior and its relationship to an experimental task. *Amer J. Ment Defic,* *69*:253-264, 1964.

Francis, R.J., and Rarick, G.L.: Motor characteristics of the mentally retarded. *Amer J Ment Defic, 63*:792-811, 1959.

Gesell, A., and Ames, L.B.: The ontogenetic organization of prone behavior in human infancy. *J Gen Psychol, 56*:247-263, 1940.

Ingram, T.T.S.: A characteristic form of overactive behavior in brain-damaged children. *J Ment Sci, 102*:550-558, 1956.

Nunley, R.L.: A physical fitness program for the mentally retarded in the public schools. *J Amer Phys Ther Ass, 45*:946-954, 1965.

Nunley, R.L.: The physical therapist at home with the mentally retarded. *J Amer Phys Ther Ass, 47*:926-932, 1967.

Schaltenbrand, G.: The development of human motility and motor disturbances. *Neurol and Psychiat, 20*:720-730, 1928.

Zuk, G.H.: Overattention to moving stimuli as a factor in the distractibility of retarded and brain-injured children. *Train Sch Bull, 29*:150-160, 1963.

Chapter Five

PROPRIOCEPTIVE NEUROMUSCULAR FACILITATION: THE PNF METHOD

Dorothy E. Voss

A method of exercise for the child with central nervous system deficit, including perceptual deficits and mental retardation, will be effective insofar as it is based upon principles derived from normal motor development including developmental aspects of motor learning and insofar as the procedures or techniques of the method are based in neurophysiology and can be used to enhance motor learning. The method known as "proprioceptive facilitation" (Kabat and Knott 1953) or as "proprioceptive neuromuscular facilitation" (Knott and Voss 1968) was first used in the treatment of patients having cerebral palsy, although its use was very soon extended to the treatment of many types of patients having neuromuscular disabilities.

The treatment of children whose development has been arrested or impaired requires that emphasis be given to the developmental aspects of the approach. The developmental aspects are grounded in normal motor behavior. Some of the guide lines which are used in treatment can be related to or drawn from studies of animal behavior (which were carried out to further understanding of human behavior); others are clearly based in normal human development.

Beyond the developmental aspects, the approach includes specific procedures which can be used to promote motor learning, some of which can be used without the patient's voluntary effort, and some of which are more dependent upon the cooperation of the patient. The specific procedures may be used singly, or may be combined as necessary according to the needs and abilities of the patient.

Note: Partial support for the preparation of this chapter was provided by the Physical Therapy Fund, Inc., 1156 15th Street, N.W., Washington, D.C. 20005.

Application of the method, as with any method, requires that an assessment of the child be made, and that treatment be designed for the individual child. Assessment reveals the level of the child's ability, his specific abilities and disabilities, and how he organizes his abilities toward success or failure. Assessment tells us where to begin. We have then to select appropriate activities and appropriate procedures so as to favorably influence his motor behavior, and, hopefully, to improve his ability to function at the highest possible level in keeping with his potential.

Guide Lines from Animal Behavior

Numerous researches by physiologists and experimental psychologists have had a singleness of purpose: to contribute to understanding of the human species, of how the central nervous system functions and of how learning occurs. A superficial consideration of only a fragment of the work done yields certain broad guide lines for the treatment of the child having central nervous system deficit with or without mental retardation.

In stating that "it takes more than a baby and a box to make a normal monkey," Harlow (1960) implied that the infant monkey had experienced normal prenatal development. While observations of developing animal behavior, of the responses of animals to various learning situations and to alteration in the environment, add to our knowledge of developing human behavior, the hazard of direct extrapolation is usually expressed. Few would deny, however, that it takes *more than* a normally developed human infant and a crib (or a playpen) to make a normal adult. Studies conducted with animals reveal some of the "more thans" that have to do with the promotion of development and of learning.

Levine's studies of infant rats and their responses to stress imposed through handling and electrical shock showed that stress promotes maturation (Levine 1960, 1962). Infant rats subjected to either form of stress developed more rapidly in all respects than did those that were not handled and were not stimulated by electrical shock. The infant rats who were subjected to stress became normal active adults. They explored their surroundings and defecated and urinated less frequently than did those rats which were not handled as infants and which as adults crouched in a corner. Normal prenatal development can be assumed, and it took "more than" a nest to make a normal adult rat.

According to Harlow and Harlow (1962) in a discussion of principles of primate learning, the monkey becomes able to solve increasingly complex problems as he grows older. This progressive improvement is a matter of maturation and not of learning by practice. The sequence from simple to complex is conditioned responses, ability to discriminate between objects, ability to transfer information from one problem to another, and ability to solve quite complex problems requiring concept formation. Learning ability in infant monkeys increases progressively with age over a considerable period of time. Once an ability matures, it is retained without exercise. As learning ability is taxed by complex problems, the individual can learn the more difficult tasks through the use of "stepwise procedures" and carefully planned training schedules. These workers pointed out that for each species and for each individual within a species there is a limiting line, or asymptote, of ability, the point beyond which no learning occurs in spite of training procedures. In the Harlows' studies the infant monkeys were responsive to shock stimulus in conditioning procedures and to rewards (food) in more complex problem solving. Again, it can be assumed that these infant monkeys had experienced normal prenatal development. Most of these infants were separated from their mothers at birth, but their experiences were not limited to those provided by the environment of a "box."

Pavlov (1927) in his writing on conditioned reflexes stated that "It is obvious that the different kinds of habits based on training, education, and discipline of any sort are nothing but a long chain of conditioned reflexes." Pavlov's original concept that the cerebral cortex is the essential organ for conditioned learning has been modified according to Buchwald (1965) who stated that "While the cortex is considered important in facilitating motor learning, it is not essential for the development of simple conditioned responses." Buchwald (1965) pointed out that brain, spinal cord, and feedback mechanisms all make important contributions to motor learning, and that proprioceptive feedback plays a significant role in simple conditioned responses. Furthermore, the learning capacity following deletion of any part of the nervous system (deafferentation to cortical ablation) varies between species and according to the age of an individual within a species. Following deletion of the cortex, simple motor acts can be learned but more complex acts requiring discrimination of sensory cues cannot. For learning to occur, appropriate methods of training must be paired with the available nervous mechanisms. Again, in the many studies cited by Buchwald, the kittens and cats and other animals used as subjects doubtlessly had experienced normal prenatal development. Too, they were subjected to many repetitions of the appropriate stimulus in an appropriate environment.

Studies by Travis and Woolsey (1956) revealed the monkey's ability to recover motor function and to learn "to care for himself again" following ablation of cortical areas. Mature, normal monkeys were used as subjects. In the postoperative care of these monkeys, "more than a box" was used to promote recovery. The animals were not permitted to remain in the postures they preferred; they were placed in various positions. They were handled and were given "passive exercise" through full ranges of trunk and limb musculature. They were assisted in the performance of motor acts for which some capacity seemed to be present.

What is the "more than" which is necessary to development and learning in the human infant and child? The "more than" must include the wide range of sensory and social experience to which the normal infant is exposed. The range includes contact with and handling by the mother, stimulation of the special senses by light, sound, and odor, and opportunity to explore an ever-expanding environment. The environment and experiences are not limited to a physical setting and a collection of toys. Interaction with mother, father, siblings, and playmates provides frequent stimulation through handling. Handling ranges from comforting to bouncing and trouncing, from situations which are stressless to those which are stressful.

What broad guide lines for treatment can be drawn from these studies on development and learning? The following are some of them:

1. An understanding of normal behavior is necessary to the understanding of deficient behavior. (In these studies normal individuals were used as a kind of basic control.)

2. Stress promotes maturation and learning. (These studies involved the use of stressful stimuli ranging from handling and electrical shock to the presentation of choices.)

3. Stress promotes the capacity for exploration of the environment. (Levine's rats which were handled or shocked explored their surroundings; the nonhandled rats crouched in a corner.)

4. Stress promotes recovery after trauma to the cortex. (Travis and Woolsey relied upon handling to hasten recovery of motor function.)

5. Learning is a feature of development and maturation; the capacity to solve increasingly complex problems also matures. (Harlow and Harlow found that learning occurred at an optimum rate when the task was appropriate for the age.)

6. Learning that is coupled with maturation has a motor component. (The monkeys studied by Harlow and Harlow were engaged in motor acts.)

7. Conditioning of responses is the simplest form of learning and would seem the most appropriate for the immature. (Harlow and Harlow classified conditional responses as the simplest form. Pavlov indicated the importance of conditioning of reflexes in the formation of habit patterns. Buchwald's discussion tells us that the interplay of neural mechanisms is not simple and that methods of training must be geared to the available nervous mechanisms.)

8. Learning to solve complex problems which tax the learner's ability can be facilitated by the use of progression and carefully planned training. (Harlow and Harlow used "stepwise procedures" in training when the individual was unable to master the total problem as a whole.)

9. Learning, or the ability to learn, is an intraindividual characteristic. Each individual has his limitation beyond which he cannot proceed. (Harlow and Harlow indicated that there is

a limiting line for each individual. Buchwald pointed out that capacities for learning, or for relearning, vary from individual to individual, especially in terms of age.)

These guide lines are "built-in" features of the development of the normal infant and child. The "normal" parent (whether cat or human) of the "normal" child (kitten or human) understands something of normal motor development and behavior. The infant is coddled but is also subjected to stress. The infant and child are conditioned in many ways. The child is permitted and encouraged to explore and to experience new situations. The child is "shown" how to perform more difficult tasks. The child is led toward independence in appropriate ways at appropriate times.

Guide Lines from Human Behavior

The guide lines drawn from animal behavior are compatible with the concepts of proprioceptive neuromuscular facilitation. Because human beings vary from other species both as to structure and function, additional guide lines may and must be drawn from observable events in human development. Overlapping will be evident and many of these guide lines could be drawn from animal behavior as well. Underlying all guide lines, or principles, and treatment itself is the belief that *all* human beings have potentials that have not been fully developed.

1. Normal development, structure and function, proceeds in a cervicocaudal and in a proximodistal direction (Hooker 1952, McGraw 1962, Gesell and Amatruda 1947). In treatment, the direction of development is heeded. Attention is directed toward activity and development of the superior region, head and neck, upper trunk, shoulder-girdle and upper extremities in order that this region may lead and favorably influence the inferior region. In the inferior region emphasis is given to movements of the pelvis and hips before becoming specifically engrossed with movements of feet and ankles.

2. Developing fetal behavior is characterized by a sequence of reflexive responses to exteroceptive stimulation (Hooker 1952). The sequence reflects expansion of the receptive area, and thus

the expansion of responses in keeping with the direction of development, and the derivation of individuated patterns, or localized responses, from total patterns. The sequence reflects that flexion precedes extension (head and neck); extension of shoulders is combined with flexion of head and neck; adduction precedes abduction of shoulder; internal rotation precedes external rotation; hand-closing precedes hand-opening; plantar flexion precedes dorsiflexion of foot; and participation of thumb and hallux lags or appears later than does that of other digits. Whereas in the beginning the response to a unilateral perioral stimulus is a turning of the face away from the stimulus, the response becomes that of turning toward the stimulus. The sequence in which movements of lips, tongue, sucking, and swallowing appear is apparent and has been summarized (Twitchell 1965). In treatment, where deficiency is profound, the reflexogenic sequence provides a guide as to which movements may be elicited first, and clues as to the developmental level of the patient.

3. Early motor behavior is dominated by reflex activity (Hooker 1952, McGraw 1962). Mature motor behavior is reinforced or supported by postural reflex mechanisms (Hellebrandt et al. 1962, Hellebrandt and Waterland 1962). In treatment, where deficiency is profound, reflexes are stimulated to initiate movement and to promote postural control. Wherever possible, reflex mechanisms are harnessed to promote and reinforce voluntary effort.

4. Developing motor behavior is intertwined with developing sensation and the development of the special senses or distance receptors, visual and auditory (Gesell and Amatruda 1947). Vision and hearing give direction to movement; movement proceeds toward the stimulus in approach or pursuit, or away from the stimulus in avoidance or withdrawal. In mature motor behavior volition may modify responses to stimulation of the special senses. In treatment, tactual, visual, and auditory cues are used to promote the desired response and to reinforce the patient's voluntary effort.

5. Early motor behavior is characterized by spontaneous and rhythmical movements through full ranges or extremes of flexion

and extension (McGraw 1962). This characteristic reversal of direction of movement is used throughout life. In treatment, reversing movements are used to establish interaction between antagonistic movements, reflexes, and muscle groups.

6. Developing motor behavior is expressed in an orderly sequence of total patterns of movement and posture (McGraw 1962, Gesell and Amatruda 1947). Most infants and children proceed through the various stages rather than bypassing several activities (Ames 1966). Mature motor behavior includes these total patterns in the vast repertoire of motor acts; total patterns may be used at will. Movement and posture are adjusted as necessary to the task at hand and both have their dynamic aspects. The ability to maintain posture matures so that while posture is readily disturbed for agility in movement, responses to disturbance by external forces are quite predictable. Equilibrium reactions have been identified as having proprioceptive components and labyrinthine components (Weisz 1938). Slow disturbance elicits proprioceptive responses; quick disturbance elicits labyrinthine responses. The responses are in keeping with the quality and rate of disturbance. In treatment, the developmental progression of total patterns is followed with the recognition that each phase, including acts of assumption and maintenance of posture, must contribute to the organization of the whole (Gesell 1954).

7. Developing motor behavior is characterized by the combining of extremity movements in increasingly complex ways (Gesell and Amatruda 1947): bilateral, symmetrical, ipsilateral, and bilateral asymmetrical, alternating reciprocal, and diagonal reciprocal. Throughout life, movements are combined in these basic ways with selectivity as to range, rate, and intensity. In treatment, movements are combined for organization of a total pattern of movement, and for reinforcement of deficient movements by more effective movements. In a total pattern, all component movements, or individual patterns, contribute to the direction of the total pattern.

8. The growth of motor behavior has cyclic trends which result in the organization and reciprocal interweaving of opposing

or antagonistic functions (Ames 1966). These trends include shifts between flexor dominance and extensor dominance of total patterns of posture and movement (Gesell and Amatruda 1947). The rocking movements observable in the normal child (McGraw 1962) promote reciprocalness. In mature motor behavior, shifts between flexor and extensor dominance are used as necessary to the motor act. In treatment, total patterns may be initiated with flexor dominance or with extensor dominance. Dominance is altered by changing direction (creeping forward, flexor dominance; creeping backward, extensor dominance). More advanced patterns have flexor phases and extensor phases which depend upon ability to shift dominance. (Rising to standing from sitting requires that flexion be used to initiate the total pattern and that extension be used to assume an upright position.)

9. Developing motor behavior reflects a sequence as to direction of movement which is apparent in developing vision, eye-hand coordination, vocalization, percept-concept formation, and postural behavior (Gesell 1954). The sequence is from vertical (representing flexion and extension) to horizontal (representing adduction and abduction) circular (representing rotation), and oblique (representing combined vertical and horizontal and circular or combining flexion or extension with adduction or abduction and rotary components). Thus, movements in an oblique or diagonal direction are the most advanced. Mature motor behavior permits selectivity as to direction with the combining of components as necessary. In treatment, total patterns, such as those of prone progression, are performed in all appropriate directions: forward, backward, sideward to left and right, turning in a circle, and diagonally forward and backward toward the left and toward the right. Performance of a total pattern in a diagonal direction requires use of the spiral and diagonal patterns of proprioceptive neuromuscular facilitation (Voss 1967).

10. Mature motor behavior is characterized by selectivity in voluntary and skilled movement. The normal person is selective as to the motor acts he undertakes. He selects an appropriate posture, selects appropriate combinations of movements, selects the direction of the movement, selects the rate, the degree of

effort, and the range of movement. As he learns a skill, his movements become stereotyped and selectivity becomes automatic; he no longer needs to give his full attention to the motor aspects of a task. In treatment, selectivity is promoted by the performance of many combinations of movement. In the training of a skill, repetition is used to promote automatic use of appropriate movements so that attention need not be centered on the motor aspects of the task.

These guide lines, as with those drawn from studies of animal behavior, are built-in features of normal motor development. The normal infant and child in a normal environment may reflect individual differences as to rate of maturation and as to variations in motor performance. Nevertheless, by the time he is mature, his motor behavior is essentially normal.

In summary, the guide lines drawn from studies of animal behavior are primarily concerned with learning and include factors that can be used to promote motor learning. The guide lines drawn from studies of human behavior are primarily concerned with motor-learning aspects of development or the growth of motor behavior. They include factors which must be considered if the handicapped child, whether mentally retarded or not, is to be led along the path that leads toward mature motor behavior. Many of the guide lines from animal behavior and from human behavior are universally followed; others are more specifically used in the method of proprioceptive neuromuscular facilitation. They reflect features which are unique and which distinguish this method from others.

Unique Features of the PNF Method

The first unique feature is the *concept of human motion* which is inherent to the method. The spiral and diagonal patterns of facilitation were first referred to by Kabat as "mass movement patterns" (Kabat and Knott 1953) and more recently have been termed "irradiation patterns" (Kabat 1961). These patterns of facilitation, or irradiation patterns, are specific movements wherein each joint of a body segment contributes three components of motion. That is, flexion and extension are combined with abduction and with adduction, and with external *or* internal rotation.

In the upper extremity, with the scapulohumeral joint as the frame of reference, external rotation is always combined with flexion, and internal rotation with extension. In the lower extremity, with the hip joint as the frame of reference, external rotation is always combined with adduction and internal rotation with abduction. The patterns of facilitation with their spiral and diagonal characteristics may be observed in sports activities where skill and power are demanded (for example, in serving a tennis ball and in the arm and leg movements of a highly skilled baseball pitcher). As stated in the guide lines on direction of movement, the patterns become evident when a total pattern such as creeping, or walking, is performed in a diagonal direction. Diagonal, or oblique, direction is the most advanced in the sequence of development as pointed out by Gesell (1954).

The patterns of facilitation permit easy elicitation of stretch reflexes because the topographically related groups of muscles are subjected to maximum tension when a segment is positioned in the extreme lengthened range of the desired or agonistic pattern. The lengthened range of the agonistic pattern is the shortened range of the antagonistic pattern. Thus as movement proceeds from lengthened toward shortened range, the antagonistic pattern is subjected to stretch and is thereby prepared to respond. This sequence of events occurs in normal motor acts which require reversal of direction. In treatment the stretch reflex is used to initiate movement in the agonistic pattern and to promote inhibition or relaxation of the antagonistic pattern. The patterns have been analyzed as to major muscle components and components of joint motion and have been described by Knott and Voss (1968).

A second unique feature is the *training of coordination* within patterns of a segment and between segments. Coordination is fostered through the use of timed sequence of muscle contraction (Knott and Voss 1968). That is, in the freely moving segment the sequence is from distal to proximal; in the stable segment the sequence is from proximal to distal. Coordination between segments is promoted by combining movements of the segments in keeping with those of normal motor development: bilateral symmetrical, ipsilateral, bilateral asymmetrical, alternating reciprocal (upper or lower extremities), and diagonal reciprocal (four extremities). The coordination, or organization, of a total pattern is promoted by combining appropriate patterns in appropriate ways so that each component pattern contributes to the direction of the total pattern at an appropriate time. The coordination of component patterns is considered in the analysis of motor performance and in the planning of a treatment program.

The third unique feature is the *use of maximal resistance* and adjusted resistance to promote irradiation of impulses within a pattern, and from head and neck and trunk to the extremities, or in a reverse sequence. The technique used to promote irradiation within a pattern is referred to as timing for emphasis. Promotion of irradiation from one segment to another is referred to as reinforcement although timing is a necessary ingredient of the procedure (Knott and Voss 1968). Irradiation and reinforcement occur in normal motor acts performed under stress. The sequence of events within a segment has been studied by Gellhorn (1947). Patterning of irradiation beyond the moving segment has been observed by Hellebrandt, Schade and Carns (1962) and by Hellebrandt and Waterland (1962).

A fourth unique feature is the *battery of techniques* or procedures which are superimposed upon movement or posture to enhance performance and to promote motor learning. These techniques have been described most completely by Knott and Voss (1968). The patient's voluntary effort is enlisted insofar as it is possible. If a patient is unable to cooperate, or prefers not to do so, use of positioning, manual contacts for handling, stretch, traction and approximation, and resistance can be used to promote the desired response. Handling appropriately provides the stress necessary to enhance movement or posture, the ability to move and the ability to maintain a position.

The fifth feature which seems unique is the *use of tone of voice* to increase or decrease stress. According to Buchwald (1967), tones of moderate intensity can easily evoke gamma motoneuron activity and louder tones can alter alpha motoneuron activity. In treatment, loud tones of voice are used to promote movement; softer tones are used to encourage stability. In this method of treatment, the "quiet" atmosphere, which has prevailed in the traditional methods used with children who have cerebral palsy, is not a standard rule. The needs of the child determine the tone of voice to be used.

ASSESSMENT OF MOTOR PERFORMANCE

The developmental scale as outlined by Gesell (Gesell and Amatruda 1947) has been used almost universally for evaluation of the child with central nervous system deficit. Thereby the child's achievements in terms of his chronological age may be determined. Attempts to design a test which permits accurate measurement of minimal degrees of progress have often resulted in rating scales patterned after manual muscle testing (Daniels et al. 1956). Such a scale has been devised by Zausmer and Tower (1966). Factors of "quality of performance, independence, speed and endurance" are used as criteria. In this test, and in the vast majority of others, emphasis is centered on achievement.

McGraw's studies (1962) extended beyond the listing of achievements and identified the changing form and configuration of total patterns of movement and posture from initial stages to mature or stable forms. Achievement is but one factor. Organization of motor behavior has to do with how the child coordinates or organizes his movements, how he combines component patterns in the performance of a total pattern. McGraw's observations as

Note: Illustrations included in "Assessment of Motor Performance," and in "Primary Problems and Suggested Procedures," present two children. The first child (Figs. 5-1, 5-3, 5-4–5-9) was, at the time of photography, four years of age. The diagnosis is spastic diplegia of lower extremities with mild spasticity of upper extremities as the result of head injury.

The second child (Figs. 5-2 and 5-10–5-14) was, at the time of photography, 45 months of age. The diagnosis is choreo-athetosis secondary to erythroblastosis with profound deafness.

The series of illustrations should not be interpreted as reflecting an appropriate program for either child. These children were used only to illustrate selected points. Therefore, complete case histories are not included nor are specific comments made as to the programs of treatment and progress made.

to the quality of performance, the sequence from automatic to deliberate use become, it would seem, important in the assessment and treatment of children with central nervous system deficit, especially those with mental retardation.

Gesell's observations (1947) of flexor dominance and extensor dominance and of reciprocal interweaving are of value in the analysis of movement and posture. Flexor and extensor dominance have to do with directionality of movement as well as with the configuration of posture.

According to this method of treatment organization of total patterns is assessed in terms of ability to do the following:

1. Respond to visual, auditory, and tactual cues.
2. Move in timed sequence leading with the superior region of body—head and neck, upper trunk, and upper extremities, and with the inferior region—lower trunk and lower extremities. (The dorsolumbar junction is the frame of reference for division of superior and inferior regions.)
3. Move in all possible directions, forward and backward, sideward, circular, and diagonal.
4. Initiate movement with flexor dominance and with extensor dominance as related to direction of movement, and to shift dominance as related to acts of assumption and maintenance of upright postures.
5. Select and combine appropriate patterns of facilitation so that the total pattern is reinforced in regard to direction.
6. Sustain a total pattern of posture and combine mobility with stability as necessary for a total pattern of movement.

Sensory Cues

As with any method, observation of the child's responses to sensory stimuli appropriate to his age yields information useful in the identification of specific problems. This information provides clues as to what extent vision, hearing, and tactual sensation can be relied upon to favorably influence movement and posture, and conversely, clues as to which total patterns and which patterns of facilitation need emphasis in order to enhance responses. The following questions in no way replace tests for vision, hearing, and sensation; they simply may help to assess the child's coordination of sensory input as a means for reinforcement of movement and posture.

VISION. Questions include the following:

1. Do the eyes follow an object moved in all possible directions? As the object is moved through extreme ranges, does the head proceed in the same direction?

Eye Movements	Related Head and Neck Movements
Downward	Flexion
Upward	Extension
Lateralward, L/R	Rotation, L/R (chin to shoulder)
Oblique, upward, L/R	Diagonal, extension to L/R
Oblique, downward, R/L	Diagonal, flexion to R/L

Note: Oblique upward movement toward left is antagonistic to oblique downward movement toward right. Because oblique diagonal movements are the most advanced, eye movements should be assessed in the suggested sequence.

2. Can movement of the eyes be facilitated by placing the related head and neck pattern in the lengthened range? Does the use of stretch and resistance stimulate eyes to lead movement of head?* (See Fig. 5-1.)

Comment on vision: In the performance of total patterns, eyes should lead movements of head and neck. Eye movements reinforce and are reinforced by related head and neck patterns. Failure of the eyes to participate will distort or delay performance of a total pattern.

HEARING. The following are important questions:

1. Do the eyes, head and neck move toward an enticing auditory stimulus of moderate tone, and away from the threatening stimulus louder in tone? Is the startle response (Moro reflex) hyperactive in view of chronological age?

2. Is the child able to follow spoken instructions for perform-

---

*If, for example, the left eye maintains a posture which is inward toward the nose, it is the following eye during head and neck rotation from left to right while the right eye leads. First resisting head and neck rotation to the right may prompt the left eye to lead during resisted head and neck rotation to the left. (The antagonistic pattern, to right, was resisted first for stimulation of the agonistic pattern, to the left.) Head and neck rotation to the left is the pattern in need of emphasis through repetition so that the left eye moves lateralward to the left.

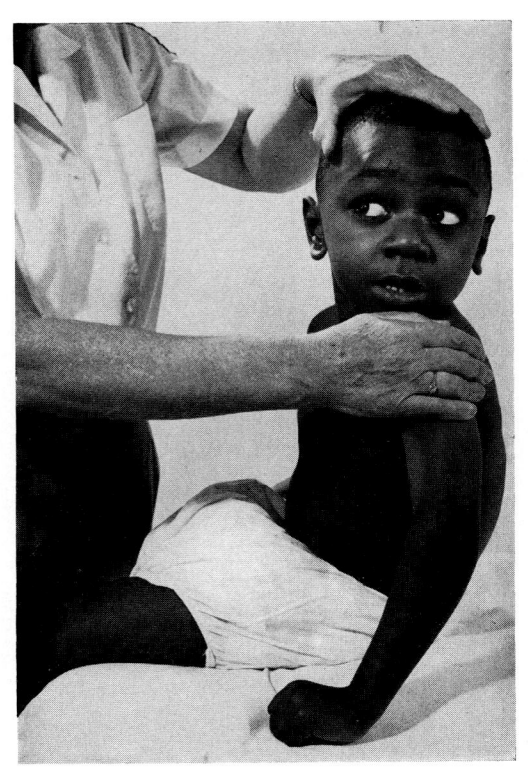

Figure 5-1. Head and neck rotation to the left is the lengthened range of head and neck rotation to the right. Eyes move laterally toward right as stretch and resistance are used to facilitate head movement to right. Test may be performed in any position, supine or prone, that permits the desired movement to occur. Note that here and in Figure 5-3 extensor tone prevents assumption of erect sitting.

ance of a motor act? Can he follow brief commands appropriate to his chronological age and appropriate for his level of motor ability?

3. If the desired motor response is facilitated by use of pressure, stretch, and resistance, does the child then respond more readily to verbal commands?

Comment on hearing: If the child does not respond to auditory stimuli, then visual, tactual, and proprioceptive stimuli must be used for communication and for training of the ability to follow spoken instructions and commands.

TACTILITY. These questions are important:

1. Do the eyes, head and neck move toward or away from appropriate tactile stimuli? With the child supine, areas to be touched include midline near umbilicus, anterior surfaces of shoulders and thigh, palms of hands, and soles of feet, in turn from left to right.

2. Does deeper pressure with repetitive stretching of underlying muscles attract attention of the eyes, or withdrawal from the stimulus with overt movement of the segment? (See Fig. 5-2.)

Comment on tactility: If tactile responses are deficient, the use of visual and proprioceptive stimuli becomes of great importance. Developmentally and functionally, these mechanisms are interrelated. One may be used to influence the other.

Timed Sequence of Movement

The timing of movement is one of the most important ingredients of coordination. Mature coordination of a total pattern requires that head and neck lead, that upper extremities reach toward the goal and that lower extremities proceed toward the goal. Thus, the superior region leads and the inferior region supports the direction by following the superior region. While the inferior region may lead—as for example, in thrusting of the lower extremity against the surface to initiate rolling toward prone—such initiation is not acceptable as an only approach. Within the freely moving segment, movement is timed in a distal to proximal sequence. This is to say that in reaching for an object, the hand opens before the act is accomplished and not after the object has been approached.

Specific questions related to timed sequence include the following:

1. Do head and neck move in advance of the extremities?

2. Do upper extremities move in advance of the lower extremities?

3. When movements of intermediate joints (elbow and knee)

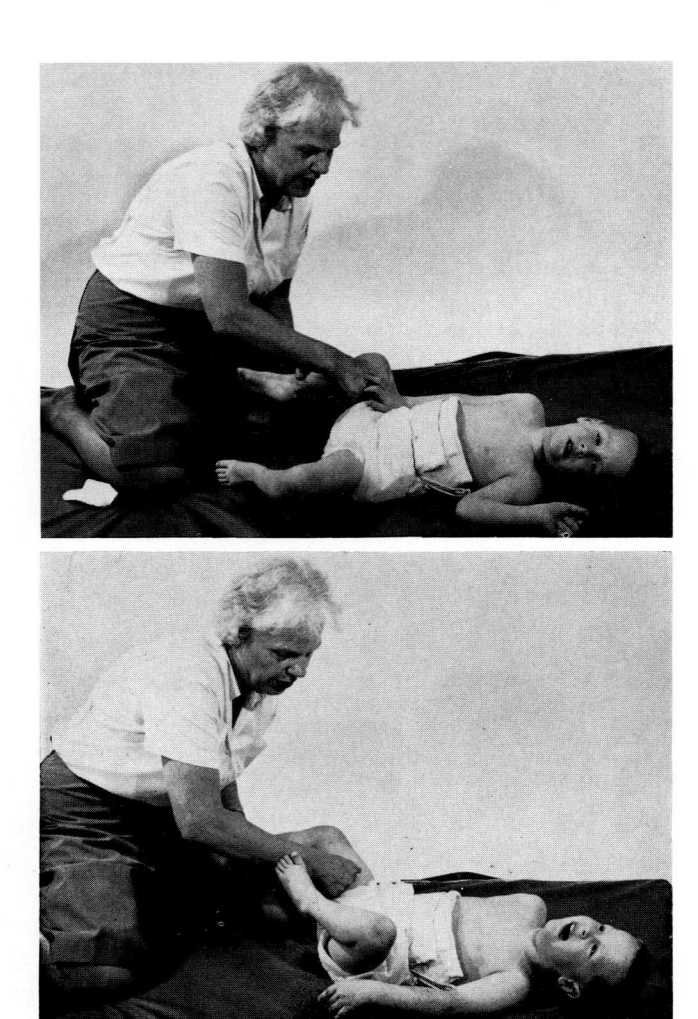

Figure 5-2. Use of varying degrees of repetitive manually applied pressure. *Top,* stimulus of moderate pressure prompts child to use right hand while eyes and head turn toward left in gesture of withdrawal from stimulus. *Bottom,* stimulus of more vigorous pressure elicits protest and an organized attempt to remove stimulus. Head and neck extend, which reinforces use of left foot; arms extend in a position for reinforcement. Note changing positions of head and neck: *Top,* partial rotation to left with eyes turned toward left; *Bottom,* extension toward left with eyes turned toward right. See Figures 5-10 through 5-12 and 5-14 and note that child's hands open when elbows are extended. When elbows are flexed, hands tend to close. Actually this child can voluntarily open and close his hands but his spontaneous responses are interesting.

are used, do distal parts (hand and foot) precede or follow? (See Fig. 5-3.)

4. When movements of intermediate joints are used, do proximal joints (shoulder and hip) follow, or does movement of elbow or knee proceed through range before shoulder and hip begin to participate?

5. Is interaction of segments smooth, or is there a lag or premature movement of one segment?

Direction—Flexor and Extensor Dominance

The normal child and the normal adult can move in all directions including forward, backward, sideward, in a circle, and diagonally forward and backward. In normal development there is a reciprocal interweaving of flexor and extensor dominance (Gesell and Amatruda 1947). In general, forward direction is flexor dominant; backward direction is extensor dominant. The rocking movements used by the developing child promote reciprocal interweaving in that in this activity the child "finds" his balance for a newly acquired posture (Fig. 5-4). In order to maintain posture, there must be a balanced antagonism between flexion and extension, between flexor and extensor reflexes. In mature motor behavior, dominance shifts as necessary to the performance of a total pattern.

Specific questions as to flexor and extensor dominance and direction of total patterns include the following:

1. Is the child able to move in all possible directions and in so doing, engage upper and lower extremities as necessary to the total movement?

2. Does the child move toward the left and toward the right in those total patterns which involve or permit sidedness?

3. In the assumption of an upright posture, does the child initiate with flexion and then adjust appropriately toward extension? Or, does he remain in a flexed posture?

Organization of Total Patterns

The sequence of developmental activities as used in this method have been described (Knott and Voss 1968, Voss 1967).

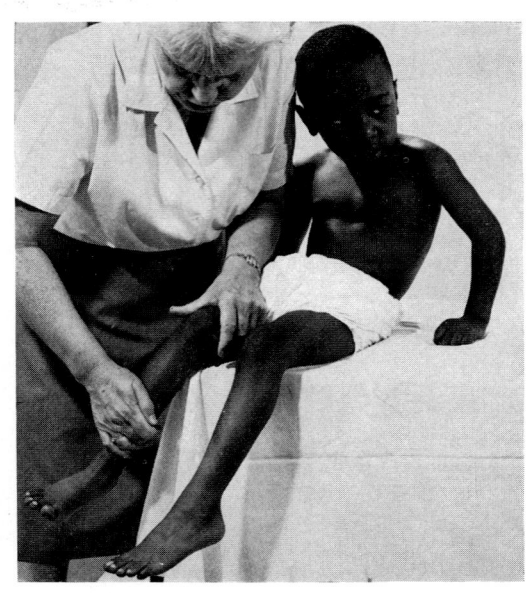

242   *Physical Therapy Services in the Developmental Disabilities*

Figure 5-3. Child attempts to extend knee against resistance. By restraining hip flexion and movement at the knee, dorsiflexion of foot and ankle occur. Child is not able to extend knee beyond this point because of dominant mass flexion and mass extension patterns; thus, when he tries to flex hip, knee flexes automatically. When he tries to extend hip, knee extends automatically. He has not learned the more advanced patterns wherein hip flexion is combined with knee extension, and hip extension is combined with knee flexion. Thus, he cannot maintain balance while kneeling because he cannot extend his hips while knees are flexed. In standing, his feet are plantar flexed. With braces maintaining feet in dorsiflexion, mass flexion of hip and knees results.

Timed sequences cannot be developed with this child in the sitting position; it is too advanced. See Figure 5-4 through 5-6 and 5-8 and note varying degrees of hip and knee flexion with dorsiflexion of foot and ankle in prone postures. See Figures 5-9 and 5-13 and note that in the lateral or side-lying position, lower extremities are in extension. The lateral position is favorable for flexion of the uppermost extremities and for extension of the undermost extremities. Yet, child's right lower extremity remains extended. There is need to promote use of the first diagonal (flexion-adduction external rotation pattern with knee flexion, Table 5-I) during rolling (Knott and Voss 1968, Voss 1967). This may be done by resisting at pelvis, for reinforcement, and at foot and ankle demanding dorsiflexion with flexion of hip and knee while undermost extremity extends appropriately. The total pattern of rolling from supine toward prone promotes de-

The sequence includes acts of assumption, posture or position, the various postures used for the development of balance, and modes of progression or locomotion. Flexor and extensor dominance have been ascribed according to direction. The eyes, head and neck give direction to the total pattern as the extremity movements are combined in appropriate ways. A sample of selected combinations of patterns of facilitation used for rolling, crawling, and creeping are summarized in Table 5-I. The combinations for plantigrade walking, an often neglected activity, and for upright walking are the same as for creeping.

Head and neck patterns are the key to the combining of extremity patterns. For example, the selected combinations for rolling from supine toward prone are designated by numbers, 1-4, which also indicate the relative ease of performance. Thus, head and neck rotation, 1, is the least difficult and is combined with the flexion-adduction external rotation patterns of the contralateral extremities, 1-C. The normal child acquires the ability to roll or to turn over using all of these combinations. If, in assessment of the handicapped child, it is learned that he can perform rolling toward prone only by using head and neck flexion with rotation, 3, with extension patterns of contralateral upper extremity, 3-C, the child is rolling with flexor dominance. The next combination to be attempted is head and neck rotation, 1, because rotation has a component of extension, and, finally, head and neck extension with rotation, 2. Whatever combination is available to the child is used at first. He is then led to performance of other combinations. Thus, in assessment, the place to begin is identified and the enlarging of the child's repertoire of combinations becomes a goal.

The various forms of combined extremity movements extend from those used in rolling to those used in bipedal or upright

---

velopment of reciprocation of lower extremities which is lacking in this child. When this pattern has been learned, first diagonal flexion may be performed with knee extension (hip flexes, ankle dorsiflexes), a more advanced combination. Then, after the advanced combination is developed in this *less* advanced posture or position, the child should be more able to perform the desired movement.

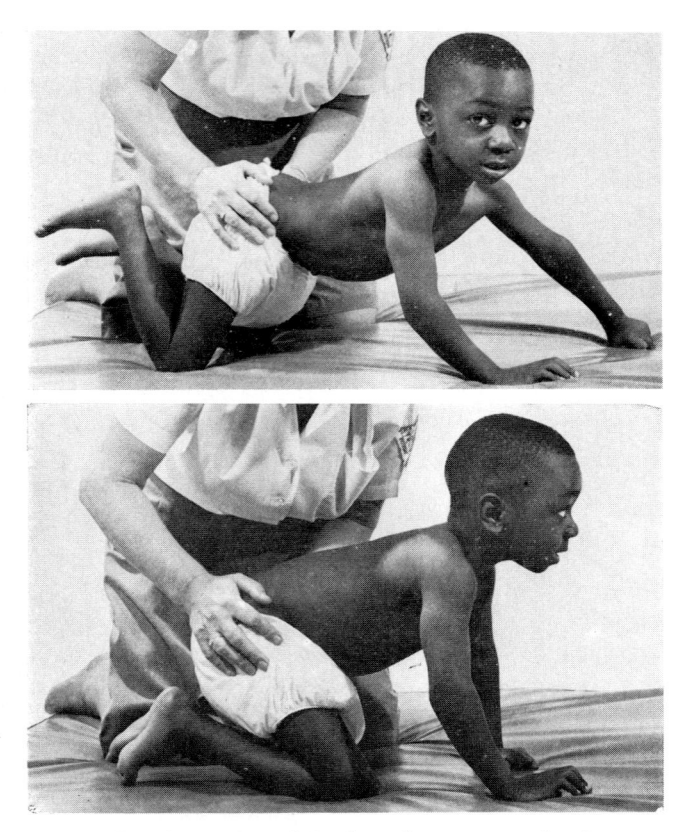

244 *Physical Therapy Services in the Developmental Disabilities*

Figure 5-4. Rocking forward and backward promotes development of balance. Resistance is given at pelvis but alternatives include resistance with manual contacts at head or at shoulders. Therapist must then take a position at child's head.

This child does not rock adequately. Symmetric tonic neck reflex dominates so that flexion of hips and knees fails to release as he attempts rocking forward *(Top)*; rocking backward *(Bottom)* is done easily. Actually, child is able to creep forward. He is not able to creep backward, nor sideward, nor in a diagonal direction. See also Figure 5-8 regarding child creeping in diagonal direction and position of therapist. To improve ability to rock with inferior region of body participating, head and neck flexion should be resisted during rocking backward *(Top)* into total flexion; head and neck extension should be resisted during rocking forward *(Bottom)* toward total extension. Adversive rotation of superior and inferior regions (Fig. 5-10) may be a useful preliminary activity.

TABLE 5-I
TOTAL PATTERNS PERFORMED WITH SELECTED AND
APPROPRIATE COMBINATIONS OF PATTERNS OF FACILITATION

Patterns of Facilitation	Total Patterns				
	Rolling			Crawling†	Creeping‡
	Toward Prone	Toward Supine			
Head and neck Rotation	1	1		1-forward direction, head *rotates* side to side	1-diagonal direction, head and neck *extension* with *rotation* in direction of total pattern
Extension with rotation	2		2, 3	2-circular pivot, head *rotates* in direction of pivot	2-as in 1
Flexion with rotation	3, 4				
Upper extremity First diagonal					
Flex.-add. ext.rot.	1-C, 2-C	1-I	3-B(C)	2-Cb	1-Cb, 2-Cc
Ext.-abd. int. rot.		4-B(I)			
Second Diagonal					
Flex.-abd. ext.rot.			2-I, 3-B(I)	1-Ia, 2-Ia	1-Ia, 2-Ia
Ext.-add. int.rot.	3-C, 4-B(C)				
Lower extremity* First diagonal					
Flex.-add. ext.rot.	1-C, 2-C, 3-C, 4-C	1-I, 2-I, 3-I			1-Cb, 2-Cb
Ext.-abd. int.rot.					
Second diagonal					
Flex-abd. int.rot.		4-B(I)		1-Ia, 2-Ca,b	1-Ia, 2-Id
Ext.-add. ext.rot.			3-B(C)	2-I, inactive	

Key: 1-4 denote extremity patterns as combined with head and neck patterns.
C—Contralateral extremity; I—Ipsilateral extremity; B—Bilateral asymmetrical combination.
a—d denote sequence for extremity patterns during prone progression, initial phases.
*The first diagonal of the lower extremity is used in rolling but is not used in crawling. The second diagonal of the lower extremity is not used in rolling unless both lower extremities move in bilateral asymmetrical combination; it is used in crawling.
†In 1, ipsilateral extremities flex, while contralateral extremities extend. In 2, the contralateral lower extremity flexes (a), then extends (b) while the ipsilateral lower extremity is relatively inactive.
‡In 1, ipsilateral extremities move together, homolateral pattern. In 2, extremity patterns are combined for diagonal reciprocation, cross pattern.

walking. Their use extends throughout normal motor development with the symmetric tonic neck reflex supporting symmetrical postures and movement, and with the asymmetric tonic neck reflex supporting ipsilateral and asymmetrical movements and postures. Their use extends beyond normal motor behavior into the combining forms from which various crutch-gait patterns and supported walking patterns are derived. An analysis of commonly used crutch-gait patterns (Buchwald 1952, Deaver and Brown 1945, 1946) is presented in Table 5-II.

Thus, the assessment of motor performance includes *organization* of total patterns as well as achievement. Those combinations which are present will be reflected in each total pattern that the child attempts. This is to say that if, for example, a child is limited to ipsilateral combinations, he will be able to roll but cannot use bilateral symmetrical and asymmetrical combinations. He will crawl and creep with ipsilateral combinations and if walking is attempted, he will use ipsilateral combinations rather than using symmetrical or reciprocal combinations. He relies upon the asymmetric tonic neck reflex for support.

Mobility and Stability

Coordinate movement and the ability to maintain or sustain posture are complementary abilities. An immobile state may reflect a kind of stability but it is stability without purpose. Mobility without stability also reflects lack of purpose. Mobility and stability as features of normal motor behavior become interwoven in the developmental process from elevation of head and control in the prone posture to standing on one foot in the upright posture. Assessment of motor performance should reveal the ability or inability to move and the ability or inability to stabilize. Both abilities are essential ingredients of any motor act whether it be one of locomotion, assumption of a position, or a manipulative skill.

Specific questions to be answered as to acts of assumption and maintenance of posture include the following:

1. Does the child organize an act of assumption of a position

TABLE 5-II
CRUTCH-GAIT PATTERNS: COMBINING MOVEMENTS

Name	Sequence	Combining Movements (and Quality of Movement)
Swing-to[1]	Both crutches; then, feet clear floor and then contact floor between crutches (tripod initially)	Bilateral symmetrical of upper extremities; bilateral symmetrical of lower extremities (deliberate to moderately rhythmical)
Swing-through[1]	Both crutches; then, feet clear floor and then contact floor in front of crutches (tripod, then reverse tripod)	Bilateral symmetrical of upper extremities; bilateral symmetrical of lower extremities (moderately rhythmical to rhythmical)
Two point Amputation[2]	Right crutch and right foot simultaneously; then, left crutch and left foot simultaneously	Alternating ipsilateral of left extremities, then of right extremities (deliberate to moderately rhythmical)
Three point[2]	Both crutches and the weaker lower extremity simultaneously; then, stronger lower extremity	Bilateral symmetrical of upper extremities; alternating reciprocal of lowers (deliberate to moderately rhythmical)
Tripod alternate[2]	Right crutch; left crutch; then, shuffle or drag feet to tripod, or new starting position	Alternating reciprocal of upper extremities;; bilateral symmetrical of lower extremities (deliberate)
Rocking chair[2]	Both crutches; then, one foot then other foot	Bilateral symmetrical of upper extremities; alternating reciprocal of lower extremities (deliberate)
Four point[1]	Right crutch; left foot; left crutch; right foot	Diagonal reciprocal (deliberate)
Two point[1]	Right crutch and left foot simultaneously; then, left crutch and right foot simultaneously	Diagonal reciprocal (rhythmical)

[1]Buchwald, E., *Physical Rehabilitation for Daily Living.* New York, Blakiston Co., 1952.

[2]Deaver, G. G., and Brown, M. E.: The challenge of crutches. Reprinted from *Arch Phys Med,* July 1945, Aug. 1945, Sept. 1945, Dec. 1945, March 1946, Nov. 1946.

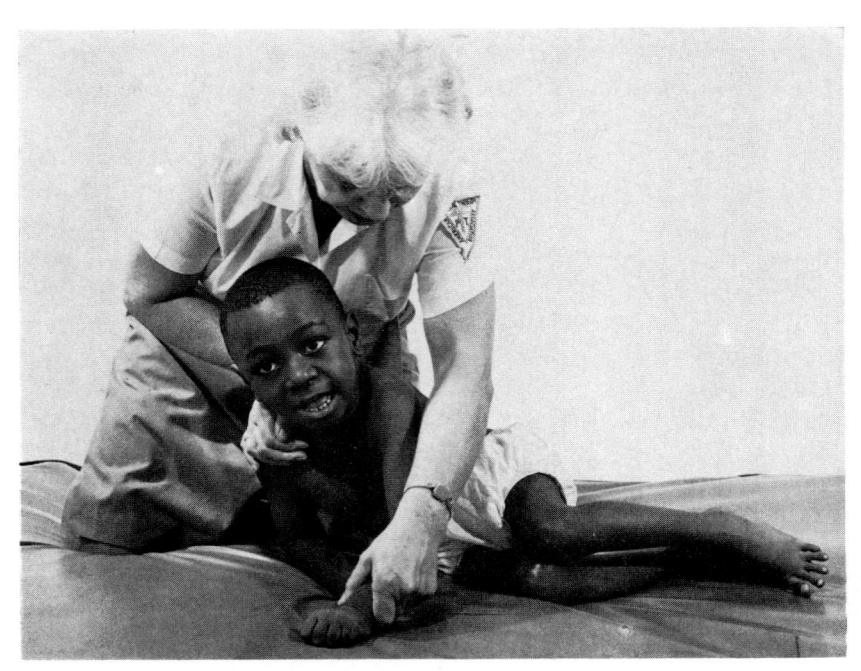

248 *Physical Therapy Services in the Developmental Disabilities*

Figure 5-5. Rising to sitting from prone. Child's left hand is held in contact with mat while approximation is given at right shoulder in attempt to promote elevation of superior region by use of bilateral asymmetrical extension of upper extremities to right. As superior region elevates, inferior region should adjust with bilateral asymmetry so that child is in side-sitting position supporting weight on hands. However, this activity is too advanced for this child. See Figures 5-9 and 5-13 for less advanced activities which should promote ability to rise to side-sitting. Rolling in Figure 5-9 is from supine toward prone. Reversal of direction, rolling from prone toward supine, should be emphasized. Manual contact for upper extremity is as shown in Figure 5-13, and second contact should be on posterolateral aspect of hip and pelvis. Note that child's inferior region remains flexor dominant as is true in all of his prone postures. Note too that whenever weight is borne on the left hand, the hand is closed. In side-lying position and in sitting (Fig. 5-6) hand is relaxed or open. The right hand is open except in one instance (Fig. 5-13) when attempt is made to push superior region toward supine. Child can voluntarily open and close both hands. He feeds himself with his left hand; his right hand is said to be his dominant hand. Other than feeding he is dependent for all self-care.

(as in rising to sitting from prone) by combining movements in appropriate ways? (See Fig. 5-5.)

2. Are preparatory movements (such as positioning of lower extremities in rising to sitting) appropriate in that they promote movement?

3. Are compensatory adjustments (such as altering position of head or trunk toward a symmetrical sitting posture) following an act of assumption appropriate in that they promote stability of posture?

4. Having assumed a posture, is flexor or extensor dominance evident—as in sitting with hands supporting in front of the body (flexor dominance) or with hands supporting behind the body (extensor dominance)?

5. Having assumed a posture, are responses to disturbance appropriate?

    a. Upon quick disturbance (labyrinthine) is the recovery of equilibrium quick so that equilibrium is immediately restored?

    b. Upon slow disturbance (proprioceptive) is the compensatory movement adequate so that equilibrium is recovered? (See Fig. 5-6.)

6. Having assumed a posture, can it be maintained while head and neck move in all directions? Will unsupporting extremities move in all possible directions while reaching for objects?

Rate of Movement

The combining of appropriate patterns of movement and the timed sequence have to do with coordination and organization of a total pattern. The rate of movement, too, must be appropriate. Movement of the total structure is slower than movement of a distal part. Movement of a segment which involves flexion or extension of elbow or knee is slower than movement which does not. These features of normal motor behavior deserve consideration.

Specific questions related to rate of movement include the following:

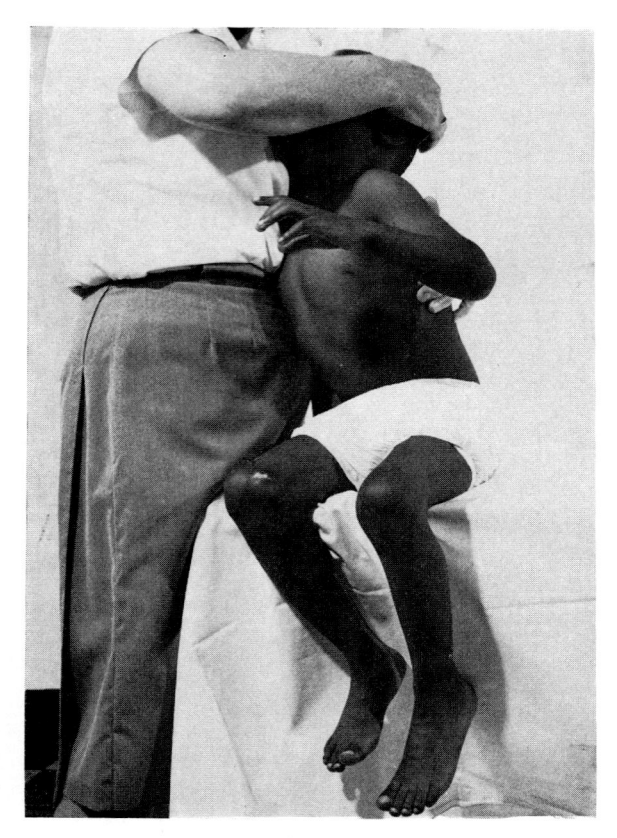

Figure 5-6. Disturbance of equilibrium for proprioceptive response. Child has been pulled diagonally forward toward right and attempts to recover upright position. Head and neck extend appropriately but left upper extremity fails to reach toward supporting surface. Therapist could resist head and neck extension with left hand, and extension of left upper extremity fails to reach toward supporting surface. Therapist could resist head and neck extension with left hand, and extension of left upper extremity with right hand placed on child's wrist. Preparatory activities include total flexion, head toward right knee with knees flexed, and total extension, superior region returning toward upright as knees extend. As can be seen in Figures 5-1 and 5-3, child is unable to voluntarily assume upright sitting because of extensor tone in this position. Yet, in this figure as head and neck and trunk are extended, lower extremities assume flexed postures, right more than left, in which flexion has released slightly. Again, rolling will prepare for erect posture during sitting (McGraw 1962).

1. Is movement of adequate rate, or is it slow and laborious?
2. Is the rate more rapid than is appropriate so that stability of posture is disturbed?
3. Is the rate of all component patterns or combining movements harmonious and consistent, or does the rate of a moving segment interfere with performance of a total pattern?

Muscle Contraction

The normal person is able to perform voluntary isotonic muscle contraction through a complete range of motion with good strength and endurance. He is able to voluntarily maintain the posture of the body and its segments with isometric-hold or static contractions of antagonistic muscles in a state of cocontraction. If his attempt to move is prevented, he will select a circuitous route in order to escape. If the normal person's attempt to "hold" is stretched or is defeated by supramaximal resistance, he will readily recover his position as soon as resistance is lessened. The normal person exhibits a balance of power between antagonistic muscle groups and is capable of smooth performance of any desired movement and of various combinations of movements in appropriate postures.

Specific questions as to the ability to perform the various types of muscle contraction include the following:

1. Is the patient able to initiate movement with isotonic contraction for the assumption of a posture and the performance of patterns of facilitation? In the lengthened, or stretch range? In middle range?
2. Is the patient able to maintain posture, total or of a segment, in all parts of the available range?
3. Does resistance applied to the antagonistic movement enhance the patient's ability to initiate movement?
4. Does resistance applied to simultaneous isometric-holding of agonist and antagonist promote cocontraction and thereby enhance his ability to maintain posture? When the isometric-hold is stretched so as to disturb balance, is he able to recover the initial position?

Recording Results

Regrettably, an appropriate form for recording which combines the developmental scales and observations according to this method of treatment has not been devised. Notations as to the child's performance may be made. Such notations will usually provide clues as to emphasis of certain patterns, the need to promote use of appropriate combinations, the need to promote flexor or extensor dominance, the need to promote mobility or stability, the need to promote movement in certain directions, and, of course, observable deficiencies and alterations in the child's responses to sensory cues.

In this method, information gleaned from assessment will provide guides for the physical therapist working with the child. The information should guide the way for achievement of goals as indicated by developmental scales. In a sense, the developmental scales constitute a test. Practicing the items on a test do not constitute the means to the promotion of development. A test is not a treatment.

THE PROBLEM

Recently expressed views of the child with central nervous system deficit tend to reflect a broad perspective. Twitchell (1965) has pointed out that these conditions are not static and that separation of patients into categories such as spasticity, rigidity and athetosis is artificial and that the physiological substrata for such phenomena can be demonstrated in all patients. Ames (1966) has stated that ". . . abnormal behavior is often not entirely different from normal behavior but is often merely normal behavior at a level much lower than the one which would be suitable for the individual in question at the age in question." Such attitudes lead us to consider the total patient, to consider his total motor performance rather than fragments of the whole, to begin where he *is* and not where we think he *should* be.

All will agree that there is a wide range of normalcy and that there is a wide range of abnormalcy. Motor deficiency may be profound and coupled with severe mental retardation; motor deficiency may be moderate with low or high levels of intelligence;

motor deficiency may be minimal with various levels of intelligence. It seems that all variations and combinations can occur. It is a commonplace, too, that motor and mental ability are intertwined and that a deficiency of one ability may alter the other. Normal persons who function at a high level of motor and mental ability must have experienced normal prenatal development; they must have been endowed with the potential for a high level of development; they must have been permitted or encouraged to explore; and they must have been subjected to appropriate degrees of stress during their developmental years.

In considering children having neuromuscular handicaps either with or without mental retardation, several factors defy alteration. The prenatal development—faulty, arrested or delayed—cannot be changed. The quality of the endowments of heredity cannot be changed. If handicapped children are to be led toward more mature behavior, we must rely, it seems, upon environmental influences including appropriate degrees of stress.

General Suggestions

If this approach is to be used, there are certain suggestions that should help to avoid disenchantment with the approach since a full description is not possible. Certain pitfalls, some of which are grounded in tradition, should be avoided. Suggestions are as follows:

1. Handling and frequent stimulation are of paramount importance in the provision of adequate stress. This is to say that the time that the physical therapist devotes to the individual child is inadequate. The members of the family or the substitute family must be involved appropriately. Appropriately, in this instance, means that a very few activities will be selected for frequent stimulation and repetition. Often, "home programs" and programs carried out by ward personnel have failed because too much detail was included, too many things were to be done. If *one* activity in need of emphasis, or even *one* phase of an activity for which the child is ready and is attempting is used as the basis, more will be achieved in the long haul. The child who is mentally retarded will respond better if he is required to repeat one or two activities

than if he is exposed to so many demands that he fails to learn anything thoroughly. When parents and their substitutes are trained to promote total patterns, the activity has meaning because they themselves have had this experience.

Beyond the one *activity* which is to be emphasized, frequently changing the child's *position* to one which is antagonistic to his preferred position will foster a balance of reflexes. Also, parents and their substitutes should be reminded of the bouncing and trouncing the normal child undergoes. If the patient is manageable insofar as size is concerned, lifting him in midair, turning him this way and that, and inverting him by the heels all become a part of the bouncing and trouncing. Such activities, of course, must be done within the limits of safety, and the more specifically such stimuli are used the more helpful they will be. Frequency of stimulation is important to motor learning; several brief periods of activity will have more value than will one prolonged period.

2. Development of perception has motor components that are ingrained and intertwined with the total patterns of the developmental sequence. The training of perception as such probably cannot be isolated and fragmented with effectiveness anymore than can the whole patient be fragmented—for example, sending the arm and hand to occupational therapy and the leg and foot to physical therapy. Common sense tells us that the normal infant is soon exposed to a variety of stimuli including firm and yielding surfaces, hardness and softness, smoothness and roughness, stickiness and slickness, warmth or heat and cold. The not-so-fortunate infant is coddled and may experience only firmness and softness and warmth; he is overprotected and deprived of experience. In this approach to treatment, as many favorable influences as can be used and combined should be brought to bear on the child. The eyes, the ears, the hands and feet are used to promote the desired response. Specific manual contacts are used; they are the key to adequate elicitation of specific patterns. The approach designed by Rood (Stockmeyer 1967) is complementary to proprioceptive neuromuscular facilitation and the two approaches should be combined in practice. The selective brushing (Stockmeyer

1967) and use of cold (Levine et al. 1954, Knott 1966) are useful preliminaries to the procedures of proprioceptive neuromuscular facilitation.

3. Vital and related functions such as breathing, sucking and swallowing, facial motions, tongue movements, bladder and bowel function deserve high priorities in treatment. Where problems exist, these functions receive emphasis (Fig. 5-7). Application of the procedures and techniques specifically directed toward these functions has been described (Knott and Voss 1968). These functions have motor components and if the specific motor problems of the child are identified and attacked, vital and related functions will be influenced favorably although secondarily. Again, the approach of Rood (Stockmeyer 1967) is a complementary approach.

4. Motor learning is retained through repetition and use of the activity. Just as with frequency of stimulation, repetition of activities that can be independently performed under supervision should supplement the child's individualized treatment. Group activity provides for interaction and social experience as well as having a built-in motivating factor. Some patients can be of specific help to other patients. In this light a group is composed of individuals with various levels of ability.

Repetitive use in occupational therapy, in play therapy, and in all situations amenable to control should be implemented. Such integration of total treatment, of course, demands that goals for the patient and activities in need of emphasis be clearly defined. Unless communication is an open and frequently used line, what one discipline contributes, another may contradict. Imbalances of antagonistic functions may be fostered and reinforced and the child arrives at a plateau far sooner than his potential might warrant.

5. The use and development of total patterns is necessary before individual patterns are emphasized in treatment. This is to say that attempts to work with an individual segment in the performance of a single pattern will rarely be successful, especially where spasticity is the dominant problem. The cephalocaudal and proximodistal direction of development must be heeded.

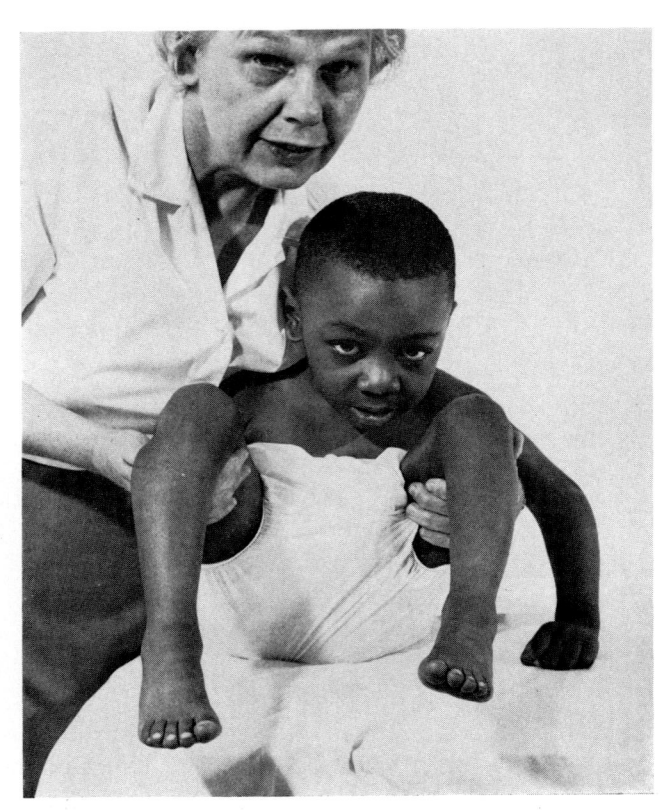

Figure 5-7. Stimulation of perineal muscles to promote bladder and bowel control. With hips flexed in abduction, internal rotation stretch is applied repetitively and child is urged to push legs down and together. Resistance is given, primarily to external rotation, and the lengthened range or beginning of the movement is emphasized or stressed. For purposes of photography child is in sitting position. As he extends head and neck, extension-adduction external rotation of hips will be reinforced. However, supine position would have permitted greater range of desired position of hips, especially internal rotation. Crawling with lower extremities participating in second diagonal (Table 5-I) is the best preparatory activity. Lower extremities may be resisted at feet and ankles (Knott and Voss 1968, Voss 1967). Creeping on hands and knees does not satisfy the need because perineal muscles are not stimulated by stretching during this activity.

There is little to be gained by direct attention to apposition of the thumb and fingers when an imbalance of scapular muscles exists. Proximal imbalances of head and neck, shoulder-girdle, and upper trunk must be corrected first. For the severely handicapped child without and especially with mental retardation, the performance of a single specific pattern is usually too advanced. Gross motor ability must be developed first. Those who have ignored this concept have become disenchanted with this approach in a short time. The use of less advanced total patterns will be far more fruitful.

6. Where there is profound deficiency of motor ability and mental ability, a desired response may seem unattainable. Usually, repetitive stimuli are required so that a "try, try, try again" situation exists. Where the patient's voluntary effort is of little or no help in facilitating a desired response, repetitive use of the stretch reflex may be necessary to activate a pattern of movement. Moving the patient passively through complete range and reversing the direction repetitively results in activation of antagonists through the stretch reflex. For example, in the side-lying position the patient may be rolled to and fro, but purposefully and through complete range; he may then become "aroused" to participate in the movement. Adversive or counter rotations of upper and lower trunk may be of help. When a response is achieved, repetition is necessary to condition the response and repeated training sessions are necessary.

The stretch reflex is a potent force and unless care is taken to balance antagonistic reflexes, flexion and extension, an imbalance may be created. Other favorable stimuli such as resistance to promote irradiation should be coupled with the stretch reflex as should the patient's voluntary effort whenever possible.

7. Where there is inability to sustain posture, emphasis should be given to the *assumption* of posture. If a child learns to assume a posture, he is likely to be able to maintain it. Too often children have been positioned in an advanced posture when compensatory responses are very inadequate. Rolling in all directions and elevation of the head and trunk from prone should be accomplished before expecting the child to learn *sitting balance.*

8. Because of the close contact between therapist and patient in this approach, the position of the therapist in relation to the patient is highly important. During activities having symmetry, the therapist assumes a symmetrical position, at the head or at the feet (Fig. 5-8A). During asymmetrical activities, diagonal direction, the therapist takes a position in line with the diagonal, near the left shoulder or the right hip and so on (Fig. 5-8B). In this way, visual cues and manual contact will be more appropriate and resistance can be more specifically applied. In working with children where the therapist may serve as a lure or as a threat, the position of the therapist greatly influences the response.

9. In this approach, effective movements are harnessed to promote reinforcement of less effective movements; thus the therapist must be organized and must have a motor plan in mind. The therapist's attention must be directed to the part that is expected to respond. For example, if the patient is to roll, the therapist's commands, hands, and control of component patterns must be synchronized toward the goal—rolling. In learning the method, the therapist often becomes engrossed with a detail which attracts attention and so forgets to move with the patient, or to allow a segment to move, and all is to no avail. The therapist's thoughts affect the patient's response.

10. Because this approach demands close interaction between therapist and child, and because a child's response and the therapist's performance during a treatment period are not completely predictable, and because there are innumerable choices as to specific reinforcements and procedures, the way must be left open for the therapist to make decisions. The physician, who is responsible for the patient, must, with the cooperation of others who contribute to the development of the child, delineate long-term objectives for the child. The prescription for treatment which reads "Stretch the adductors and the hamstrings and get the child to walk," is in itself a contradiction. It implies that, hopefully, by demanding lengthening of two individual muscle groups, some miracle will result whereby the complex neuromuscular activity of walking, which requires integration of postural and righting reflexes and balanced antagonism from head

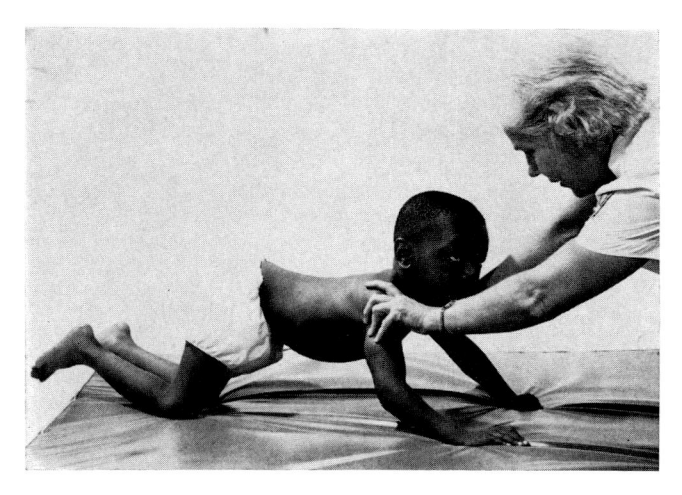

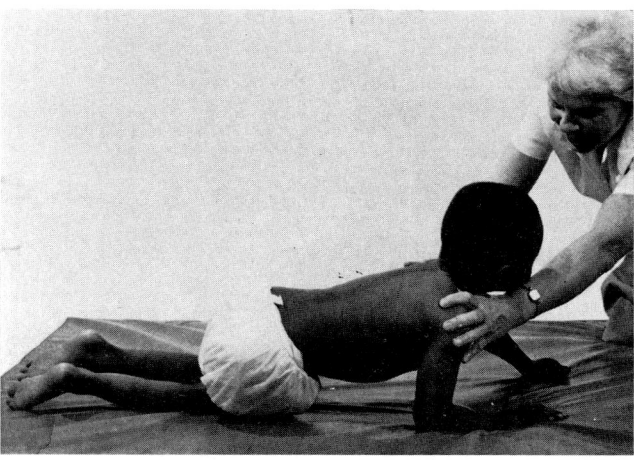

Figure 5-8. Creeping forward and diagonally forward to the left. The therapist assumes a position in line with the direction in which the child is to move. *Top,* child is relatively stable as a straight forward direction is attempted. *Bottom,* as a diagonal direction is attempted, the child's balance is immediately disturbed; the inferior region fails to support the total pattern of movement. Preparatory activities include rolling to promote reciprocation of lower extremities and development of the patterns of the first diagonal (Fig. 5-9), and crawling to promote development of the patterns of the second diagonal (Table 5-I). Child must learn to creep in all possible directions, but less advanced activities must be used to prepare him and to coordinate superior and inferior regions.

to foot, will be achieved. The neuromuscular mechanism is complex; methods for facilitation are complex. There are few shortcuts to the achievement of a goal. A too-stringent prescription will limit the success of all—the child, the physical therapist, and the physician.

11. Because the child's potentials for development are frequently obscure, the limiting line, or asymptote, beyond which the child cannot proceed is also frequently obscure. The philosophy that holds that treatment must be delayed until the child is old enough to cooperate is incompatible with the philosophy of methods for facilitation. "Old enough to cooperate" implies that nothing can be done for the child unless he can voluntarily contribute. The normal infant is not left "in a box" until he is old enough to understand what tying his shoelaces means. Years of experience have contributed to his ability to learn to tie his shoes. If a child has not had normal prenatal and postnatal experiences, the longer treatment is delayed, the more difficult it will be to develop his potentials. Imbalances will be firmly established and may defy correction. An asymptote is imposed upon him by others.

Asymptotes may be imposed in other ways. Surgery such as neurectomies, tenotomies, and tendon transferences may be necessary, providing the child and the physical therapist have first been given a chance. Surgery frequently limits what can be achieved in attempts to balance antagonistic movements and reflexes. Movement is patterned, spasticity patterned, and athetotic movements are patterned in the central nervous system. The release of one muscle or tendon rarely solves the larger problem and sometimes intensifies it. Rigid bracing, too, may impose an asymptote. Normally, the superior region leads during total movement; the inferior region follows and supports the superior region. Rigid bracing of the inferior region demands that the superior region accommodate to the inferior region. Imbalances in the superior region may be intensified. This is not to say that surgery is *never* necessary or that braces are *never* necessary. It is to say that *if* methods for facilitation are to be used under optimum conditions, the timing of surgical procedures and of the application of braces must be based on considered judgment of the whole child and not of one or two segments.

The child's asymptote for learning will become evident after all that can be done to promote his maturation has been done—after repeated attempts to condition and balance reflexes have failed, after repeated attempts to train total patterns of the developmental sequence have failed, after repeated attempts to train self-care skills and gait patterns have failed, after everyone has done his part—not before. Realism and economics are intertwined and may impose an asymptote on everyone. These facts of life demand that the most be done in the least possible time. The child's asymptote may be a lesser barrier than the combined asymptotes of the rest of us.

PRIMARY PROBLEMS AND SUGGESTED PROCEDURES

While the goal of all treatment is to develop insofar as is possible the patient's potential, more often than not primary problems loom and must be attacked. More often than not a part of the total problem is in knowing *how* to begin as well as *where* to begin. Obviously if a child cannot move, effort must be directed toward developing the ability to move. If he cannot sustain posture or is unstable in his movements, efforts must be directed toward developing the ability to sustain posture. In a broad sense, the goal is to balance antagonistic functions. In this light, immobility (posture) is antagonistic to movement; instability (movement) is antagonistic to posture. In the normal child, a balanced antagonism develops and remains until an advanced age unless disease or injury interfere.

The guide lines drawn from human behavior must be followed. The guide lines drawn from animal behavior, which were learned or observed on behalf of humans, can be helpful. The foremost of these is that stress promotes maturation. Stress includes handling, manipulation, and resistance. Stress includes the direction of choices, the channelling of effort and energy. Secondly, the method of training must be appropriate for the level of the patient in terms of motor ability and mental ability. Methods of training extend from conditioning of responses to the use of stepwise procedures in the learning of a difficult task such as rising from a chair or climbing stairs.

Risking oversimplification, the primary problems may be identified as related to hypertonia and to hypotonia with recognition that the vast majority of patients may reflect the presence of both problems with dominance of one, and that some patients may be handicapped primarily by impairment of special senses. Primary problems may be considered in terms of flexor dominance or extensor dominance with an imbalance of antagonistic reflexes favoring the dominance that is present. Primary problems may be considered in terms of lack of control of movement and posture and lack of selectivity as to direction, degree of range, and rate of movement. Primary problems may be coupled with deficient ability to learn tasks such as self-care activities. Whatever the primary problem, the procedures used to alleviate it must be suitable for the individual patient when his ability to cooperate and to learn is considered.

Hypertonia with Imbalance of Antagonistic Reflexes

The following are suggested methods:

1. Position the patient so that gravity will *assist* the weaker movements. Such a position will have the support of tonic labyrinthine reflexes, the stretch reflex can be elicited readily throughout the desired pattern of movement, manual contacts with skin overlying the agonistic patterns can be achieved (as compared with assistive-active exercise where manual contacts are favorable for the antagonistic pattern), and a weak movement may be resisted so as to foster a balance between antagonistic reflexes.

Example: A patient who cannot voluntarily flex head and neck because of extensor spasticity may be positioned in prone with support on forearms and pelvis. Head and neck flexion with rotation patterns and those of the upper trunk may be stretched with hands placed on the flexor surface, and the response to stretch may be resisted. Reversal of antagonists techniques including rhythmic stabilization (Knott and Voss 1968) may be used to develop head control. Rhythmic stabilization is a technique whereby stability is promoted through manually resisting a patient's efforts to maintain the body or a segment in a stable position. The patient is told to "Hold still. Don't let me move you." Pressure is applied alternately to antagonistic muscle groups so that a cocontraction of all muscles is encouraged. For example, in the standing position the therapist may place the hands on the patient's shoulders and while the left shoulder is pressed forward, the right is pressed backward. By such a maneuver an impasse is reached so that stability results.

2. The rotation component is "locked" by spasticity. Use the rotation component to reduce spasticity. In patterns of facilitation the rotation component is used to achieve maximal stretch of the muscles responsible for the pattern. The rotation component can be used to promote a balance between flexor and extensor reflexes.

Example: A patient who is limited by hyperactive symmetric tonic neck reflexes maintains the head in midline. Rotation components are deficient in head and neck and severely imbalanced in the extremities. The head and neck rotation pattern requires movement from lateralward extension on one side, chin to shoulder, through flexion to lateralward extension on the opposite side, chin to shoulder. Head and neck rotation, supported by the asymmetric tonic neck reflex, is used in rolling from supine toward prone (Fig. 5-9) and from prone toward supine. Through rolling from supine toward prone (flexor dominant) and from prone to supine (extensor dominant) using the head and neck rotation pattern, the two sides of the body are stimulated to interact in a sideward direction with rotation of the total body. When rolling is used toward both sides, ipsilateral combinations of upper and lower extremities are activated to offset the limitation of symmetry imposed by the symmetric tonic neck reflex. If rolling cannot be initiated from supine, the patient should be positioned side-lying toward prone. If the patient is able to cooperate, he should be told to "Stay there," while he is pulled back toward supine by manual contacts at head and pelvis, and then at shoulder and pelvis. The technique of repetitive stretching, repeated isotonic contractions, and, as ability improves, re-

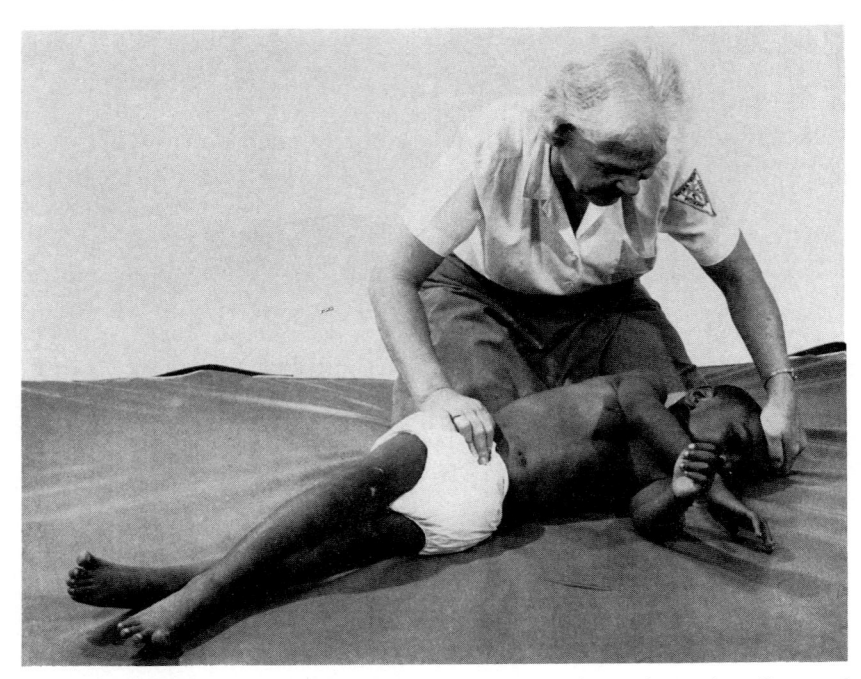

264 *Physical Therapy Services in the Developmental Disabilities*

Figure 5-9. Rolling is supported by the asymmetric tonic neck reflex and promotes development of patterns of the first diagonal (Table 5-I). Rolling prepares for diagonal reciprocation of lower extremities in that the uppermost extremity flexes while the undermost extremity extends. While other combinations of head and neck and upper extremity patterns may be used (Table 5-I), the lower extremity consistently performs patterns of the first diagonal (Voss 1967). Note that child's right hand is open and is prepared to contact surface so as to reverse direction toward supine. Note that in Figure 5-13 during adversive rotation of shoulder-girdle and pelvis (shoulder pushes toward extension, pelvis pulls toward flexion), child's right hand is closed. For Figure 5-13. child was positioned on his side rather than actively rolling from supine toward prone which might have caused him to open his hand to contact surface as in this figure.

versal of antagonistic techniques may be used (Knott and Voss 1968).

Example: A patient who, while supine, lies with hips and knees flexed has need to develop extensor dominance in the inferior region. Head and neck rotation pattern, which activates the

Proprioceptive Neuromuscular Facilitation 265

homologous pattern of the upper trunk, may be combined with lower trunk rotation to activate lower trunk and hip extensors (Fig. 5-10). Lower trunk rotation is performed with hips and

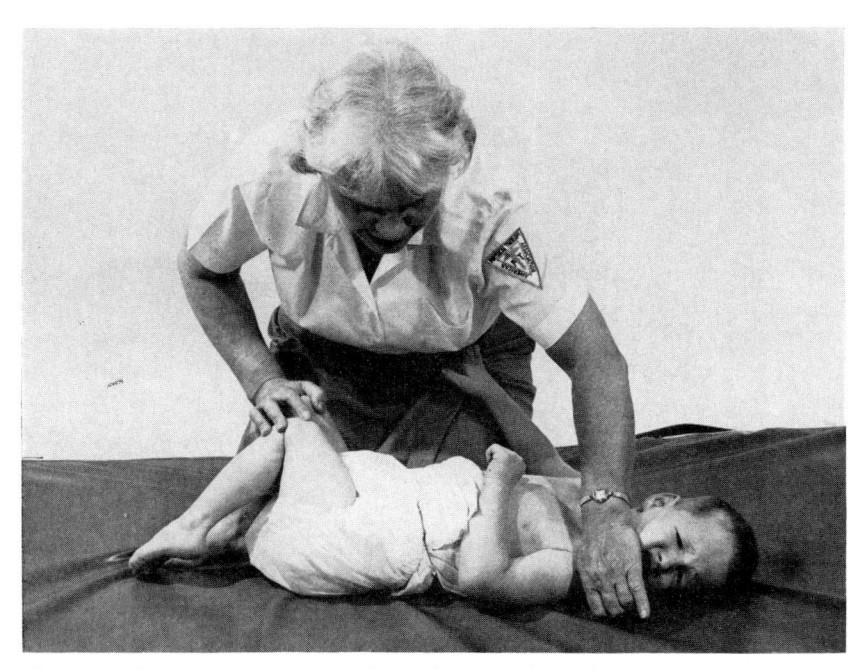

Figure 5-10. Lower trunk rotation with rotation of head to the opposite side. As child moves knees from right to left, abdominal muscles contract and as left thigh approaches surface, the extensors of lower trunk on the left and those of left hip contract. This activity prepares for "bridging," pelvic elevation while supine, and for kneeling (Voss 1967). Head may rotate to same side rather than to opposite side in which case the child would roll toward prone with bilateral asymmetrical flexion of lower extremities. Head-turning to opposite side provides stability.

knees flexed so that soles of feet are in contact with the surface. The lower extremities are held in close contact with each other so as to obtain influence on the trunk. Again, as with head and neck rotation, movement proceeds from lateralward extension on one side, through flexion, to lateralward extension on the other side. This is achieved by moving the knees toward one side as far as possible so that stretch is superimposed on lateralward extensors of the opposite side. The child is told to pull his knees toward the opposite side as stretch is superimposed and resistance is graded throughout the range. If the child cannot follow instructions, repetitive stretching should be used, reversing passively from side to side until response is achieved. Head and neck rotation should be performed, head leading, at the same time toward the same side (this will produce rolling or turning on the side), and toward the opposite side. As lower trunk rotation is resisted, elevation of the hips from the surface with hips and knees tending toward extension occurs. Manual contacts are made with one hand on lateral side of face, the other on lateral aspect of thigh of leading lower extremity or with knees held together.

Lower trunk rotation may be carried out in the prone position if stimulation of lower trunk flexion is desired. The hips are then in extension while the knees are maintained in flexion. Manual contacts may be made at knees, posterior aspect, and at ankles, dorsal aspect.

3. Use approximation to promote postural responses where flexor reflexes are dominant. Approximation as a technique is performed by compressing the joint surfaces; it is the opposite of applying traction to a joint or segment (Knott and Voss 1968). For example, in the standing position the therapist may place the hands on the patient's shoulders or laterally on the brim of the pelvis, and then suddenly apply pressure in a downward direction. This maneuver promotes extension of hips and knees and is often combined with rhythmic stabilization for encouraging stability of posture. (See "Hypertonia with Imbalance of Antagonistic Reflexes," No. 1.) Approximation, as a technique, is directed toward joint receptors through compression of the joint surfaces (Knott and Voss 1968). The joints to be compressed must be positioned so that extension is as complete as is possible. A certain degree of stretch of related antagonistic muscle groups will necessarily occur and cocontraction will be promoted.

Example: The child who habitually flexes the elbows can be assisted toward voluntary extension by the use of approximation in the hand-knee or creeping position. Resisting elevation of head and upper trunk will promote the desired posture. Approximation may be done bilaterally or for one upper extremity. If a unilateral approach is used, the head should be turned toward the extending elbow to achieve support by the asymmetric tonic neck reflex. Manual contact is made at the scapula lateralward enough so as to superimpose pressure downward throughout the extremity. Pressure is abruptly given and if the child is able to cooperate, he should be told to "Hold still." The procedure should be repeated until a response of elbow extension is felt or observed. If response lags, resistance applied simultaneously to neck extensors may assist bilateral elbow extension. A bilateral approach is preferable because of the bilateral symmetrical posture and a good response on one side may facilitate the response of the lagging side. Another maneuver may be used as preparatory. In the same position, placing the hands in the axillary space so as to abruptly disturb the posture by lifting the extremity from the supporting surface may facilitate elbow extension as the hand reaches for the surface. This also may encourage hand opening. Approximation should be applied immediately after the hand contacts the surface to further activate the extensors.

Example: The child whose standing posture is dominated by flexion can be assisted by the use of approximation at several levels—head, shoulder-girdle bilaterally, pelvic-girdle bilaterally, or by placing the hands in various combinations such as shoulder and pelvis on opposite sides. Again, the procedure should be repeated, and, if necessary, the posture should be adjusted and assisted toward as much extension as possible.

Example: The child who sits with head and neck flexed may be assisted in the development of head control by using approximation at both shoulders. The head will "bounce" toward extension. As the head lags toward flexion again, the procedure should be repeated. (The need for frequency of stimulation should never be overlooked. This particular procedure can be taught to other personnel or members of the family, so that each time they approach the child who is sitting in a chair, they can promote a better posture in this way.)

4. Use stretch to aid initiation of movement and to increase

rate of movement. While the stretch reflex is coupled with resistance to facilitate response and the initiation of voluntary movement, both may be used to increase the rate thereby reducing the labored quality of the child's efforts. Resistance is lessened so that movement proceeds at a more rapid rate and so that movement may be repeated a great many times.

Example: The child who has need to learn to extend the lower trunk and hips may be positioned supine as for lower trunk rotation with soles of feet in contact with the surface. The child is guided and resisted in "bridging," which is elevation of hips from the surface. Stretch is used upon initiation, resistance is given through the available range and, as the child attempts to maintain the position, the pelvis is pushed down toward the surface thereby again stretching the hip extensors. As the child resumes bridging, resistance is lessened so that more range may be achieved at a quicker rate. The procedure should be repeated with light resistance but with repetitive stretch to hasten response. With hips elevated as far as possible, if some flexion of hips remains, the pelvis may be rotated during rhythmic stabilization as the child attempts to maintain the position. Again, the rotation component is used to promote reduction of spasticity.

Example: As the child laboriously attempts to rise from prone to side-sitting he may achieve partial range with incomplete extension of the elbows. Repetitive stretch coupled with resistance should be given with manual contacts for the head and neck extension with rotation pattern toward the side or direction of the movement and for approximation given at the scapula of the upper extremity toward which the head and neck are extending. Lower extremities must adjust by lower trunk rotation toward the opposite side. (Preparatory activities therefore include lower trunk rotation as discussed previously.) With the lower extremities appropriately positioned, the child may be moved passively through the necessary range of upper trunk rotation so that stretch is superimposed alternately for rising from the surface and lowering toward the surface. Again this rotation of upper trunk will reduce the spasticity so that movement may become brisker. Then, as the child attempts elevation against resistance, and as he proceeds through range, quickly pushing him down toward the prone position will promote response through stretch. Resistance should be lessened so that movement occurs at an increased rate and so that a greater number of repetitions can be carried out.

Hypotonia with Deficient Postural Responses

Procedures are as follows:

1. Use "threat" to increase tonus and response to stretch. In severe hypotonia, hypermobility is a characteristic feature. Response to a stretch stimulus is inadequate. Within the limits of safety, quickly moving the small child in space as if "throwing him away" while supine and prone, inverting him so that his head approaches the surface and lowering him suddenly and briefly onto a turkish towel wrung from ice water may increase tone. Threat includes loud tones of voice interspersed with moderate tones. If the child cries, tonus may be increased.

Example: If a child appears to be generally hypotonic and immobile in the supine position, he may exhibit a slight increase in tonus during "throwing away" maneuvers. While held in prone posture by hands in contact with the thorax (and if necessary, the chin) and the pelvis, stretch of all trunk flexors can be quickly given. If the child has reacted to the maneuver by extensor response, so much the better because the flexors will be better prepared to respond.

2. Use total flexion and total extension to promote response to stretch. Although placing an individual pattern under tension with stretch quickly applied may fail to elicit a good response, applying stretch to head and neck, upper and lower trunk patterns at the same time may produce a far greater response. If both flexion and extension responses are deficient, attempts should be made to activate flexion first, because in the sequence of normal development, flexion precedes extension.

Example: With the therapist sitting, preferably on a mat, the child may be placed prone across the lap. Head and neck, and upper trunk pattern (one hand placed on anterior surface of thorax so that chin is in contact with therapist's forearm), and lower trunk patterns (other hand placed on anterior surface of lower trunk and in contact with pelvis) may be stretched by lifting the child toward complete extension (Fig. 5-11). With tension maintained at lower trunk, repetitive stretch of head and neck and upper trunk flexors may be given. Although at first no response may be felt, the child should be permitted to flex with

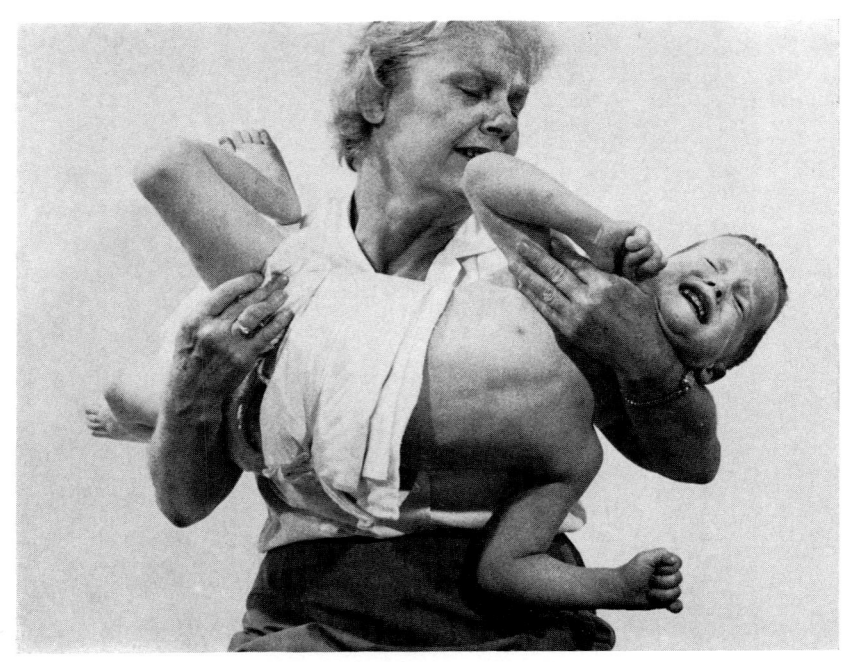

Figure 5-11. Child lifted in total extension of head and neck and trunk so as to stimulate total flexion. Child will flex toward the left because he is extended toward the right. Direction is diagonal so that the right external oblique and left internal oblique abdominal muscles are stimulated rather than rectus abdominis. To achieve balance by flexing toward right, child must be repositioned with head on therapist's right arm. As the child flexes, upper extremities should extend toward the left in a bilateral asymmetrical movement as can be seen in Figure 5-12. If a child's size or weight prohibits the therapist from performing this maneuver, the child's inferior region may be made stable by strapping him on a padded bench or table so that therapist can support and stimulate by controlling the superior region. This compromise position may be less effective because therapist cannot contact and stimulate inferior region.

Proprioceptive Neuromuscular Facilitation 271

the assistance of gravity and then should be brought back toward extension and the procedure repeated. In a like fashion, repetitions of lower trunk flexion may be done.

Example: Again with the therapist sitting, the child may be held supine with the entire body flexed so that the forehead or nose contacts the opposite knee; or, if range permits, head is taken beyond the knee (Fig. 5-12). This maneuver produces stimulation of the extensor pattern of upper trunk toward one side and of lower trunk extension toward the opposite side. Again, repetitive stretching may be used, allowing the child to move into

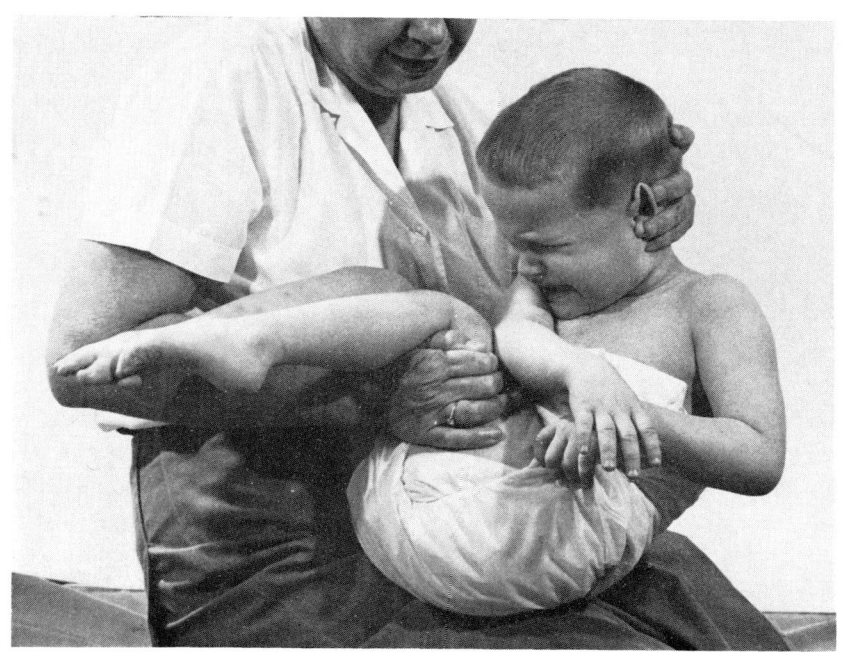

Figure 5-12. Child positioned in total flexion so as to stimulate total extension. Child will extend toward left because he is flexed toward right. As in Figure 5-11, child must be repositioned for stimulation of extension toward left. Note that in Figure 5-11 child's extremities have automatically flexed with hands fisted. In this figure, child's lower extremities are prepared to extend; feet have plantar flexed. Upper extremities have automatically assumed extended position with hands open. As child extends, upper extremities should move toward flexion, or should at least release from extension if normal reinforcement is to occur.

some range of extension before stretching is repeated. This entire maneuver stimulates inspiration during extension which may be helpful in increasing tone.

3. Use total patterns of posture to promote postural response. Although response to stretch in individual patterns may be deficient, a total pattern may promote response.

Example: With the child positioned on hands and knees, the therapist standing astride the patient's pelvis, and if necessary, gripping with the knees to maintain the posture of the inferior region, "bouncing" may be used with the superior region. The therapist places the hands in the patient's axillary spaces having reached downward and across the pectoral regions, and alternately lifts and lowers the child's hands from and toward the surface. As the hands contact the surface, the therapist may quickly shift his hands to the posterior surfaces of the scapulae and apply approximation. If necessary, the approach may be unilateral rather than bilateral; or, one hand may remain in the axilla of one side, with lifting away from the surface carried out while approximation is used on the opposite side.

Example: With the child side-lying, adversive movements of upper trunk rotation and lower trunk rotation may increase the response to stretch. The therapist places one hand on the scapula and shoulder, the other is placed on the pelvis. The superior region may be pulled toward supine while the inferior region is pushed toward prone and the direction reversed (Fig. 5-13). Repetitive stretching of both regions may be done simultaneously, the inferior region may be held under tension with repetition given to the superior region, or the superior region may be held under tension while repetitions are directed to the inferior region. As the child begins to respond, movements should be resisted to further increase response.

Deficient Control of Movement and Posture

The following are suggested procedures:

1. Use diagonal patterns of head and neck to promote balance and control of head and neck and upper trunk. The development of control of head and neck is necessary to the functions of breath control, jaw control, swallowing, and speech.

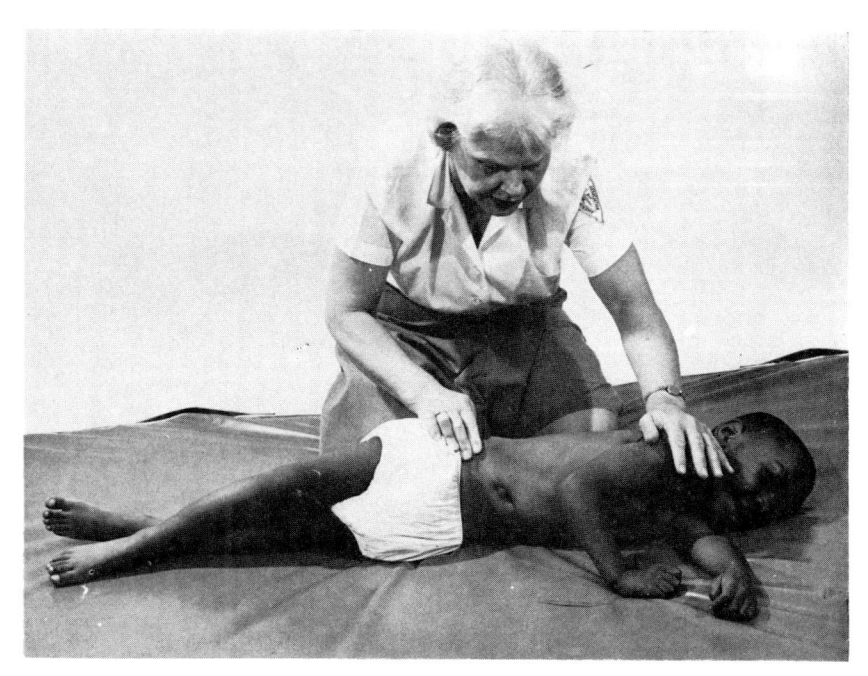

Figure 5-13. Adversive movements may increase response to stretch. Stretch may be applied repetitively, or, if the child is able to cooperate, he is told to push back at the shoulder and to pull forward at the hip. Direction is reversed by the therapist shifting hands so as to resist shoulder pulling forward as hip pushes backward. This activity prepares for diagonal reciprocation in walking which requires that shoulder-girdle and pelvic-girdle rotate in opposite directions (i.e. shoulder-girdle forward on arm swing and pelvic-girdle backward during stance phase). Rhythmic stabilization may be performed to promote stability (See "Hypertonia with Imbalance of Antagonistic Reflexes," 1. for description of technique. See also Fig. 5-9 and legend regarding opening of hand.)

Example: A child who lacks control of movement often exhibits an imbalance of antagonistic patterns of head and neck. Extensors may be hyperactive and flexors may reveal marked weakness so that flexion patterns cannot be performed from the lengthened or stretch range. Placing the chin on the chest so that nose is in line with the opposite hip and gently and repetitively lifting and lowering the chin may elicit a response in the flexors in the shortened range. The range through which flexion may be performed may be gradually increased from shortened to lengthened range.

2. Use both diagonals of extremity patterns to promote balance of antagonists and control of movement. The first diagonal is developed or promoted by rolling, the second by crawling. The development of both are necessary to control of movement and posture.

Example: A child who exhibits involuntary motion during voluntary effort, as in athetosis, may have a deficiency of one diagonal of movement as well as hyperactive tonic neck reflexes and avoidance responses. Involuntary movements of hand and wrist may oscillate between radialward extension of wrist and ulnarward flexion, components of the second diagonal of the upper extremity. Emphasizing radialward flexion and ulnarward extension of the wrist, components of the first diagonal, may promote development of control. Control of proximal joints, scapular and shoulder movements, should be fostered through rolling with appropriate combinations of head and neck patterns. Control of supination and pronation and movements of wrist and hand must be developed by use of specific patterns of facilitation.

Involuntary movements of foot and ankle may oscillate between dorsiflexion with inversion and plantar flexion with eversion, components of the first diagonal of the lower extremity. The second diagonal, with its components of dorsiflexion with eversion and plantar flexion with inversion, may be promoted by crawling with ipsilateral combinations with head and neck rotation pattern.

3. Use isometric-holding in the shortened range to increase ability to perform from lengthened range, to correct severe imbalances in distal parts, and to control range, timing, and rate of movement.

Example: The child with athetosis lacks control of direction, timing or sequence of movement, and rate of movement. Irradiation of nerve impulses is abnormal so that voluntary movement is not well controlled (Kabat and McLeod 1959), and, as mentioned previously, imbalances between diagonals may exist. When the child moves, there is an oscillation between extremes of range, and the proximal joints (i.e. knee and hip) complete their range in advance of distal joints (i.e. foot and ankle) where movement appears to lag as if it were an afterthought.

Since all movement proceeds toward the shortened range, eliciting a "hold" contraction in the shortened range may provide the means to improving the timing and rate. Each component of a given pattern may be emphasized beginning with proximal joints and proceeding toward distal, and proceeding from isometric contraction in the shortened range to isotonic contraction from the lengthened range. As an example, the upper extremity may be placed so that the arm is across the face in the flexion-adduction external rotation pattern, elbow flexed, hand closed toward the radial side. The hold is elicited first at shoulder, then elbow, then wrist and hand. With the hold secured, repeated contractions, with increasing decrements of range, may be performed first at shoulder, then elbow, then wrist and hand. Following the procedure, the part may be moved to the lengthened range and movement attempted toward shortened range with proximal joints prevented from moving until the distal part, hand and wrist, have moved in accordance with normal timing, distal toward proximal. The child's voluntary effort to cooperate is highly important.

4. Use approximation and rhythmic stabilization (Knott and Voss 1968) to promote control of posture. These procedures promote cocontraction or isometric-holding of agonist and antagonist.

Example: The hyperactive child lacks control and exhibits movement without purpose although the configuration of movement and posture may appear to be quite normal. His lack of control results in clumsiness. Repetitive movement with isotonic contractions of muscle may make him worse. The child may be approached in any of the total patterns such as creeping position, kneeling, sitting, or standing (Fig. 5-14). Manual contacts may be made with head and shoulder, both shoulders, both hips, head and opposite hip—all possible combinations. Approximation is applied and the child is told to "Hold!" Resistance is given to the hold contractions, primarily to the rotation components. Thus, for example, with hands at the level of the child's shoulders, one

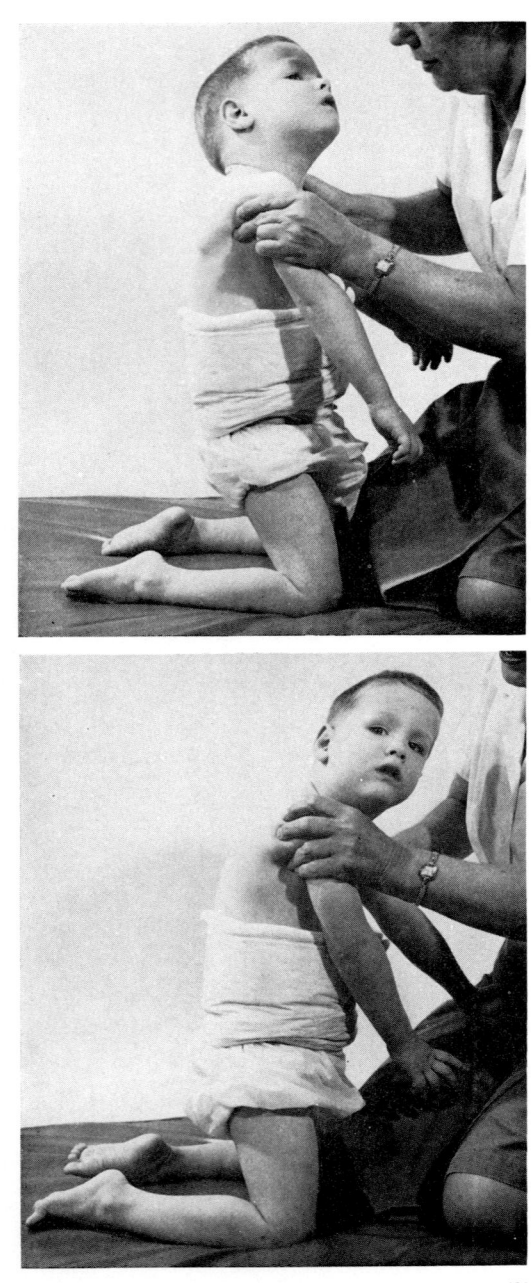

Figure 5-14. Approximation used to promote postural stability. *Top,* child is assisted to kneeling. Head extends but hips remain partially flexed.

hand pushes him forward while the other pushes him backward. An impasse is reached so that the child's stability is increased.

Example: The child with ataxia lacks control of the flexion and extension components while the rotation component appears deficient. Again, resisting active movement with isotonic contraction of muscles may only increase his problem. He may be positioned in various postures and, again, approximation and rhythmic stabilization are the procedures of choice.

Neuromuscular Deficiency with Deficient Learning Ability

The following procedures are used:

1. Use procedures which promote motor learning through repetition. Repetitive use of stretch coupled with isotonic contraction against resistance to promote movement, and repetitive use of approximation with resistance applied to isometric-hold contractions of antagonistic muscle groups to promote stability of posture may foster automatic responses with little or no voluntary effort by the child. Communication is achieved through manual contacts although vocal commands are used so that the child may learn to follow commands.

Example: A child who has not learned to turn himself in bed may be conditioned to do so by the therapist placing hands at head and scapula or head and pelvis so as to stretch appropriate patterns of head and neck and trunk. The child may be placed in the side-lying position and may be rolled quickly toward supine or prone with appropriate commands. The procedure should be repeated until the tactile stimuli and vocal commands acquire meaning and until response becomes automatic. Ward personnel may be taught the appropriate cues and procedures. Lures and

---

Bottom, approximation is given at shoulders; hip extension is somewhat better; head assumes a forward position as child reaches for support with left hand and decides to look at camera. Verbal commands to hold are given, but child cannot hear. Nevertheless, giving commands assists therapist in timing pressure at shoulder-girdle. In a sitting position, this maneuver helps the child whose head lags into extension or flexion. A lag in response may occur but with repetition of approximation head assumes upright position.

rewards, especially "love-pats" and praise should be used as necessary.

2. Use stepwise procedures and repetition in the training of more difficult tasks. Repetition of a whole task which has several phases, one of which is inadequately performed, does not promote learning at an optimum rate; the unsatisfactorily performed phase detracts from performance of the whole task. Repetition of a phase may enhance performance of the whole task. Because self-care activities and gait activities are essentially whole tasks requiring total patterns of interaction of the body and its segments, the phases which make up the whole may be identified and emphasized as necessary to learning.

Example: A child may have failed to learn to rise from a chair by pulling on parallel bars. This activity has the following phases: (1) Place feet in symmetrical position with knees flexed appropriately, (2) lean body forward and reach for and grasp bars, and (3) rise to standing by pulling on bars and elevating head to lead toward total extension.

Phase 1: Resist flexion of both knees from a fully extended position. If one leg lags in movement, resist more strongly the opposite leg to promote irradiation and to time for simultaneous movement. Repeat several times and then request child to place feet from a too-far-forward position.

Phase 2: Resist at forehead and at wrist of a lagging arm, or at both wrists. Repeat with hands placed at head and one arm, head and the other arm, then at wrists for both arms. As child approaches bars, push him back so as to repeat the phase and complete it by successfully grasping bars. This phase is flexor dominant.

Phase 3: Resist at back of head on one side and at front of pelvis on opposite side as child pulls to standing. Give approximation at shoulder and pelvis, or through head and pelvis as phase nears completion. Repeat activity by pushing child back to sitting so that neck and upper trunk extensors are again activated by stretching. This phase is extensor dominant.

When possible, the child should be taught to push to standing by placing hands on arm rests of chair. Flexor and extensor phases may be emphasized more completely.

If phases (1) and (3) are adequate but phase (2) poses a problem, this phase should be emphasized as a step in the total procedure rather than simply repeating the whole task. Finally, the whole task, or total pattern of pulling to standing, may be repeated, hopefully with success. If the potential is adequate, facilitating and emphasizing the various phases may produce a very good response. If the potential is low, less advanced activities such as rolling and rising from prone to side-sitting may need perfecting, or repeated training sessions may be necessary.

Closing Comment

Proprioceptive neuromuscular facilitation as a method of treatment includes a concept of human movement and specific procedures designed to hasten motor learning. Sophisticated application of the specific procedures requires the development of skill. For the inexperienced or unskilled person the guide lines from human behavior become of paramount importance. Many facets of this method seem to be in direct contradiction with more traditional methods. While the professional person who has had habit patterns and concepts instilled through use of traditional methods may have difficulty in learning spiral and diagonal patterns of facilitation and specific procedures, the lay person, the family and members of the substitute family, have very little difficulty. These persons can learn without the deterrent of having to unlearn a previously ingrained habit or attitude.

The child with central nervous system deficit, with mental retardation, with a combination of several problems any one of which seems insurmountable, has been accepted as a challenge. The challenge, simply stated, is to find ways to promote his development and maturation. If the child and his parents could do it alone, it would be done. But those most vitally interested need help. Those who have accepted the challenge to help have only begun to learn how best to help. The lack of success in the past can be and has been attributed to the family's lack of cooperation, to the patient's lack of motivation, to the lack of time, to the lack of money, and to sundry other lacks. Lacks promote a seeking for shortcuts, a tending to begin with where the child *should* be in terms of chronological age rather than where he *is*. At a time when he *should* be able to tie his shoes the child may be able only to respond to the simplest form of training—conditioning of reflexive or automatic responses. If the method of training is inappropriate or too advanced, whatever time is given, whatever money is used, will have been used unwisely. Any learning which results will be due largely to the maturation process itself, the process which those who want to help hope to promote and hasten. A method of treatment will be successful only if it is grounded in development of normal motor behavior, if it has a firm basis in neurophysiology, and if it includes procedures which will hasten motor learning by providing appropriate stimuli and appropriate degrees of stress.

BIBLIOGRAPHY

Ames, L.B.: Individuality of motor development. *Phys Ther, 46*:121-127, 1966.

Buchwald, E.: *Physical Rehabilitation for Daily Living.* New York, McGraw, 1952.

Buchwald, J.S.: Basic mechanisms of motor learning. *Phys Ther, 45*:314-331, 1965. Reprinted in: The Child with Central Nervous System Deficit. Washington, D.C., U.S. Department of Health, Education and Welfare, Welfare Administration, Children's Bureau, 1965.

Buchwald, J.S.: Exteroceptive reflexes and movement. *Amer J Phys Med, 46*:121-128, 1967. (Proceedings of Exploratory and Analytical Survey of Therapeutic Exercise held at Northwestern University Medical School, July 25-August 19, 1966. Baltimore, Williams and Wilkins, 1967.)

Daniels, L., Williams, M., and Worthingham, C.: *Muscle Testing: Techniques of Manual Examination,* 2nd ed. Philadelphia, Saunders, 1956.

Deaver, G.G., and Brown, M.E.: The challenge of crutches. Reprinted from *Arch Phys Med,* July 1945, August 1945, September 1945, December 1945, March 1946, November 1946.

Gellhorn, E.: Patterns of muscular activity in man. *Arch Phys Med, 28:* 568-574, 1947.

Gesell, A.: Behavior patterns of fetal-infant and child. *Genetics, Proceedings of Association for Research in Nervous and Mental Disease, 33*:114-123, 1954.

Gesell, A., and Amatruda, C.S.: *Developmental Diagnosis*, 2nd ed. New York, Paul B. Hoeber, 1947.
Harlow, H.F.: The nature of love. In Haimowitz, M.L., and Haimowitz, N.R. (Eds.): *Human Development. Selected Readings*. New York, Crowell, 1960.
Harlow, H.F., and Harlow, M.K.: Principles of primate learning. In *Lessons from Animal Behavior*, Ch. 5. Little Club Clinics in Developmental Medicine, No. 7. The Spastics Society. London, Heinemann, 1962.
Hellebrandt, F.A., Schade, M., and Carns, M.L.: Methods of evoking the tonic neck reflexes in normal human subjects. *Amer J Phys Med, 41:* 90-139, 1962.
Hellebrandt, F.A., and Waterland, J.C.: Expansion of motor patterning under exercise stress. *Amer J Phys Med, 41:*56-66, 1962.
Hooker, D.: *The Prenatal Origin of Behavior*. Lawrence, Kansas, U of Kans, 1952.
Kabat, H.: Proprioceptive facilitation in therapeutic exercise. In Licht, S. (Ed.): *Therapeutic Exercise*, 2nd ed., Ch. 13. New Haven, Licht, 1961.
Kabat, H., and Knott, M.: Proprioceptive facilitation technics for treatment of paralysis. *Phys Ther Rev, 33:*53-64, 1953.
Kabat, H., and McLeod, M.: Athetosis; neuromuscular dysfunction and treatment. *Arch Phys Med, 40:*285-292, 1959.
Knott, M.: Neuromuscular facilitation in the child with central nervous system deficit. *Phys Ther, 46:*721-724, 1966.
Knott, M., and Voss, D.E.: *Proprioceptive Neuromuscular Facilitation: Patterns and Techniques*. 2nd ed. New York, Harper and Row, Hoeber Medical Division, 1968.
Levine, S.: Stimulation in infancy. *Sci Amer, 202:*5:80-86, 1960.
Levine, S.: Some effects of stimulation in infancy. In *Lessons from Animal Behavior*, Ch. 3. Little Club Clinics in Developmental Medicine, No. 7. The Spastics Society. London, Heinemann, 1962.
Levine, M.G., Kabat, H., Knott, M., and Voss, D.E.: Relaxation of spasticity by physiological technics. *Arch Phys Med, 35:*214-223, 1954.
McGraw, M.B.: *The Neuromuscular Maturation of the Human Infant*. New York, Columbia, 1943. Reprinted edition, New York, Hafner, 1962.
Pavlov, I.P.: *Conditioned Reflexes*. London, Oxford U. P., 1927.
Stockmeyer, S.A.: An interpretation of the approach of Rood to the treatment of neuromuscular dysfunction. *Amer J Phys Med, 46:*900-956, 1967. (Proceedings of Exploratory and Analytical Survey of Therapeutic Exercise held at Northwestern University Medical School, July 25-August 19, 1966, Baltimore, Williams and Wilkins, 1967.)
Travis, A.M., and Woolsey, C.N.: Motor performance of monkeys after bilateral partial and total cerebral decortications. *Amer J Phys Med, 35:* 273-310, 1956.

Twitchell, T.E.: Normal motor development. *Phys Ther, 45:*419-423, 1965. Reprinted in: The Child with Central Nervous System Deficit. Washington, D.C., U.S. Department of Health, Education, and Welfare, Welfare Administration, Children's Bureau, 1965.

Voss, D.E.: Proprioceptive neuromuscular facilitation. *Amer J Phys Med, 46:*838-898, 1967. (Proceedings of Exploratory and Analytical Survey of Therapeutic Exercise held at Northwestern University Medical School, July 25-August 19, 1966. Baltimore, Williams and Wilkins, 1967.)

Weisz, S.: Studies in equilibrium reaction. *J Nerv Ment Dis, 88:*150-162, 1938.

Zausmer, E., and Tower, G.: Quotient for the evaluation of motor development. *Phys Ther, 46:*725-727, 1966.

Chapter Six

FACILITATING FEEDING AND PRESPEECH

Helen A. Mueller

THE APPROACH

Speech is an important tool for communication and self-expression. Where hand use is limited, as may be the case for the brain-damaged individual with a motor handicap, speech may be the only tool for communication and self-expression. Yet, speech calls for the finest and fastest motor coordination. Motor involvement quite frequently affects the speech organs. It is especially obvious when spasticity or intermittent spasms interfere with breathing, phonation and articulation, and when control of the motions of the head, jaw, lip, tongue, velum and pharynx is affected. The result is a combination of speech problems, abnormal breathing accompanied by dysphonia, hypernasality and dysarthria. Sometimes, but not always, we find language problems in addition. Speech is not just retarded, it is distorted; speech development is not only delayed, it is pathological.

Mental retardation also may cause speech difficulties. The mentally retarded are often known to have "a heavy tongue"; their articulation and voice are likely to lack refinement. However, their speech is primitive rather than pathological.

A child suffering from both motor involvement and mental retardation is not only doubly handicapped but multiply so; he has to live not with two isolated but with two interwoven problems and they affect and stamp the entire personality. Faced with such grave difficulties, must we resign, or is there actually a way to change the facts (Mueller 1966b)? Speech therapists who have worked with these children know about the long-term treatments and the unsatisfactory results. Yet, what becomes of these handicapped individuals when they do not receive help in respect to their speech development?

1. Every child, including the mentally retarded who seemingly might not have much to say, feels the urge to communicate and/or express himself. If he is not successful in making himself understood, he will get more and more frustrated. This in turn will tend to increase his difficulties in society and may lead to psychological problems.

2. The speech organs are not only insufficiently coordinated for speech but also for the more simple functions of feeding. Without treatment, the difficulties in mastering liquids and food are not lessened through the years. On the contrary, they are very likely to become more abnormal by daily use, making the care of such children increasingly difficult and frustrating.

3. Incoordination of the speech organs usually is followed by lack of automatic control of saliva. Drooling is common among these children and becomes a real social problem as the child gets older.

Facing the facts, we cannot overlook the problems and close our eyes to the future of the multiply handicapped; their problems are and will remain our problems all through their lives.

The neurodevelopmental approach to the treatment of the motor handicapped associated with central nervous system (CNS) deficit has opened up new and more effective possibilities for influencing motor development, especially within the first ten months of life (Kong et al. 1967). It seems logical to use the same approach in treatment for motor patterns of speech.

Speech development begins with birth, as Gesell illustrates (Gesell and Amatruda 1960), and is very intense during the first few months (Herzka 1967). Abnormalities can be detected during these very early months. In reality, differential diagnosis in early infancy presents considerable difficulties because of the variation of the normal. Breathing, for example, may be recognized as abnormal when each expiration is blocked by a spasm, yet finer deviations are harder to detect as the very young infant's breathing follows his emotions and activities and is thus very irregular when he is awake. A thorough sensorimotor speech evaluation is based upon good knowledge and broad practical experience of normal development, exact observation of the handicapped individual in various situations, and careful analysis of the motor behavior.

SENSORIMOTOR EVALUATION

Since the results of the evaluation provide the outlines for treatment, good assessment and responsible interpretation are essential (Mueller 1967). Careful observation of the child at rest and during spontaneous motion is very important since knowledge of gross motor behavior will help in understanding fine motor abnormalities. The baby is watched best while on the mother's lap or arm and while she talks and plays with him. He is also observed in supine and in prone position and during locomotion or attempted locomotion. It is better to observe the child before manipulation and testing so that one is sure of spontaneous behavior.

The functioning of the speech organs has to be seen in relation to the whole body since the cerebral-palsied child usually reacts in more or less total movement patterns at any age. The normal child, through maturation, gradually inhibits the total motor patterns and acquires isolated and refined movements. Thus, the extent to which the cerebral-palsied child is functioning in relation to total reflex patterns and how exaggerated these responses are in comparison to the normal expected at age level will help to determine whether and to what degree motor abnormality is responsible for the feeding and speech problems. To differentiate pathological patterns from primitive patterns we watch for and compare (1) consistency of abnormal muscle tone, (2) motor quantity, quality, and symmetry at rest and in spontaneous motion, and (3) motor, mental, and social development with actual age.

To determine the language level and outline treatment, language reception and expression have to be evaluated in addition to the sensorimotor speech evaluation. Tests have been developed (D'Asaro 1961) and guides written (Wood 1964) which we have found of great interest and practical help. The important role which learning and vision play in speech development is well known. It will suffice here to refer to representatives of the existing literature who focus on very early diagnosis (Jones 1965, Lowe 1962).

It is important to bear in mind that generalized motor involvement from birth on distorts and limits normal sensory input and feedback, thus affecting language. For this reason it is important to bring to such infants the stimuli normally obtained through the infant's own exploratory efforts (another reason for early diagnosis) rather than to diagnose mental retardation.

Feeding Behavior

Feeding is the forerunner of speech, and the spontaneous feeding behavior of a child tells much about his oral development (Bosma 1963a, 1963b). Speech problems are likely to follow abnormal oral development. In the child with cerebral palsy, this abnormality is very frequently evident from birth. In fact, incoordination of jaws, lips, tongue, palate, pharynx, and larynx are among the earliest, and perhaps the easiest detectable signs of CNS deficit, where such deficit is due to prenatal or perinatal factors. These signs can best be observed during feeding. When asked about feeding behavior, the mother of such a child will usually answer in a positive sense if she has managed to get some nourishment down within a reasonable time. We must be interested in the *how* of feeding, and it is always wiser to watch the feeding behavior with our own eyes.

Testing the Oral Reflexes

This should be done first because these reflexes give a picture of the basic functioning of the oral structures. For procedures we refer to Prechtl and Beintema (1964).

ROOTING REFLEX. In the normal child the rooting response is present from birth, except when urinating, and gradually becomes weaker until it disappears at around three months of age. The child with cerebral palsy might show remnants of the rooting response much longer than that; in some cases he never has one. This latter finding might be a deception, however. We have found cases who reacted to testing in a seemingly negative manner; however, upon most careful observation, very weak signs of a reaction in the tongue or lips in the direction of the stimulus were noticed. It should be noted that the head never moved at all because of the influence of a tonic labyrinthine reflex. Inhibition of this reflex, using the shoulders as a key-point, immediately resulted in a classical rooting response. Experience has taught us that testing, as well as interpretation, cannot be undertaken with too much care, and that the entire child must be kept in mind at all times.

SUCKING-SWALLOWING REFLEX. This reflex appears in the normal baby (Baliassnikowa 1965) within the first or second day of life and remains until about two to five months. With cerebral palsy, it may continue much longer—in several cases for a number of years. In some cases, especially of hypotonia, it seems to be absent. In those with cerebral palsy, this reflex quite frequently goes along with protrusion of the tongue over the lower jaw or in severe cases, over the lower lip. A clicking sound of the soft palate can often be heard, and choking occurs more frequently than usual, leading us to suspect incoordination. Additional abnormalities of oral function during sucking are discussed later in the section on "Drinking, Sucking, Swallowing," and others can be seen during the observation of the sucking-swallowing reflex.

BITE REFLEX. The bite reflex is normally present from birth, gradually becoming weaker and disappearing at about three to five months. This reflex may continue throughout the life of an individual with cerebral palsy if he has not been helped to overcome it. It can become so exaggerated that the slightest stimulation will set it off, thus interfering with any of the child's activities. Such a dominant bite reflex makes feeding and dental care most difficult, unpleasant, and frustrating.

GAG REFLEX. Normally, the gag reflex can be elicited from birth, but becomes much weaker after about seven months when chewing has begun. Individual differences are normal but the posterior half of the tongue and the soft palate are the usual reflexogenic areas. It is considered exaggerated or abnormal if the gag reflex can be obtained by stimulation outside of the described boundaries. There seems to be a close relationship between the gag reflex and oral tactile sensitivity.

Oral Tactile Sensitivity

The threshold to tactile stimulation in the mouth very often is abnormally low in the person with cerebral palsy. It is seldom too high. This is called tactile hypersensitivity, a phenomenon which can be demonstrated especially clearly in the hemiplegic. The normal child might dislike testing within his mouth and turn his head away, but the oral muscle tone remains relaxed upon palpation. Those with cerebral palsy, however, often react in a total pattern of hyperextension or even with a startle response. In addition, the muscle tone differs from that found in the nonhandicapped. The lips, cheeks, tongue, or soft palate may offer considerable resistance to palpation. The gag reflex may be brought into action immediately or with delay as in cases with an ataxic component. Oral tactile sensitivity is, in our experience, highly exaggerated in children fed through a nasal gastric tube, yet seems to improve if the child is taken off the tube feeding before a prolonged period. This leads us to the conclusion that gavage feeding causes strong oral overstimulation.

Oral tactile hypersensitivity is always followed by feeding problems, as the child reacts to each stimulation of the spoon, cup, food or liquid in his mouth. Gagging, choking, or a total extensor thrust are very frequent consequences.

Tactile hyper- or hyposensitivity is not restricted to the oral structures. It can often be traced over the rest of the body, namely the head, trunk, and upper extremities (Rudel et al. 1966). Occasionally it is accompanied by oral hypersensitivity to taste and/or temperature.

Drinking, Sucking, Swallowing

The child with cerebral palsy often cannot adjust his lips to seal the sides for leaks while drinking (Fig. 6-1) and cannot close his jaws and coordinate his tongue for proper swallowing. This is true whether he is sucking from a bottle or drinking from a glass or cup. For the same reason, he cannot manage his saliva and often continues drooling throughout life. The tongue often protrudes over the mandible (Fig. 6-2) and in severe cases over the lips. Retrusion of the tongue is found less often. In children

Facilitating Feeding and Prespeech 289

with severe motor involvement, especially in those who have had gavage feeding, rhythmical tongue protrusion and mandibular retrusion can be observed almost without exception. This is a

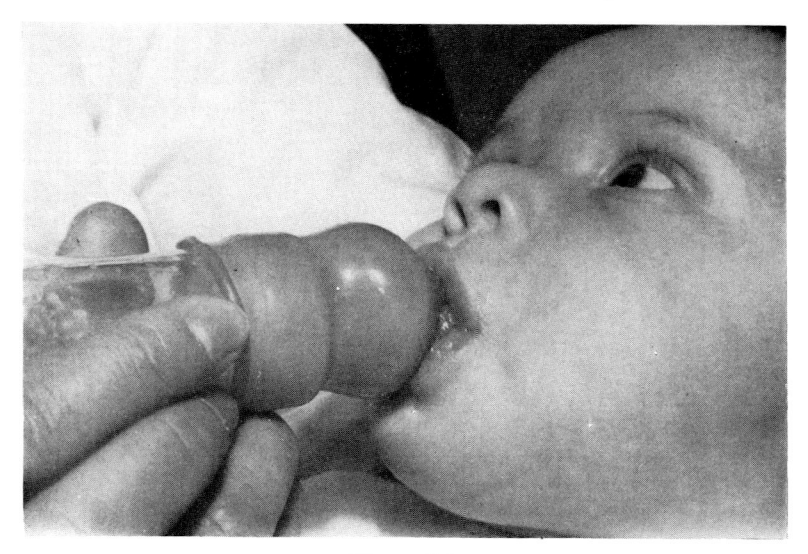

Figure 6-1.

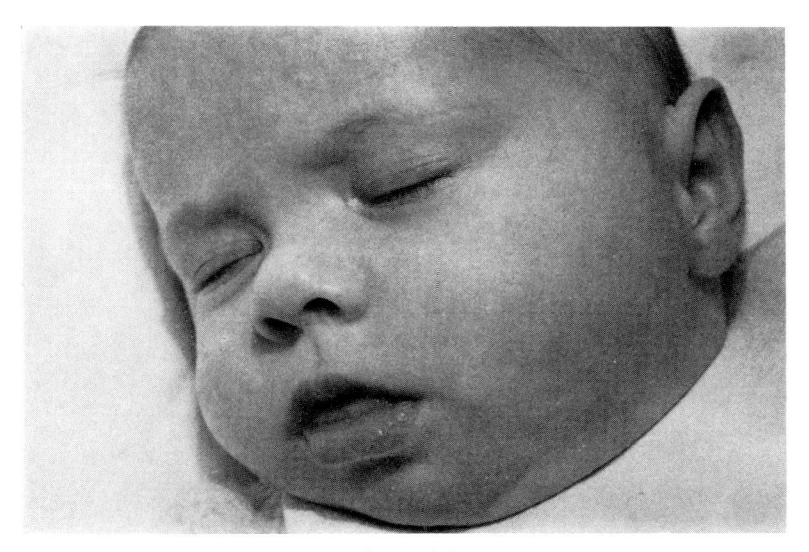

Figure 6-2.

primitive pathological motion which occurs in place of the sucking-swallowing reflex and includes a further opening of the already half-opened jaws and lips and no actual sucking or swallowing. Tactile hypersensitivity and an exaggerated gag reflex accompanies this phenomenon. There is absolutely no swallowing coordination, and the motions are in opposition to those needed for sucking, drinking, and swallowing. The abnormality seems more pronounced in children with an epileptic component, regardless of the mental status. It can become so overdeveloped that any stimulation, whether tactile, acoustic, visual, or proprioceptive may bring it into action.

FEEDING SOLIDS. Oral incoordination becomes even more obvious when spoon-feeding solid or semisolid food is presented. Mothers or nurses sometimes struggle up to an hour or more to get one meal down. When the food keeps being pushed out by the tongue or a strong gag reflex, the child is usually tilted back to let the food go down passively. Semisolids are used to make this easier. This is a torture for everybody involved, and it is not surprising that such children sometimes are kept on the bottle (if any type of sucking is possible regardless of how pathological it may be) long past the usual age or, if problems are drastic, tube feeding is introduced to keep the weight up.

Difficulties with the spoon may be less severe however. The child with cerebral palsy, after considerable initial problems, may begin to adjust but still lose parts of the bolus. He bites but does not chew what stays in the mouth because the jaws lack the rotatory movements and the tongue the fine motor control necessary for transference. The bolus may get partially stuck in the highly arched palate, and get partially gulped down the throat, frequently accompanied by some choking and/or gagging and coughing. We have met older children who used their extensor thrust to get the food back down, a way of self-help which certainly makes the pathological gross motor behavior continuously worse.

Mothers cannot be blamed for giving strained food in the most adequate feeding position for years if their child chokes on solids, although this is certainly to no advantage to his teeth, gums, and further oral development. Even then, it might still remain a time-consuming and unesthetic duty which has to be done regularly and reliably since the child's health largely depends on it. It may easily become a source of tension between mother or nurse and child.

Breathing, Voice, Phonation

Breathing

The next step in evaluation consists of observation of breathing at rest and under stimulation. In the normal child, it is regular and deep at rest. Under stimulation it is adaptable; changes in rate and volume are made rather smoothly and immediately if necessary. The cerebral-palsied individual's breathing under stimulation as well as at rest may be shallow and irregular and is often blocked by intermittent spasms. His flexor pattern fixes the arms against the sides of the rib cage; deep inhalation is impossible in this posture. When the extensor pattern is dominant, the chest is drawn flat and breathing is superficial.

Voice

Voice is largely based on breathing. Where breathing is abnormal, voice will be abnormal in volume, fluency, initiation, and adaptability. In addition, the neuromotor-handicapped child is likely to show spasms of the diaphragm, pharynx, and velum causing aphonia and/or dysphonia. Voice might be heard on inhalation instead of exhalation. The pitch often is too low or too high; under sudden or extreme excitement it may switch to the other extreme. Spasticity or hypotonia limit the range of voice, keeping it monotonous and short-winded, while intermittent spasms interfere with fluency and loudness. Constant or intermittent hypernasality is found in the majority of these children and is almost always based on insufficient velum and tongue control, making the voice sound whiny.

In normal development, the nasal monotonous cry of the newborn becomes continuously more oral and the range of voice begins to grow during the first week, although in crying it remains nasal longer than in laughing.

The voice of the individual with cerebral palsy often is forced out to make it heard. The air stream exits all at once, barely using the resonance of the oral and nasal cavities and the sinuses. The result is poor timbre, lack of volume, volume changes, and fineness—components which make speech lively and aid in the transmission of thoughts.

All the above-described abnormalities of breathing and voice can be observed in the young infant. The child need not be at the "talking age" to make evaluation of speech development possible. Crying, (Illingworth 1955) laughing, and babbling are early forms of speech, (Herzka 1967) and tell us much about development of facial expression, gesture, breathing, voice, and phonation. At three months, the normal baby makes a difference in crying depending on the reason (for example, hunger or pain). The smile first consists of grimacing, soon becomes more differentiated and accompanied by a nasal vowel sound until it turns into oral giggles at three months and into laughter at four months, with increasing variations thereafter.

Phonation

Phonation (whether it consists of crying, laughing, or babbling), facial expression, and body movement form a unity in early infancy. Neuromotor deficit will therefore usually affect all three factors. Where the body is fixed in hyperextension and the baby is unable to turn over into prone (at around 4 months), often with subluxation of the mandible and protrusion of the tongue, throat sounds may be produced but labial sounds will not come as naturally. Abnormal feeding patterns then develop as described earlier. Fine motor development of these organs is not being exercised as is the case when gradually changing the normal baby from bottle-feeding to spoon-feeding. Such a child lacks motor preparations for articulation. The refinement of facial expression cannot develop under these circumstances. A persisting asymmetric tonic neck reflex will eventually cause deviation of the mandible and tongue towards the skull side, thus restraining the articulatory structures in asymmetrical position. In neither case will dental development take its normal course.

The description of abnormal motor development due to central nervous system deficit and its influence on phonation could be continued. The relationship between intelligence quotient and articulatory development need not concern us before the age of approximately 20 months, according to corresponding studies. We merely need to learn to watch, listen, compare, and relate prespeech (Herzka 1967).

BASIC PRINCIPLES OF THE TECHNIQUE

Sensorimotor speech evaluation of individuals with cerebral palsy points out, with few exceptions, that speech developed abnormally from the very beginning affects the motor as well as the sensory part since they form a unity. Input, output, feedback, and communication are disturbed from earliest infancy. Mental, social, and motor retardation cannot but follow. The degree depends on the severity of the child's motor and associated handicaps, on the attitude of his surroundings and (we are inclined to say for a relatively small part only), on the child's capacity.

Early treatment seems to be not only a possibility but a necessity. Facilitating normal speech development must be easier and more effective at an age where the brain is at the beginning of its development and myelination has not yet been accomplished, than trying to undo set pathological patterns and to reeducate long past the stage of comparable normal development. Furthermore, the goal is the establishment of automatic habit patterns. It would be inhuman and useless for life to teach the child to swallow (saliva, liquid, food), breathe, phonate, and speak by means of constant voluntary control. He would have to center his full attention on the functioning of the tools instead of on the purpose of the function, the motivation, and the aim.

The neurodevelopmental approach to treatment has been found most adequate. Physical therapy prepares the way for gross motor control by inhibiting abnormal reflexes where inhibition by the child's central nervous system is insufficient or lacking, and simultaneously facilitating the appropriate movement patterns. Key-points are used to let the child actively, but automatically, assist and possibly complete the initiated motion. Speech therapy continues in the same fashion, making use of the improved body and head control. Emphasis is mainly toward refinement of the oral-pharyngeal movements, basically following the rules of normal development (Mueller 1966a).

Facilitating Feeding

Feeding therapy is usually practiced in the most natural and intensive way if carried out by the mother or responsible nurse, as long as her attitude toward the child is relatively healthy. Where this is not the case, it may be best to give feeding therapy a good start by the professional person before handing it over to the mother (Bosma 1963b). In either case, she needs to be instructed very carefully and in very small steps from one session to the next if treatment is to be of high quality. Regular checkups in short intervals of one week to begin with will give reassurance and encouragement and secure good up-to-date treatment. Loving consequence paired with the "know-how" make up the basis for successful therapy.

Feeding Positions

The feeding position should be such that it breaks up the motor pattern of the asymmetrical tonic neck reflex or of total hyperextension or hyperflexion of the body, and makes isolated movements of arms, head, jaw, tongue, and lips possible.

FEEDING THE YOUNG INFANT OR VERY SEVERELY INVOLVED BABY. The mother or nurse sits in front of the table, feet resting on a stool. A large pillow is placed on the edge of the table so that it covers her lap. The infant lies on his back on the pillow facing the adult. The angle at which the infant lies can be changed to a more upright position by changing the relation of the adult's lap to the table height. Through the support of the underlying table edge, the infant's head is held in slight flexion. The legs are kept apart and scissoring is made impossible by the adult's trunk. Arms are brought forward. In this position the mother or nurse then has one hand free for jaw control, the other for feeding (Fig. 6-3). She also has good face-to-face contact with

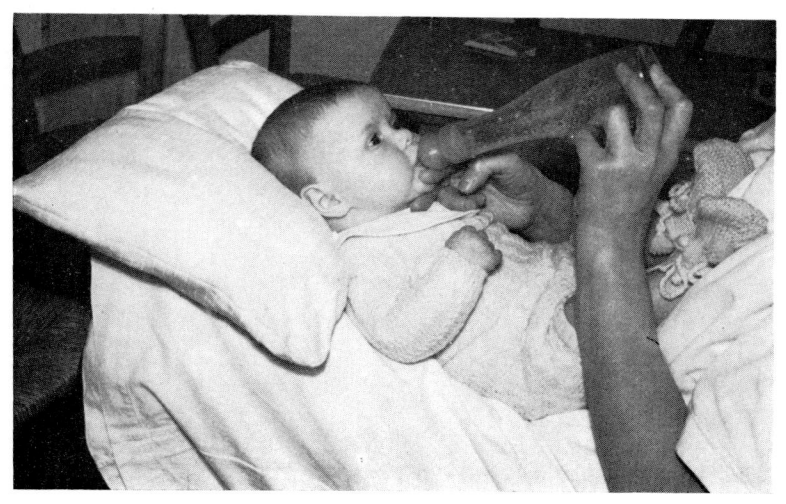

Figure 6-3.

the infant or baby and can guard against asymmetry of the head and jaw and tongue.

FEEDING THE OLDER BABY. As soon as the baby can assume the upright position or hold it if placed there, even though support is still necessary, he is best fed by placing him across the lap with hips bent at right angle and knees slightly apart. If his extensor pattern is very strong, the person feeding him should put her leg under the baby's knees. The leg should be raised by placing the foot on a stool. Thus the baby's buttocks are lowered and the flexion in the hips and knees increased. It is important to bring the arms forward to avoid hyperextension of the shoulders and the head. The adult then brings her one arm around the baby's back and with that hand can apply jaw control if needed while the other hand is free for feeding (Fig. 6-4).

FEEDING IN THE CHAIR. As soon as the baby is ready to sit in a high chair or at the table, care is taken that his hips, knees, and elbows are in a right angle position with the knees slightly apart. If the seat is too deep or wide, a wooden insert or a firm foam rubber pad will enable him to be placed in the correct position. If the child has to be fed or needs assistance, this is preferably done from the front (Fig. 6-5). In cases of poor trunk or head

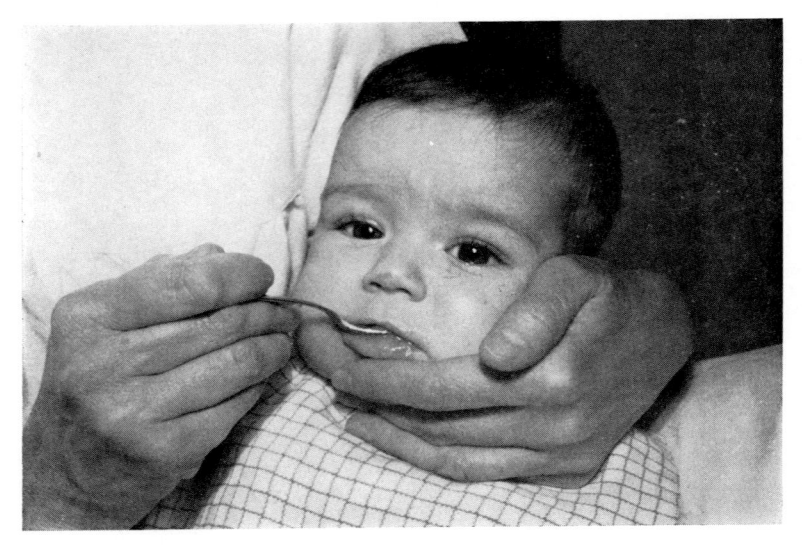

296 *Physical Therapy Services in the Developmental Disabilities*

Figure 6-4.

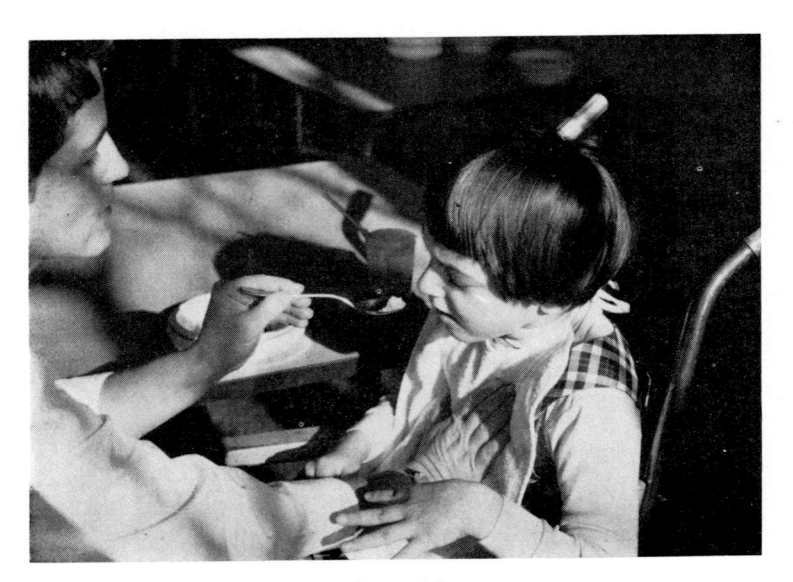

Figure 6-5.

balance and when scissoring of the legs is strong, sitting at the table in riding fashion or on a sawhorse instead of a chair will make trunk and head control possible due to the breaking up of the total extensor/flexor pattern by abduction and outward rotation of the legs. A low block attached to the sawhorse behind the child's rump will stop him from sliding back. A higher back is inadequate when aiming for trunk control.

FEEDING IN PRONE POSITION. Children with severe sucking and swallowing problems and with functional retrusion of the mandible should be put in the prone position for better coordination of these organs (Bosma 1963b). Young infants are best bundled in a receiving blanket and put on the mother's or nurse's underarm which rests against the pillow so that the infant lies at a 45-degree angle. A banana-shaped bottle might have to be used while feeding in the prone position (Bosma 1960). A bigger, stronger baby can be put across one's lap in a slanting position if one crosses one's legs or puts one's foot on a stool to bring the leg under the baby's chest up higher (Fig. 6-6).

In any of these feeding positions, symmetry of the baby's body is very important. The weight ought to be distributed evenly on both hips. If this is not the case, it may be necessary to abduct and outwardly rotate and hold one leg in this position. The asymmetrical tonic neck reflex causes asymmetry. This can be corrected by bending the extensor (face) arm across the child's chest for inhibition and by feeding him from the front (Fig. 6-12). If the baby is still being fed on the lap, he should be switched so that he has to turn his head the unused way even if this is against the mother's handedness.

Normalizing Oral Tactile Sensitivity

Exaggerated response to oral stimulation can be very destructive for feeding. Its normalization is therefore best initiated at the beginning of feeding therapy. It is attempted in one of the feeding positions described above which is most appropriate for the individual child.

Jaw control (Fig. 6-7) must be kept up from the beginning to the end of the procedure so that the lacking inhibition

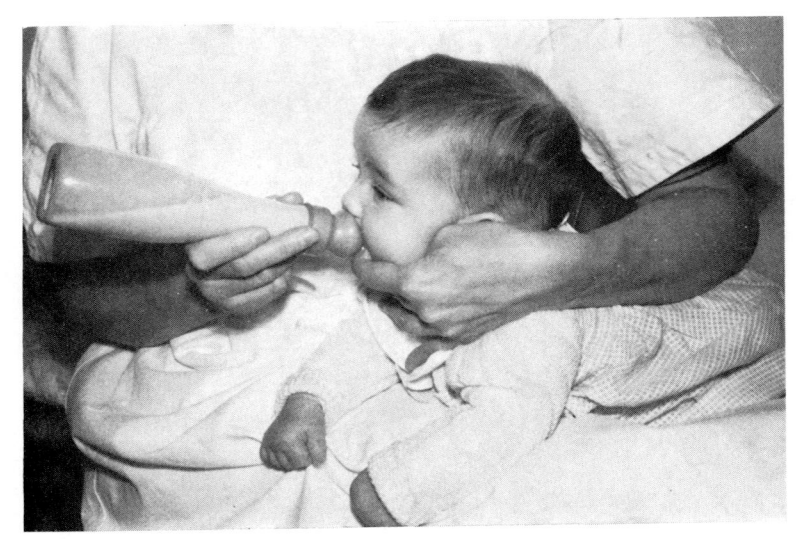

Figure 6-6.

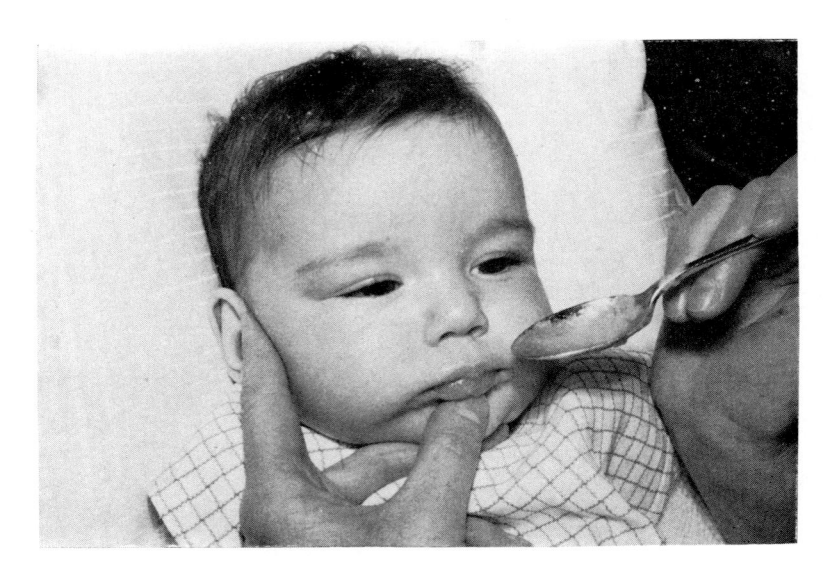

Figure 6-7.

will not cause overstimulation which reinforces the pathological response. When the jaws are held closed and in symmetry, the outer gums on one side are rubbed with a few (approximately three) firm strokes, gradually reducing the firmness later. This digital stimulation causes the production of saliva and provides an opportunity to facilitate swallowing coordination. To obtain this, we place one finger between the upper lip and nose with proximal pressure horizontally (Fig. 6-8)—this is in addition to maintaining jaw control—and leave it there until swallowing has occurred. In the beginning there might be considerable delay and/or resistance on the part of the child.

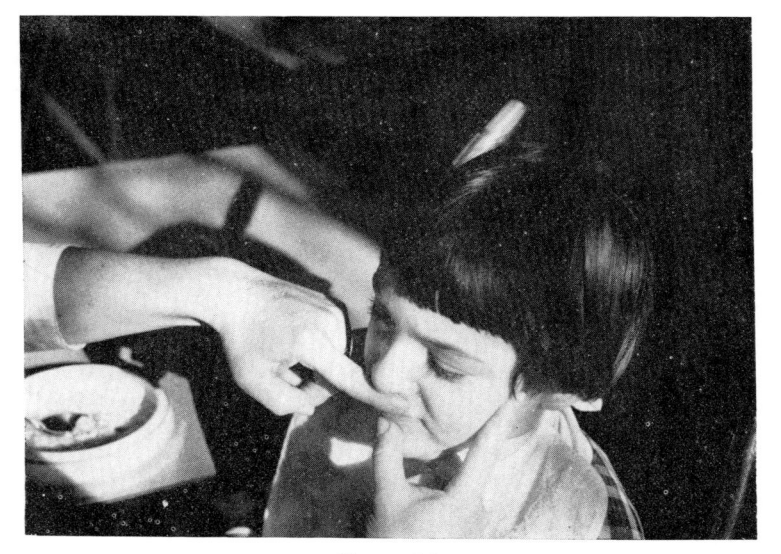

Figure 6-8.

Not until swallowing is completed do we rub the outer gum, then the gums inside the mouth on either side, and then the hard palate, alternating between the midline and lateral areas and proceeding from anterior to posterior. Lastly the tongue should be given firm strokes from front to back. Each time one of the above-named areas is stimulated, the finger should be immediately withdrawn from the mouth and the jaws and lips closed so that the gag reflex is avoided. Again, proper swallowing should be facilitated in the manner described above.

A variation for facilitating lip closure might bring a welcome change to the child. Instead of placing one finger between the upper lip and nose with proximal pressure, we may use this finger to lightly stroke the lower lip two or three times, gently pulling it out and letting it spring closed. These two ways to initiate mouth closure can also be used in daily life and eventually are much more effective and less frustrating than constant verbal reminding.

If this procedure is carried out regularly just before mealtime, feeding will become easier and hypersensitivity will decrease. Also, drooling will eventually disappear. This is due to the simultaneous improvement of swallowing coordination and oral differentiation, although this may take weeks or even months of treatment.

Facilitating Drinking

In cases of minor abnormalities in bottle-drinking (such as slight protrusion of the tongue), inhibition of the root of the tongue is indicated. The flat of the middle finger is placed under the child's mandible to decrease tongue spasticity or thrust (Fig. 6-3). If tongue and swallowing abnormalities are more severe, the child should be taken off the bottle since the tongue cannot be controlled much in bottle-drinking. Giving the liquid from a cup allows assistance in acquiring better movements. Cup-drinking is also introduced for this same reason with children who have no sucking reflex and are being gavaged. To begin with, a plastic cup with a little outward rim can be squeezed together for a spout. The jaws have to be closed first using the earlier-described jaw control. The cup is then brought to the mouth and the rim placed on the lower lip (Fig. 6-9). The cup should not be put between the teeth. This stimulates the bite reflex which is often very active in cerebral-palsied children, preventing normal oral development. Very small amounts of liquid are poured in regular intervals, leaving the cup on the lower lip during swallowing.

The same procedure is carried out when a straw is used or

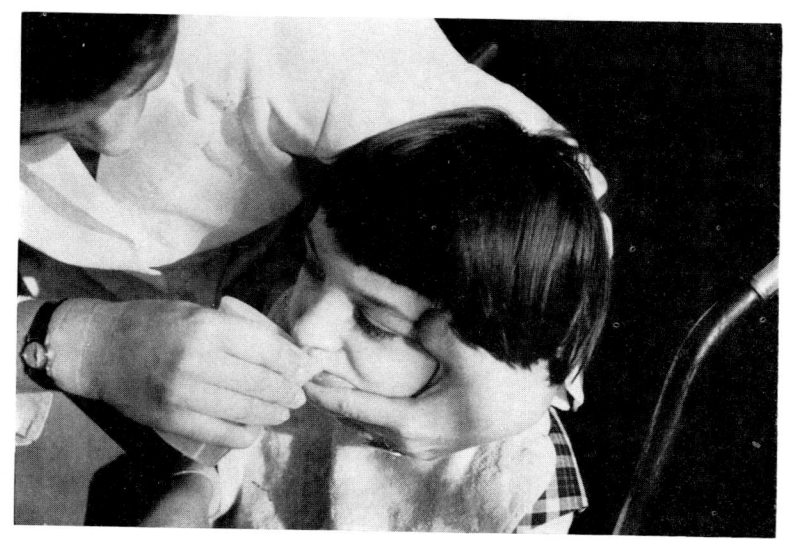

Figure 6-9.

when the child learns to drink through a straw held by the therapist. Polyester tubing serves best to teach coordinated lip-sucking, not to be confused with the much more primitive reflex-sucking. Again the child is assisted in jaw control. The tube is placed between the lips (Fig. 6-10), never between the teeth, in order to stimulate lip-sucking and to stop biting.

The child will eventually begin to take over the sucking movement (Fig. 6-11) and help is gradually withdrawn until he is able to manage alone (Fig. 6-12). Correct cup-drinking, and even more so, correct straw-sucking are excellent functional exercises for lips and swallowing coordination.

Facilitating Spoon-feeding

Head and jaw control are essential for children with feeding difficulties due to neuromotor deficit (Fig. 6-7). The adult's middle finger under the child's chin controls the opening (extension) of the mandible. The index finger on the side of the jaw regulates the horizontal deviation of the mandible. The flat of the thumb on the child's chin just below the lower lip initiates

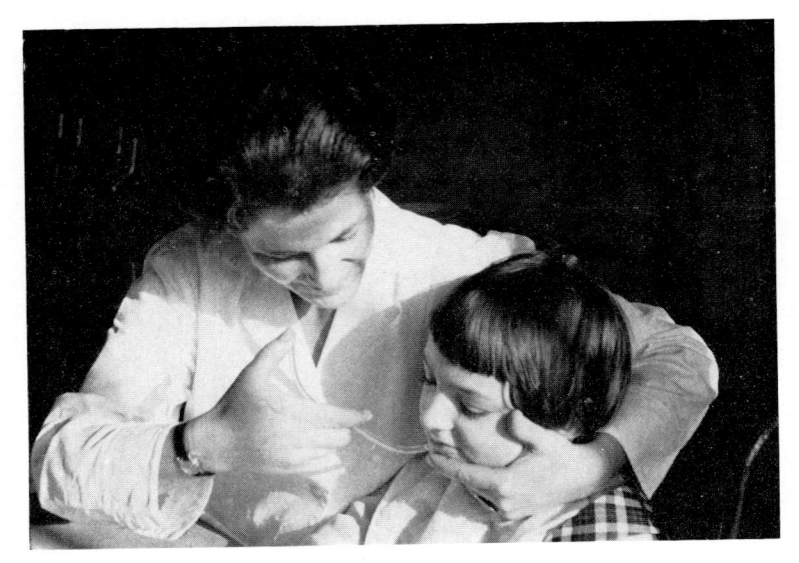

Figure 6-10.

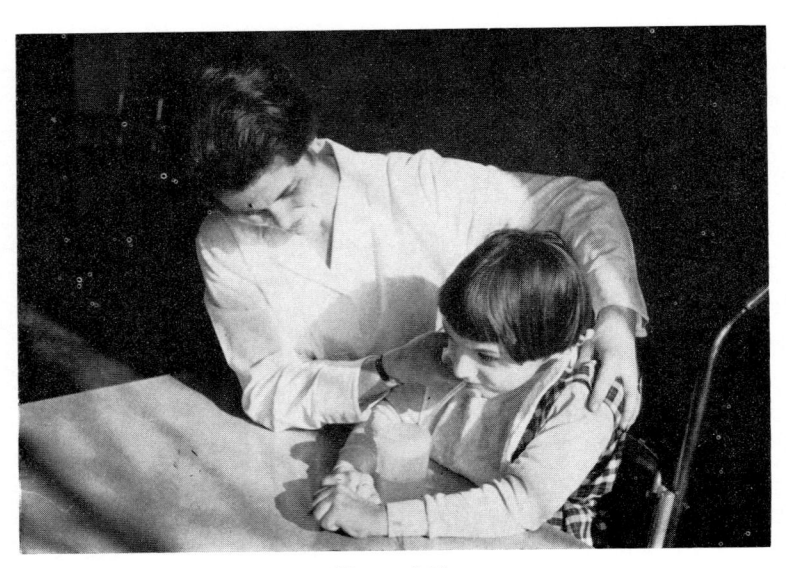

Figure 6-11.

Facilitating Feeding and Prespeech

the opening and rotatory movements in chewing and controls the closure (flexion) of the mandible. It also keeps the head in a slightly flexed position. If the child is fed from the side and the adult's arm has to go around behind the child's head to apply jaw control from the side (Fig. 6-9), thumb and index finger are exchanged in their positions.

With these three fingers the child's jaw is lightly closed. Then a metal spoon of appropriate size with just a little food on the tip is brought to the mouth in midline to keep the child in midline with visual and/or olfactory help. The jaw then is allowed to open halfway only while the spoon is placed on top of the anterior half of the tongue. Firm downward pressure is applied to the tongue with the spoon and held for a few seconds until the lips begin to close in order to take the food off the spoon. The latter is then withdrawn straight out without scraping it on the upper incisors, since the upper lip has to learn to do that job. It is most important to close the jaw immediately after the spoon has been withdrawn and to keep it closed until swallowing has occurred and is completed.

The pressure on the tongue, as well as the mouth closure,

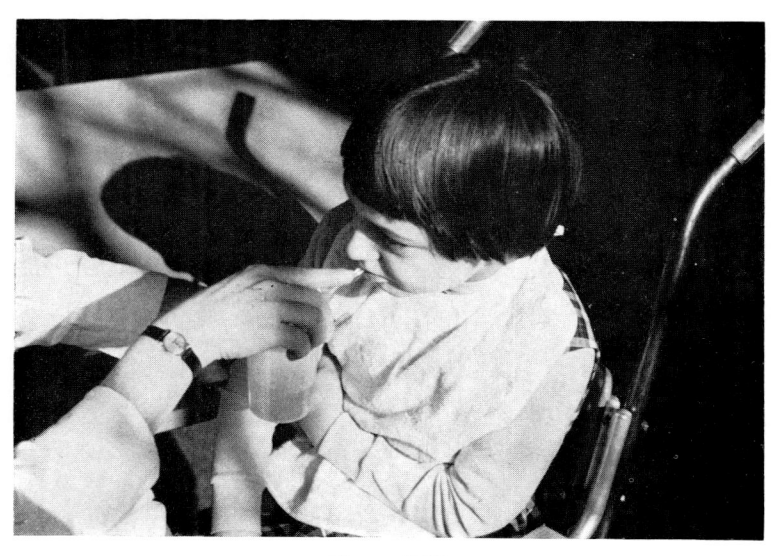

Figure 6-12.

serve to inhibit the tongue thrust and the reverse swallowing. This pressure also facilitates coordinated swallowing (Hahn 1966). This is a very important step in the development of lip, jaw, and tongue coordination and follows the primitive reflex-sucking of the very young infant. This pressure on the tongue, combined with jaw control, is introduced passively; after continuous practice, the child will take over automatically and jaw control can gradually be reduced accordingly.

The approaching spoon is a strong stimulus and frequently causes hyperextension of the head and jaw and often of the entire body. Therefore, body position and good jaw control need to be watched at all times. It is wise to reach control before approaching the stimulus, whether it is the bottle, cup, spoon, or finger. Head extension can be stopped or prevented by temporary pressure or tapping on the child's chest with the palm or back of the adult's hand (Fig. 6-5). Normalization of oral tactile sensitivity threshold will certainly pay off in spoon-feeding.

Strained but fairly dry or at least semisolid food is best chosen when introducing spoon-feeding. Liquids or very thin strained food are considerably more difficult for the child with oral dysfunction. With increasing improvement, coarser food has to be served. Food of mixed consistency, such as minestrone, will always remain the most difficult to manage.

For hand-feeding, the crust of dark bread is best. Later, apples, carrots, and similar foods may be used. White bread, buns, cookies, or similar items immediately get mixed with saliva and turn into sticky dough, usually ending up pasted onto the roof of the mouth.

For psychological reasons, children who have already been feeding themselves or are at an age when they feel a strong urge to do so should not be stopped in this self-help. In our experience, it has worked very well to assist them with a minimum of body control through key-points, such as shoulder (Fig. 6-11) and wrist (Fig. 6-13), and with jaw control and lip closure for swallowing. Sometimes it may be indicated to give the child a good start by feeding the first few bites or swallows. We may include the child's own hand until we finally can withdraw our help, partially or fully, and let the child function unassisted for awhile.

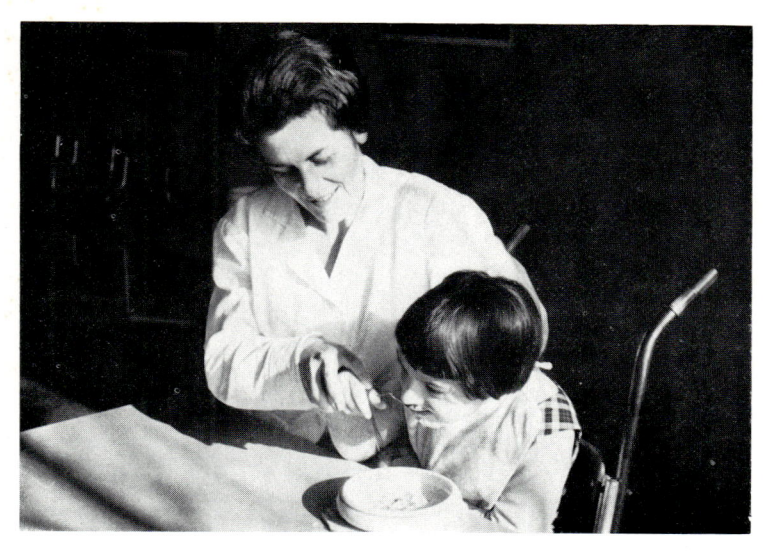

Figure 6-13.

Facilitating Prespeech

When feeding therapy is well on its way, we may proceed to this phase of treatment. To lay the ground for a useful speaking voice, attention should first be guided towards breathing. Close observation during physical therapy, if on the lines of neurodevelopmental treatment, informs us that with more normal muscle tone and motor behavior, breathing becomes more normal also. Movement, especially rotation, stimulates breathing; this means that good physiotherapy automatically includes natural breathing therapy. This preparation for speech is even more effective when facilitation of mouth closure is included to initiate nose breathing. Evaluation shows that very ׳many children with cerebral palsy lack differentiation of oral and nasal breathing and phonation.

The physical therapist can facilitate automatic mouth closure by (1) temporary pressure with one finger horizontally above the upper lip, or (2) by lightly stroking the underlip a few times, or (3) lightly stroking the upper lip if it is very spastic. In cases of strong tongue spasms (double chin) or extreme protrusion of tongue, the described facilitation may be insufficient for spontaneous mouth closure. We then need to inhibit the tongue spasm through pressure on the root of the tongue, placing the flat of our finger across and under the child's chin (Fig. 6-7) until muscle tone is felt to be more normal. If stabilization of the tongue is needed, intermittent pressure by tapping the same place is used.

This facilitation of mouth closure for nasal breathing can be attempted during any good movement pattern as long as the child's head is under control and the therapist can free one hand momentarily. No fixed position is necessary. Nose breathing is more effective still if one nostril is pressed lightly closed for awhile. This can also be done during motion. It can also be used to practice blowing of the nose, but in that case, jaw control must go along with it to prevent the air stream from taking its usual course via the mouth.

Vibration, being intense movement, facilitates voice. It therefore is an excellent means for stimulation and regulation of voice. It has proven most useful to combine it with facilitation of gross motor patterns, preferably in body rotation such as rotating from prone to supine and vice versa. Movement patterns which are geared towards dissociation of shoulder and head and facilitation of isolated head movements have an especially favorable effect on voice initiation and quality. During the child's spontaneous expiration, vibration with light pressure is applied via arm, shoulder, side of rib cage, chest or vertebrae, the latter being the most intense way in respect to voice. The palms and fingers of the therapist's hands spread pressure evenly and are never removed from the child's body; this is done in order to avoid additional stimulation. In order to get deeper and more rhythmical breathing, vibration and pressure upon exhalation is gradually increased and held longer before giving way to the next inhalation.

The therapist, possibly from the beginning of breathing-voice therapy, will make a vowel sound during exhalation and let the child experience the visual, auditory, and tactile sensation. The infant will usually react by imitating the therapist's sound. If there is no such spontaneous reaction (which may be the case in an older child), he is asked to let the sound come out rather than to make a sound since we are aiming for spontaneous automatic reaction rather than for voluntary control. For this same reason he is never asked to produce a longer, better, or louder sound. It is up to the therapist to provide the conditions for a more normal voice. The child will eventually become more aware and conscious of his own voice and phonation in a natural way, as is the case in normal development. If he does not have the correct mouth position for the vowel wanted, the therapist needs to facilitate it with one hand on the child's oral structures.

It is important to start vibration before the child initiates the sound in order to facilitate soft, relaxed phonation rather than spasm or forced voice. The therapist then changes frequency and loudness, and introduces pauses by changing the speed and intensity of vibration and pressure, thus leading into intonation of speech. All vowels are eventually practiced and used in this fashion, starting with the neutral "o" (as in father) and flexor "u" (as in food). Where voice therapy is done well, children will sometimes interpret it as playing an instrument: "I am the instrument and you are the musician." This interpretation results from a pleasant, comfortable, and valuable experience, and the child without being aware gradually turns himself into the "musician."

Consonants are then introduced in the same fashion, always using multisensory stimuli in variation. However, the consonants are never practiced in isolation but always in syllables and preferably started in medial position for soft voice initiation. They are always facilitated passively first. We may, for example, begin with vibration, and while the child sounds the vowel "o," we lightly and gently facilitate momentary mouth closure with our free hand, reopening immediately to maybe close again without interfering with the child's voicing. Thus we will have produced "obobo . . ." to his total surprise and thrill, and without voluntary effort or spasms. He will eventually take over the initiated movement.

"L" will be introduced similarly by light facilitation of a vertical movement of the tongue, with the therapist's finger under the tongue tip while the child phonates (for example, "a"). Normalization of intra-oral tactile sensitivity will then pay off.

Other consonants, such as explosives, and many lingual sounds, especially "sh," are considerably more difficult to produce for the cerebral-palsied individual. The therapist's thorough knowledge of the correct production of these consonants is necessary.

Treatment has now definitely reached the point where the speech therapist must take over. Up to now the physical therapist could very well include this prespeech facilitation in her treatment. This will be the favored procedure, especially in young infants who preferably should receive treatment from one person only. Treatment should form a unity.

All consonants will eventually have to be introduced—always in syllables and never in isolation, built into words, phrases, and sentences, using objects and later, pictures. The sequence of normal development is our guide in this prespeech therapy. Good contact between speech therapist and child is important in the dialogue which lays the groundwork for speech and language development of the physically handicapped-mentally retarded as well as for the normal baby.

Simple forms of dialogue begin soon after birth and are normally established acoustically in the eighth month of life (Herzka 1967). Emphasis should therefore be put on the learning opportunity which the dialogue offers. Mothers usually intuitively make ample use of it, but the mother of a physically-mentally handicapped infant is likely to give up if she gets poor or no reaction from him. It is wise to point out to her the importance of this combined form of visual, tactile, and auditory communication, even if it remains a monologue for some time, and to gradually teach her to facilitate sounds, thus assisting her child in prespeech. This will at the same time be a psychologically important incitation; the mother can do something for her handicapped child and usually gets some immediate result.

The sooner we start facilitating prespeech, the better are our chances. We can never make up the lost time no matter how concentrated our treatment may be. And it does need to be concentrated, even in the very young infant, to keep up with his growth. We do not, for example, wait with feeding therapy or facilitation of sounds until response to oral digital stimulation is almost normal; gross motor patterns, breathing, and oral-nasal differentiation are treated simultaneously. The same holds true for normalization of oral sensitivity, jaw-lip-tongue control and swallowing coordination in feeding. Furthermore, speech and language are always woven in naturally with the child's care and treatment to help establish concepts. The motor side alone does not make up the tools for speech and language expression; the sensory side is its mate. Prespeech therapy will inevitably outgrow the monologue and dialogue stage. A greater variety of stimuli, from a broader angle, is necessary to prepare the child for life. The adequate therapy situation will at the same time be a social and educational learning situation.

When facilitating feeding and prespeech with the physically handicapped-mentally retarded, our goal cannot be to have the child adjust to our well-planned treatment and to eventually reach perfect speech. Rather, we need to adjust our treatment to him by continuous reassessment so that it will constantly be up-to-date, meeting the child's present needs for functioning in daily living, and helping him towards the best possible development.

BIBLIOGRAPHY

Baliassnikowa, N.J.: *Zur Neurologic des Saugens.* Zeitschrift fur Kinderforschung, 1. Heft (Reprint) Springer Verlag Wien, New York, 1965.

Bosma, J.F.: Maturation of functioning of the oral and pharyngeal region. *Amer J Orthodont*, February, 1963a.

Bosma, J.F.: Oral and pharyngeal development and function. *J Dent Res*, January-February, 1963b.

Bosma, J.F.: Disability of oral function in infant, associated with displacement of the tongue. *Acta Paediat*, March, 1960.

D'Asaro, M.: "REP Scale" Rating scale for evaluation of receptive, expressive and phonetic language development in the young child. *Cereb Palsy Rev*, September-October, 1961.

Gesell, A., and Amatruda, C.S.: *Developmental Diagnosis*, 10th ed. New York, Paul B. Hoeber, 1960.

Hahn, E.: Problems in tongue behavior of children. *J S Calif Dent Ass*, July, 1966.

Herzka, E.: *Die Sprache des Sauglings.* Basel, Schwabe and Company, 1967.

Illingworth, R.S.: Crying in infants and children. *Brit Med J*, 75-78, 1955.

Irwin, O.C.: Speech development in the young child. *J Speech Disab*, 17:269-279, 1952.

Jones, M.H.: *Newer Concepts in the Diagnosis and Treatment of Visual and Related Perceptual Problems of Cerebral Palsied Individuals.* Practical implementation of rehabilitation proceedings of Third Pan Pacific Rehabilitation Conference, Tokyo, Japan, 1965. Japanese Society for Rehabilitation of the Disabled.

Kong, E., Mosthaf, U., Mueller, H.A., and Lauber, M. *Behandlung und Erziehung von Kindern mit cerebralen Bewegungsstorungen.* Schweiz. Vereinigung fur c. g. Kinder, 1967.

Lowe, A.: *Hausspracherziehung fur horgeschadigte Kleinkinder.* Berlin, Marhold, 1962.

Mueller, H.A.: *Prespeech Evaluation and Therapy.* 16 mm film, sound, black and white. University of California at Los Angeles, 1967.

Mueller, H.A.: *Spracherziehung beim cerebralgelahmten Kind.* Padiatrie und Padologie, Band 2. Heft 2/3, Springer Wien, New York, 1966a.

Mueller, H.A.: *Moglichkeiten der Sprachtherapie bei cerebral bewegungsgestorten Kindern.* Mehrfach horgeschadigte Kinder, Sonderheft 5 (also in English), Kettwig Verl., West Germany, 1966b.

Prechtl, H., and Beintema, D.: *The Neurological Examination of the Fullterm Newborn Infant.* Little Club Clinics in *Developmental Medicine*, No. 12. The Spastics Society. London, Heinemann, 1964.

Rudel, R.G., Teuber, H.L., and Twitchell, T.E.: *A Note on Hyperesthesia in Children with Early Brain Damage.* Massachusetts Institute of Technology, Cambridge, Massachusetts. *Neuropsychologia,* 4:351-356, 1966; London, Pergamon Press.

Wood, N.E.: *Delayed Speech and Language Development.* Englewood Cliffs, Prentice-Hall, 1964.

Chapter Seven

THE USE OF MOVEMENT ACTIVITIES IN THE EDUCATION OF RETARDED CHILDREN

BRYANT J. CRATTY

Introduction

IT IS APPARENT to teachers concerned with the educational needs of retarded children that they rarely give evidence of dealing with the abstract. Instead, these children are primarily absorbed by the immediate, the here and now, by what they can do motorically, and by what they observe others doing in their presence. There is an increasing amount of evidence that retarded children's educational progress may be enhanced through the use of motor tasks involving simple responses to easily discernible stimuli.

Within the past several years the writer, as a consultant to the Los Angeles City School District, has collected data and worked with teachers and students within classrooms for the retarded and physically handicapped. During this time, after inspecting the data collected in several investigations (Cratty 1966) and analyzing the observed responses of retarded children in classroom situations, it has become apparent that certain types of perceptual-motor activities may enhance their educational progress. These activities, it is believed, should not be applied in haphazard sequences, nor should they be utilized in a way which ignores extrinsic and intrinsic motivational factors such as the social rewards emanating from the teacher and the novelty and complexity of various tasks and subtasks (Cratty 1967b, 1967c).

Subdivisions of this approach to the education of the retarded include two initial stages in which the objectives of impulse control and body image are stressed; a third stage in which specific and basic perceptual-motor competencies are emphasized; a fourth and fifth stage in which seriation and pattern and letter recognition are stressed; and a final stage involving response generalization and problem solving. The following program is not believed to constitute an all-encompassing panacea which will ameliorate the intellectual, emotional, and physical deficiencies of atypical children, but at the same time it is believed that the six-phase program outlined holds promise for what is believed to be important components of a total educational program for retarded children.

Two primary advantages of a program component incorporating movement activities include the fact that the quality of the children's responses are readily evaluated by the observing teacher and the complexity of the stimulus conditions are easily adjustable to allow for increasing difficulty.

The initial stages of the program are based upon the hypotheses that (1) children must be able to place themselves under at least a moderate degree of self-control in order to learn and (2) a child must know where he is in space and where and what his body is doing before he can engage in more difficult perceptual discriminations which lead toward reading, writing, and similar classroom skills.

The intermediate stages of the program emphasize tasks which will provide additional channels through which the child will begin to organize perceptual discriminations of space and time, specifically involving the recognition of patterns, letters, and the manner in which order may be assigned to events and objects.

The final stages of the program are an attempt to lead the retardate toward a higher level of thinking. Voluntary movements of normals are, to varying degrees, accompanied by cognition (Mosston 1966). It is possible that the thought processes of retardates may be improved by encouraging them to think and then to act, rather than simply requiring them to follow another's directions without any intellectual involvement on the part of the students.

Phase I: Impulse Control

A frequent finding in the psychological literature during the past forty years is that there is an optimum level of arousal appropriate to the performance and learning of a given task (Duffy 1962). If an individual is overaroused, he is as likely to perform poorly in both intellectual and motor tasks as if he were inattentive or too passive in his approach to the task. Studies of normal children indicate that there is a high relationship between scores reflecting a good degree of impulse control, obtained as the child is asked to do various tasks as slowly as he can, and intellectual measures (MacCCoby et al. 1965). Normal male children who achieve best in classroom tasks have been found to be those who are able to place themselves under good control, while the elementary school-age girl who is slightly more vigorous in her approach to life than most is usually more creative and able when engaging in various intellectual endeavors (Kagen 1966).

It is usual to observe that children with mental and/or physical handicaps lack the ability to adjust their tension-arousal mechanisms to levels appropriate to the tasks at hand. Some may be too passive while many evidence unusual hyperactivity. They constantly function at a level of arousal inappropriate to most tasks with which they are confronted in the home and in the school. It would thus seem that one of the initial jobs for the educator is to aid the atypical child to gain better control of himself, to "slow himself down" when various tasks requiring accurate movements are called for (i.e. handwriting) and in other ways to help him to become aware of the residual tensions which plague him.

This initial phase, emphasizing impulse control, has been broken down into three subsections. One involves relaxation training which focuses upon principles first proposed by Edmund Jacobson (1938). The second section contains activities in which the child is requested to exhibit a maximum of control by performing as slowly as he can. A final section contains various motor tasks which are progressively lengthened in order to sustain his attention for increasing periods of time.

RELAXATION TRAINING. This training can be carried out with retarded and neurologically handicapped children by using a variety of techniques. Primary objectives include making the child consciously aware of the residual tensions present in his total body and its parts, and then helping him to dissipate some of this undesirable tonus. This training can be carried out using various forms of imagery or it can be applied in a more operational manner. The former approach is usually best when the children are rather severely retarded, while the latter method may also be used if the students are older, more educable retardates.

This training may be carried out while the child is standing, sitting, or lying on his back. Some of these activities may be accompanied by slow music.

1. While standing, the child can be asked to lift his arm or arms and then let them drop rapidly to his sides.

2. He can be asked to "take the bones" out of his arms or his total body and then relax into a fall on a mat.

3. When on a mat, he can be asked to "pretend to be a rag doll." The degree of relaxation he evidences can be ascertained by lifting a limb and observing whether it drops quickly to the mat when released.

4. When sitting, he can be asked to place his head (face to one side) on the desk and then let his arms swing slowly from side to side below desk level imitating the swinging of an elephant's trunk or the pendulum of a clock.

5. When standing or sitting, he can be asked to slowly move his head in circles both ways or to "drop" it quickly to the front in attempts to make him aware of residual tension in the head and neck region, a region which is usually found by experimenters to be the most reliable indicator of general bodily tension.

6. When the child is lying on a mat faceup, a number of activities can be carried out. The child can be asked to make various parts of his body "hard" (i.e. tense his feet, legs, seat, arms, etc.) in order from foot to head or vice versa. After the body is hard all over, he can be asked to become limp again. Each muscle group can also be made hard and then relaxed in turn before proceeding to the next muscle or group of muscles.

7. While on his back, the child can be asked to make his total body or one of its parts as hard as he can; then one can request that he make it almost as hard as he can, until he can adjust within fine limits the amount of tension he voluntarily evidences. This, of course, can be carried out better with children who are

capable of understanding quantitative differences of this nature and may not be possible with severely retarded children.

This type of relaxation training is appropriate after activities which usually arouse children to levels inappropriate for classroom work such as vigorous playground games, rapid exercises, and the like. Following these relaxing exercises, which may be carried out for 15 minutes or more a day, the children can be led into various coordination games—"move your arms over your head, move your legs apart, move your leg and arm on one side" —promoting body-part integration and differentiation while the children are lying on their backs. At the same time, tasks described in the next section may be engaged in following this relaxation training.

CONTROLLED MOVEMENTS. The goal of the following activities is to train the child to produce slow, controlled and accurate movements with his total body and with his limbs and in tasks involving hand-eye coordinations. These tasks can be combined with various relaxation drills and with various coordination exercises described in Phase III. Usually a class of retardates can be classified intellectually to a remarkable degree of accuracy by assessing the extent to which they are willing or able to move in a slow, controlled manner in various writing tasks, or activities involving limb movements. Examples of these activities follow.

1. Various movements involving the total body can be employed in response to the following commands:

"Let me see how slowly you can get up. Now lie down slowly."

"How slowly can you roll down the mat?"

"How slowly can you walk from this line to that line over there? (See Fig. 7-1.)

"How slowly can you walk between these two lines?"

"How slowly can you walk backward, sideways, etc.?"

At times, when performing these tasks, the child may actually have to be held back by the teacher and manually guided in order to help him gain an understanding of what "slow" means.

2. Activities involving limb movements can also be incorporated into such practice, in response to the following requests:

"How slowly can you bring your arms over your head?"

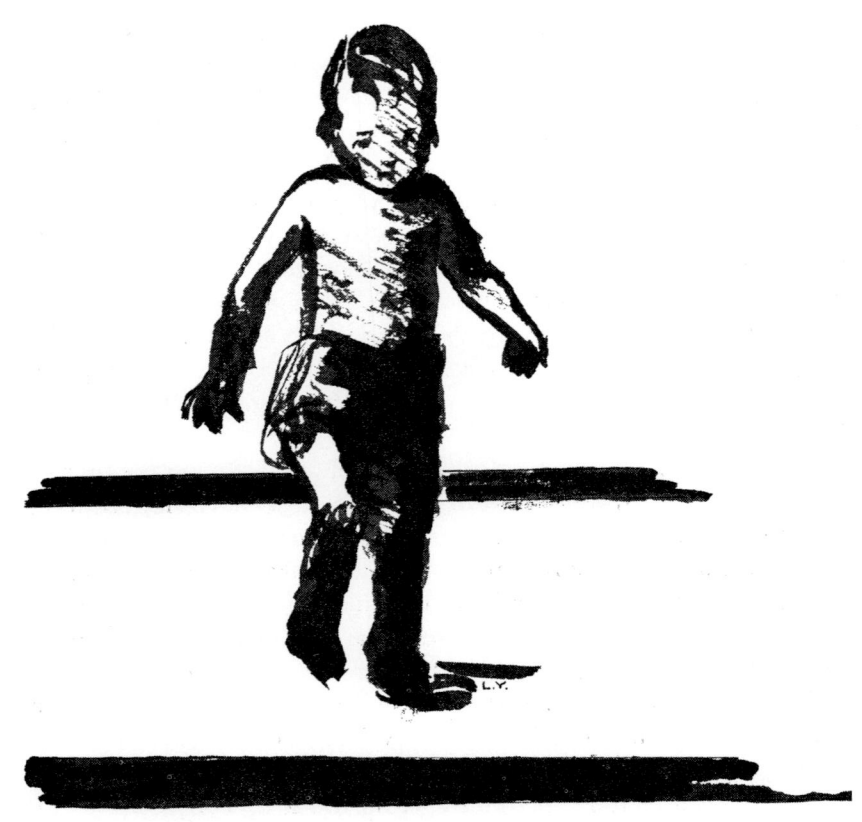

Figure 7-1. "Walk as slowly as you can from this line to that one."

"How slowly can you swing your arms to the music?"

(While lying on their back) "How slowly can you move your arms and legs apart at the same time?"

Can you just move your arms overhead slowly while pressing your legs against the mat?"

"How slowly can you pull the cart toward you (using a string)?" (See Fig. 7-2.)

3. Various drawing movements on a desk and/or blackboard are helpful in tasks involving hand-eye coordination. For example, while standing at a blackboard a child might be asked to do the following: "Draw a road from this house (point on the board) to

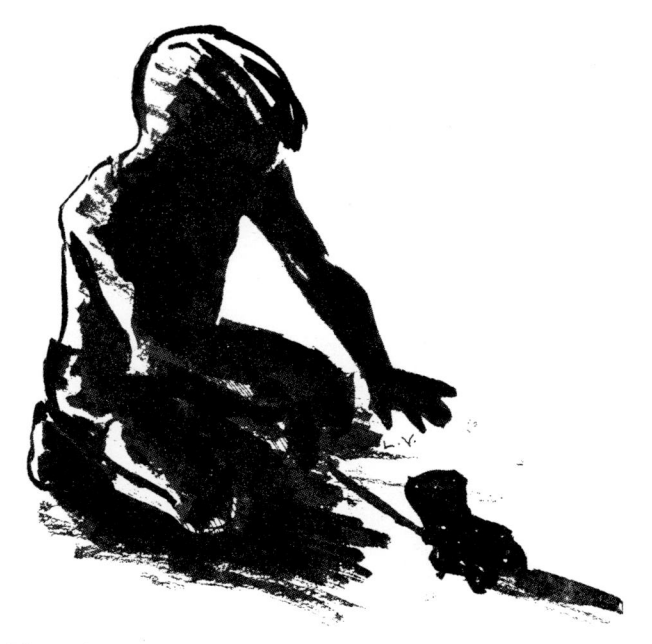

Figure 7-2. "How slowly can you pull the cart toward you?"

that one as slowly as you can." Initially, the points should be placed close enough so that the child does not have to shift his total body when connecting them. Later he might be asked to reproduce longer lines which require simultaneous movement of the body accompanying the attempt to integrate hand and eye in the drawing task, as in the following requests:

"Let me see you draw a slow line up and down these hills." (or when more accuracy seems possible) "Let me see you draw a line as slowly as you can between these two other lines" (down this street) (Fig. 7-3.)

Use of the blackboard is more amenable to group observation and effort and more than one child can be employed at a time in such tasks. For example, "While Tom is drawing his line, let me see if you can slowly draw a line over Tom's."

After a child seems to be moving with good control the teacher may alternate more rapid movements and then attempt to inter-

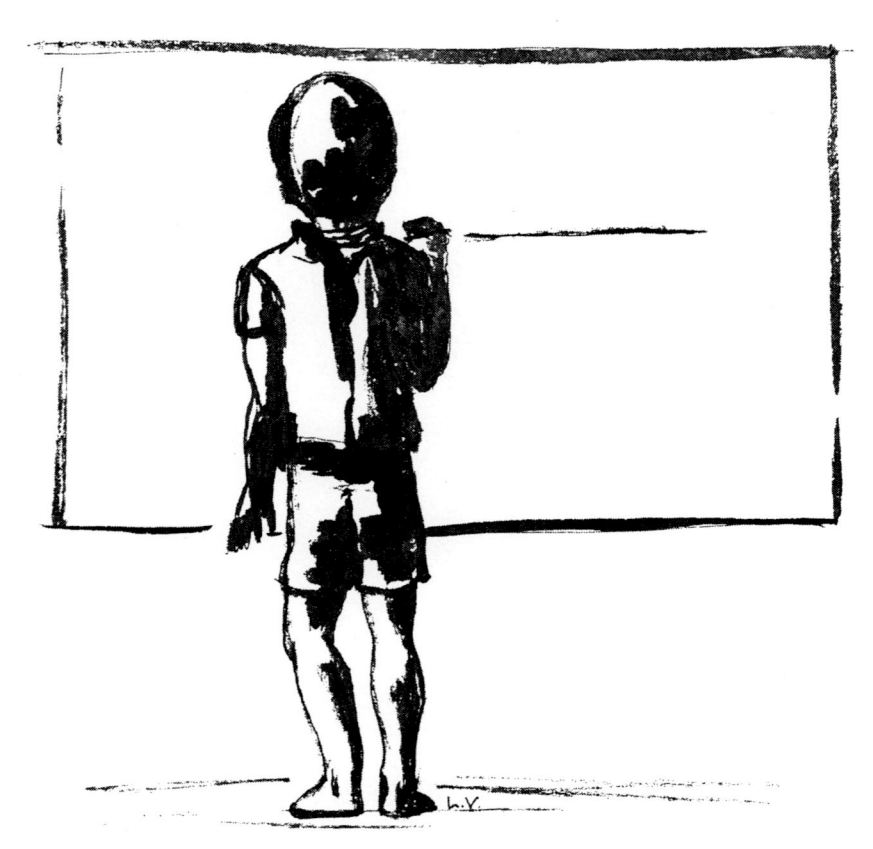

318   *Physical Therapy Services in the Developmental Disabilities*

Figure 7-3. "Let me see you draw a line as slowly as you can."

ject again a request for a slow movement to determine whether the child can alternately arouse and control himself.

PROLONGING TASKS. In a related manner, tasks can be arranged so that their performance requires increasing periods of time. For example the following:

1. After a child is willing or able to walk a line, two or more beams may be placed end to end.

2. The distances between points, delineated by a line, may be increased.

Summary

Training in impulse control involving relaxation techniques, controlled movements, and prolonged tasks would seem to form the basis for more complex learning. The attempt is made to help the child to better place himself under his own control, to become aware of and to control impeding residual tensions, and to aid him to attend to tasks for longer periods of time than he has been willing or able to do in the past. It is believed that this approach is one of the most helpful ways in which motor activities may be employed in education. For years, educators have demonstrated the ability to excite children with the traditional sports and games; some are now realizing that the movement tasks outlined above are helpful in lowering the atypical child's arousal to levels amenable to his overall progress in school.

Phase II: Body-Image Training

It seems logical to assume that basic to a child's organization of the complexities of his world is an awareness of where he is in relation to that world, cognizance of his body parts and their capacities for movement, and similar basic perceptual judgments. Substantiation of this viewpoint was recently obtained in a study by the author in which it was found that the score more predictive of the level of performance indicative of a number of perceptual-motor attributes on the part of trainable retardates was that obtained in an abbreviated body-image assessment (Cratty 1967a).

Basic to the correct placement and interpretation of letters in words is the ability of the child to place them into some context relative to the left and right and the up and down of things. The infant initially learns that a spoon is a spoon whether it be on the floor, upside down, or hanging on a wall. However, he is then faced a few years later with the fact that the innumerable shapes he must organize into letters and words are not the same unless they are arranged within certain rigid left-right up-down orientations.

But even more basic than these perceptions are ones involving simply the awareness of the planes of the body and of the locomotion and names of body parts. The normal child does not have all the "lefts" and "rights" of himself and of his movements well-organized until sometime between the ages of six and seven. Therefore, to ask a retarded youngster between the ages of three and eight years to make such discriminations is often unrealistic. The sequence which follows is somewhat abbreviated from one contained in a recent text by the author (Cratty 1967a). Simplistic developmental theories sometimes state that the child first learns about his body and then projects this body schema into related discriminations in space. The sequence which follows is based upon evidence that the child's body image involves a continuous interaction with objects in his environment and at the same time it is assumed that a child may be aided to better structure his environment only if such discriminations are taught, not left to magically occur. Transfer, we learn from experimental findings, is most likely to occur if cognitive "bridges" are constructed between two previously unrelated tasks. Thus, after a child seems able to make various left-right discriminations about his body parts and bodily movements, he must in an operational way be led to understand that words, letters, and geometric shapes may be located within a similar dimensional reference system.

An important research finding bearing upon the training of the body-image in children is that children are most often able to identify body parts correctly because they have engaged in some movement experience with them. "I remember that this is my right hand because I eat, salute the flag, and shake hands with it," is a typical response when children are asked how they make left-right discrimination (Ilg and Ames 1965).

The sequence below is divided into four subsections. The initial one involves the body plane, the second, body parts and their movements, the third, laterality, and the fourth, structuring of a stable spatial reference system.

Basic to the training of the body-image is the utilization of all available sensory input. For example, body-part identification may be enhanced with visual input by using mirrors, with tactile sensations as the body parts are stroked or touched, and verbally by pairing part and word. Attempting to use one simple body-image game in the education of a retardate will usually only result in his acquiring the ability to play only that "game" rather than the ability to generalize from and transfer to the precepts and concepts it is desired that he acquire.

BODY PLANES. Responses elicited by the following requests may be utilized in this initial phase of training:

1. "Where is your front, your back, your head, your feet, etc.?"
2. "Let's see you put your back, side, or front against the wall and stand with your back, side, or front nearest me."
3. "Let's see you jump up, go down to the floor, etc."
4. "Slide to the side, move your body forward toward me, move backwards, etc."
5. "Is that chair nearest your side, your front, or your back?"

BODY PARTS AND THEIR MOVEMENTS. The following activities are helpful in this stage of training:

1. "Touch your head, arms, legs, feet, etc."
2. "As we look in the mirror move your hands, feet, head, etc."
3. "Lie on the paper while I draw around your body. Now get up. Can you tell me where your arms, legs, head, etc. are?" (See Fig. 7-4.)
4. Can you point to your thumb, your elbow, your wrist, your thigh, your ankle, your first finger, etc.?"

During this phase emphasis is not on left-right dimensions but on simply locating and naming body parts. A normal child can identify most body parts by the age of four and by five he knows that there is a left and a right hand, ear, etc., although he is usually unaware of which is which.

Body-part training should be carried out in conjunction with training involving the body planes outlined above and should precede any attempt to establish an awareness of the left-right dimensions of the body. When training the child to identify body planes and parts, it is often appropriate to ask him to tell you how many fronts, backs, sides, ears, noses, etc. he has in order to form the basis for the laterality training which should follow.

LATERALITY. A child normally begins to utilize one hand in

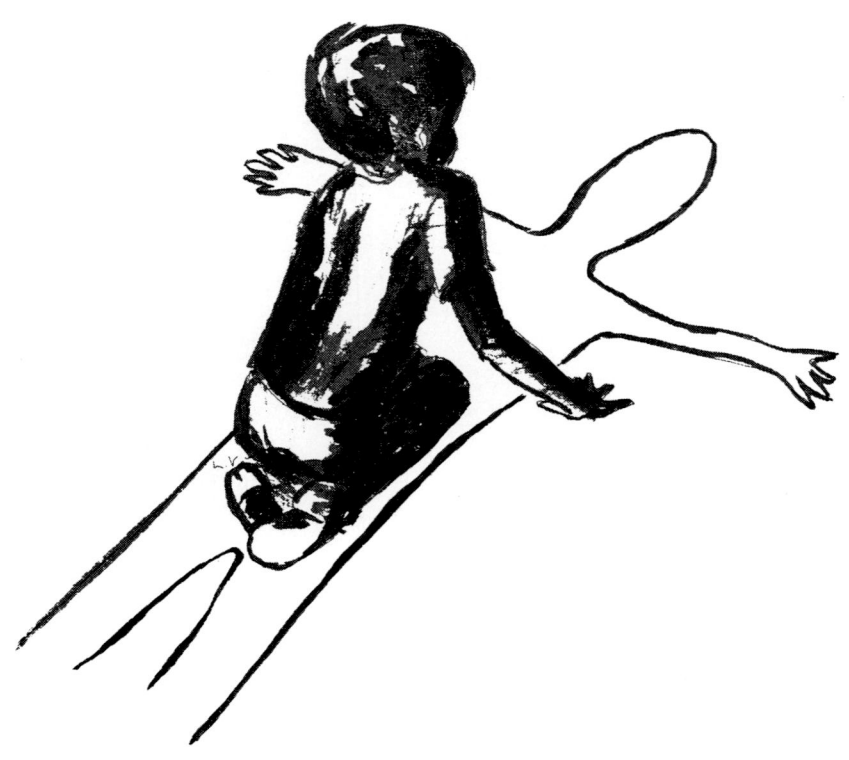

Figure 7-4. "Tell me where your arms are . . . your legs?"

preference to the other sometime between four to seven months of age; however, a cognitive awareness of which are the left and right hands, sides, and so forth of the body is not fully acquired until several years later. Unless a retarded child has a mental age of about five or six, attempting to teach the left-right differences about his body and its movements will usually lead to frustration both for the child and his teacher. The following activities should prove helpful:

1. "Touch your left hand, eye, ear, etc."
2. "Stand with your left, right side towards the wall."
3. "Can you move to your left? Now slide toward your right and jump and turn toward your left."
4. "Roll down the mat, tell us when you are on your left and right sides as you roll." (See Fig. 7-5.)

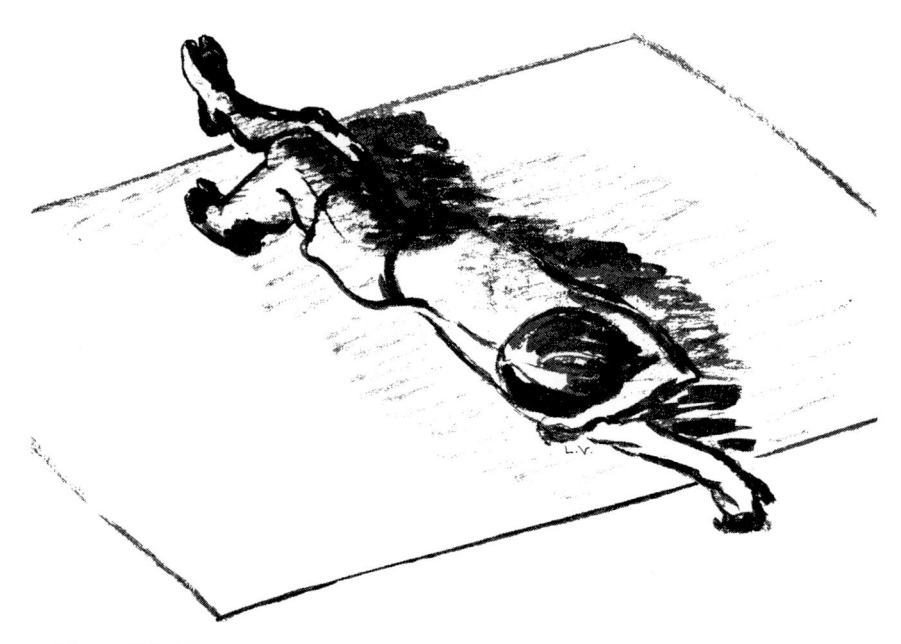

The Use of Movement Activities in Education 323

Figure 7-5. "As you roll, tell me when you are on your left and right sides."

5. "Walk around the chair. Is it nearest your left or right side? Now walk the other way. Is it nearest your left or right side now?"

6. "Close your eyes. With your right hand touch your left elbow. Touch your left ear with your right hand, etc."

STRUCTURING SPACE. After a child seems able to make correct left-right discriminations as requested above, (remember that *by chance* he will be correct 50% of the time) he may then be led to structure space, orient letters, and in similar ways utilize the concepts inherent in the tasks above to better organize his visual world. The following activities are appropriate at this stage:

1. "Which is the left and right pages of the book as it is opened before you?"

2. "What is the difference between 'M' and 'W'? Which opens up toward your head?"

3. "Which way does a 'd' face? Nearest which hand is the long part of the 'b'?"

4. "Nearest which side of your body is the 'w' in 'was'?"

These activities can be extended, if desired, by requesting that the child "project" himself into the reference system of another person. Although these latter judgments are not accurately made until a normal child is from eight to nine years of age, a teacher might desire that older retardates become able to realize that other people have left and right sides that are different from theirs, and that generally the left and right of things are relative to the manner in which two or more things are observed and/or are placed in relationship with one another.

Phase III: Perceptual-Motor Competencies

There is a considerable amount of research which supports the fact that there is a greater incidence of perceptual-motor ineptitude in populations of retarded children (Cratty 1966). Similarly, it is an ubiquitous finding that on the whole retarded children are less fit than are normal youngsters. Extensive motor training for retarded youngsters may be justified for several reasons. Achieving a moderate amount of perceptual-motor skill is the primary means through which many of them will become employable. Physical ineptitude will often lessen self-acceptance to a point wherein the retardate will totally reject himself. On the other hand, competency in motor tasks underlying recreational sports and work skills will enhance feelings of adequacy which in turn may lead toward vocational and educational improvement.

Several principles should be followed when attempting to improve perceptual-motor competencies of retarded children. These are as follows:

1. Very basic tasks involving a minimum of thought should precede more complex activities.

2. The basic attributes of balance, agility, and body-image training should precede more complex skills involving complex perceptual discriminations (i.e. catching and hitting balls).

3. The manner in which the child occupies himself visually when performing should be observed; at times more and at other times less visual inspection of the task and of his performing body parts may be required.

4. The child should be required to exercise self-control when performing, rather than simply being made excited in the situation.

5. The social complexity and pressure of the performance situation should be carefully controlled and sequenced when possible.

6. Time should be allotted for trial and error learning on the part of the retardate.

7. The manner in which the child integrates body parts—for example, his arms and legs when jumping—should be enhanced whenever possible. The manner in which the child focuses his tension in appropriate or inappropriate body parts should be observed and modifications in instructions or task conditions should be devised which will elicit more appropriate directioning of tensions when obviously called for by the characteristics of the task.

8. The child should be aided to develop better planning methods when trying to solve motor problems. For example, he might be aided in formulating a "movement program" prior to climbing a tree or when placing his work on a table for a simple assembly skill. It is often very difficult to separate the influence of innate neuromotor defects from inappropriate "work methods" when evaluating the motor performance of retardates.

9. All "channels" of input, including verbal explanation, manual manipulation, and visual demonstration, should be utilized when teaching retardates.

10. Activities should contain innate appeal. This is best accomplished by presenting novel tasks to solve and using equipment which is visually stimulating.

11. A variety of movement experiences should be provided. There is no single simple coordination task which will magically enhance all the movement attributes of children. Activities intended to enhance balance, agility, manual dexterity, locomotor skills, ball throwing and catching attributes and the like should be used. Tasks which are intended to enhance these attributes follow. A more detailed resumé of the sequences into which these tasks fall are found in a text by the writer (Cratty, 1967a).

BALANCE. Two kinds of balance tasks should be presented in a reasonable sequence based upon order of difficulty; first, balance tasks in which relative fixed positions are maintained, and then tasks in which the individual is moving along lines, balance beams, and the like. As these tasks are engaged in, the extent to which vision is involved can be modified to some degree by the teacher.

Static balance tasks can involve those in which the child is requested to balance on his hands and knees, using four, three, or perhaps two parts of his body to balance on such as a knee and a hand on the same or opposite sides. More difficulty can be achieved if the child is asked to balance statically while standing and to watch a fixed or a moving point, or to attempt the balances with his eyes closed. Standing balance can be made more difficult by asking the child to stand on a line in a heel-toe fashion, to fold his arms while maintaining the position, and later to stand on one foot while folding his arms, closing his eyes, or some combination of the above (Fig. 7-6).

Moving balance tasks are best started by asking the child with severe balance problems to walk a rather wide surface on the floor (i.e. two lines placed 8 inches apart). Later he can be asked to walk a single line and then a raised balance beam from 4 to 3 inches wide. Further difficulty can be interposed by requiring that he walk over and under an obstacle or a series of obstacles placed on the beam. The beam may be tilted to the right or left or may be raised at one end to provide further difficulty (Fig. 7-7).

After the child can traverse a balance beam with little difficulty, further difficulty can be added by requiring that he watch first stable and then moving targets placed to the front and then to the sides of the beam. These latter exercises aid the child to separate his visual system from his locomotor efforts; this is a helpful separation when the child is required to run while tracking a ball, or when engaged in similar life activities where it is not usually desirable to watch only one's feet while moving through space (Fig. 7-8).

AGILITY. Agility can be enhanced by at first simply teaching the child to fall properly on his sides, back, and front, and then to arise either rapidly or slowly after doing so. This type of training can be combined with body-image training (i.e. "Fall on your left

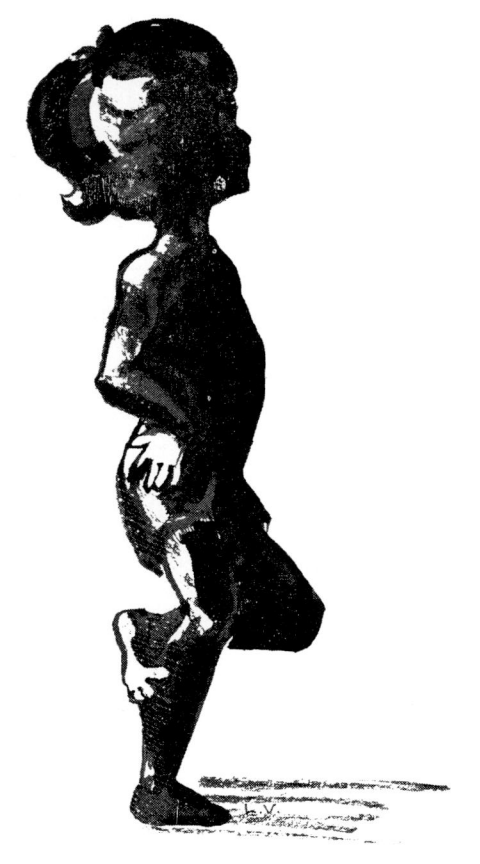

Figure 7-6. "Can you stand on one foot?"

side, roll over and stand up quickly with your right side nearest the mat"). These simple beginnings can lead toward more complicated tumbling activities. These latter tasks can be first approached by providing a hall or inclined plane for the child to roll down.

LOCOMOTOR SKILLS. Simple jumping and landing exercises should be utilized as basic exercises to enhance locomotor abilities. Emphasis should be placed on a simultaneous lift of the arms when extending the legs while jumping and upon the quick re-

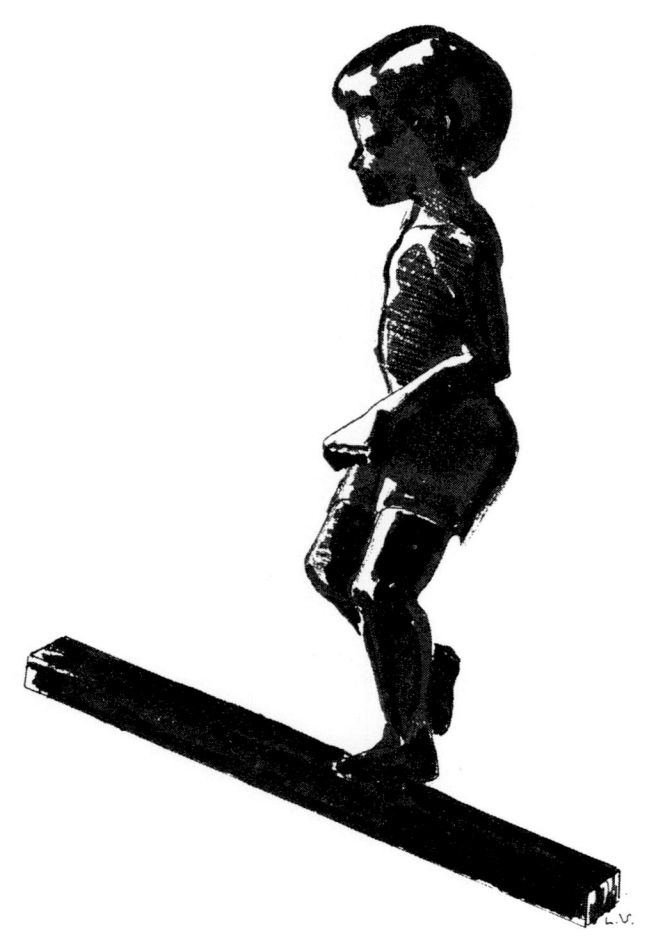

328 *Physical Therapy Services in the Developmental Disabilities*

Figure 7-7. "Can you walk the beam if I raise one end?"

laxation of the knees when landing during these initial stages. Next the child may be asked to jump and turn first one-quarter, and later half and full turns followed by the proper landing.

Proper running must be taught children with moderate to mild motor problems. Appropriate reciprocal arm action must be demonstrated and guided and the child should be taught to correctly lower his center of mass when attempting to stop his run.

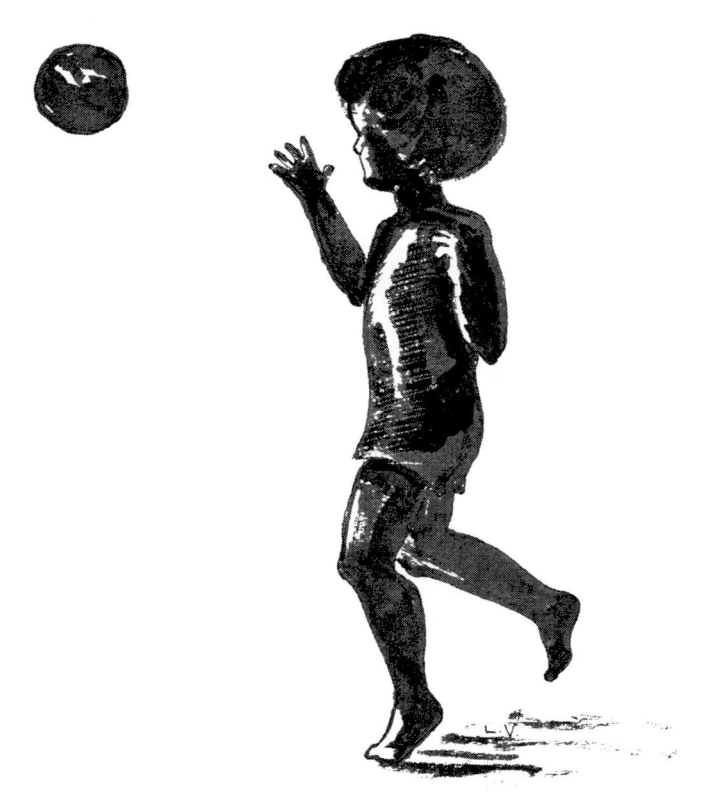

Figure 7-8. "Run and catch the ball without watching your feet."

He should be taught to run laterally and backward as well as forward. Competence in ball games requires quick locomotion in directions other than forward (Fig. 7-9).

If the child can posture on one foot for a period of time (six to eight seconds) he may be taught to hop with appropriate arm lift and then to hop rhythmically first on one and then on the other. Later he can be taught to hop and turn, to jump from one foot to a one-foot landing, and to start on one foot and land on two.

Advanced locomotor skills which are demonstrable and which are to be mastered after the previous ones include galloping, skipping, and the like. Often, practice in these can be aided by the

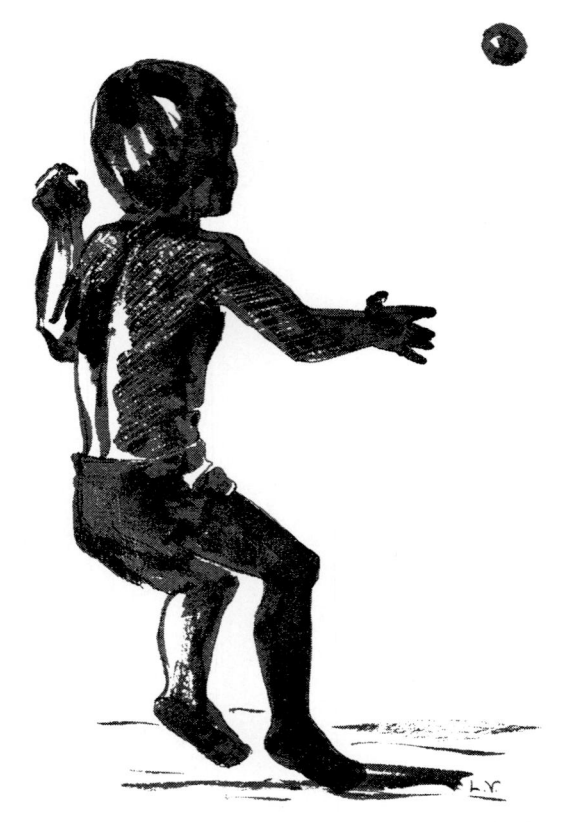

330   *Physical Therapy Services in the Developmental Disabilities*

Figure 7-9. "Sometimes you have to run backward when playing ball games."

use of footprints painted on the ground into which the child must step.

MANUAL SKILLS. Manual skills are important for many reasons, the most important of which is that the primary manner in which a child must visually express his intellect is through a hand-eye coordination (i.e. writing and drawing numbers). Most neurologically handicapped children evidence impairment in manual skills. Their improvement may be gained through four kinds of tasks: those intended to enhance the perceptions of the hands and fingers, those which promote hand-arm steadiness, those which improve finite wrist-finger dexterity, and those which resemble handwriting and promote smooth eye-hand coordinations needed when continuous movements are made with a pencil on a printed page.

The perceptions of the fingers can be improved by engaging in finger games, by naming the fingers, by engaging in clay modeling and in finger painting. The hand-image seems as closely related to their motor functioning as is the body-image and accurate bodily movement.

Aiming and steadiness of the hands can be improved, for example, by requiring that the child make tapping movements with increasing degrees of accuracy into circles of decreasing size.

Smooth visual-motor integrations in tasks resembling drawing can be improved by requiring that the child connect dots and inscribe lines between channels of lines placed decreasing distances apart.

BALL THROWING AND CATCHING. The tracking, throwing, and interception of balls are complex attributes, made even more difficult when the child is attempting them when moving himself. Throwing can be improved by attending to both the mechanics of the action as well as providing tasks in which throwing accuracy is called for. A mature throwing pattern usually evidenced by a normal six-year-old involves a weight shift by the body as the ball is released; this weight shift is carried out best if the child takes a step with the foot opposite to the throwing arm as he releases the missile. Throwing mechanics can be best improved by practicing them without a ball and practicing them in parts.

Throwing accuracy can be enhanced by throwing at targets surrounded by relatively large target areas. For example, hitting a target 1 foot in diameter is easier if it is surrounded by a larger circle of about 4 feet in diameter. The child, when throwing, should be given the opportunity to throw at targets placed on horizontal as well as vertical surfaces so that the force of his throw as well as the left-right up-down accuracy of his efforts can be improved.

Summary

Motor attributes of many retarded and physically handicapped children are relatively easy to improve if the initial tasks are easy enough and the training is carried out in a relatively tension-free motivating environment. Improvement of these attributes may help to reverse a failure syndrome often seen in the attitudes of retarded children when confronted with new and difficult tasks on the playground and in the classroom.

Phase IV: Seriation

Imperative to several components of classroom learning is the ability to attend to the order in which items are placed in a series. Children must gain a concept of a "before" and "after" when ordering their world. Rhythmic motor activities as well as activities which involve remembering the correct order of a sequence of relatively gross action patterns provide concrete situations in which a child's concept of serial order may be enhanced. Spelling and organizing thoughts in a sentence when speaking and writing are dependent upon this rather subtle attribute. Motor activities can provide important training media for the establishment of seriation.

RHYTHMICS. A mature sense of rhythm seems to be well established in normal children at about the eighth year. In children with defective nervous systems, it is usual to find the inability to integrate two or more body parts in rhythmic activities. At the same time, profoundly retarded children can often be communicated with only by imposing a vivid beat of music into their environment. Rhythmic activities for retardates should be accompanied when possible with vivid visual cues.

At the same time, rhythmic activities can be carefully sequenced by first presenting a slow beat to be duplicated initially by a simple motor response (i.e. head movement), later by a response requiring more than one body part to move (i.e. foot and hand movement), and later by faster beats involving the integration of a movement on one side of the body with a movement on the other (i.e. hop twice on one foot and then twice on the other). Still more advanced are rhythmics which require that the child "break up" a regular pattern (i.e. "Tap twice with your left hand and then three times with your right"). Usually beyond the capabilities of atypical children but seen in the movement education programs in England are tasks which require that one rhythm be established with one body part, while a separate rhythm is "picked up" by another.

SERIAL MEMORY TASKS. Using obstacle courses constructed in two or three dimensions, a child can be asked to replicate the movements of another child in two, three, four or more activities. Many trainable retardates can duplicate up to four movements seen performed by another child, while educable retardates can often duplicate six or more. These courses can be constructed of boxes, climbing apparatus, and the like, or more simply can be laid out using tape on the floor of a classroom. Hopscotch-like squares to be traversed in various ways can involve series which can be made increasingly complex and will eventually tax the ability of the most gifted child.

Phase V: Pattern Recognition

Pattern recognition is an important attribute to instill in retarded children. Innumerable training methods stemming from Marie Montessori at the turn of the century have been proposed for enhancing this ability. From an awareness of the differences and similarities in simple geometric patterns flows the ability to identify letters. Words have unique configurations whose recognition, it is felt by many authorities, is basic to reading. In addition to the usual modalities employed to enhance pattern recognition, visual inspection, tactile manipulation, and verbal discussion can be added gross movement. Within recent years, configurations other than the usual circles and squares have been added on playgrounds in schools for the physically and mentally handicapped in the city of Los Angeles. Half-circles, triangles, rectangles—when discussed, observed, played upon, and skipped around—should aid children to gain an increased awareness of the various geometric configurations with which they are confronted in classrooms.

Grids on which are placed letters and numbers have been similarly utilized to aid children to manipulate numerical concepts and to learn spelling. Such activities thus promote pattern recognition, as well as the motor attributes inherent in the task selected at the time. At the present time an investigation is being carried out which will further explore the influence of such training upon pattern recognition. Moreover, it is believed that the methodology holds much promise. It is important to remember, however, that transfer of this nature must be taught. A child cannot be expected to recognize a pattern on the playground as similar to the one drawn on the blackboard or held in his hand unless he is given structured instruction in the similarities. For example, the attributes of a triangle, after being examined tactually in class, must be followed by a request that the child find a similar pattern on the playground and then walk around it counting the sides as he goes.

Triangles can be formed into "A's" with modification, half-circles into "B's," and so forth. Letters laid out on horizontal surfaces as well as those placed in a vertical plane (as in climbing apparatus) may also provide an important learning modality for children with learning difficulties.

Phase VI: Decision Making and Problem Solving

Many experimenters interested in cognitive processes suggest that true learning does not take place unless the learner is permitted to make decisions about his actions and about modifications in the educational activities with which he is confronted (Bruner 1966). Mosston (1966), in a recent test, has outlined sequences which enable a teacher to lead a child from the usual situation in which he simply responds to the commands of a teacher to situations in which he is encouraged to make decisions about the task confronting him and about the manner in which he is evaluated; eventually, he is led to make choices about the total program in which he is engaged.

It is a truism that children in a school for the retarded, for whatever the reason (i.e. emotional problems, discipline, etc., soon assume a dependent role. It is believed that children with problems in thinking should be given every opportunity to think rather than merely be commanded, pushed, and led throughout their day. It is believed that encouraging the child to make decisions about perceptual-motor activities is one of the clearest ways in which the quality of the child's thoughts can be demonstrated. Thus, asking a child to demonstrate four ways to get over a line or perhaps six ways to get into a box on the floor seems infinitely superior to simply telling him to jump in "like this." Following this type of practice the learner may be allowed even more license by the teacher as he is asked to arrange an obstacle course or perhaps to invent games using sticks and balls and similar problems.

Whether this practice in response generalization will lead toward the tendency to assume decisions and to engage in creative thinking involving tasks unrelated to jumping over lines or into boxes is a subject for further research. At the same time, this methodology would seem to hold promise as a sound educational approach in the future. For a more thorough discussion of these concepts the reader is referred to Mosston's text (Mosston 1966).

Conclusions

That the foregoing material has been organized into six phases does not mean that the tasks must be similarly organized. Although it would seem advisable to concentrate upon stages I, II, and III prior to stages IV, V, and VI, many activity periods can include arrangements which may improve a variety of attributes. The placement of lines formed of tape on the floor will enable one to incorporate training in balance, agility, serial memory ability, laterality, pattern recognition, and decision making within a relatively short period of time (Fig. 7-10). For example, if a line 20 feet long is followed, as shown, by the other patterns, the following might be improved: "Walk the line" (balance), "Now,

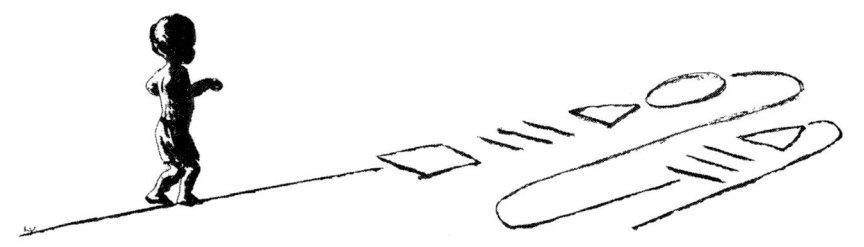

Figure 7-10. "Can you do the same six things to these patterns as Bobby did?"

jump over the line" (agility, serial memory ability), "What is that now?" (pattern recognition), "Now, jump into it left foot first" (agility, laterality), "Now, what is that pattern?" (pattern recognition), "Show me six ways of getting yourself into it" (decision making, problem solving).

Most of the activities described can be conducted with a group of from five to six children in the presence of a single teacher. If a teacher and an aide are available, from ten to twelve children may be worked with at a time.

Much is to be learned before the suggestions on the following pages are refined into exact educational practices. It is uncertain, for example, whether practice in pattern recognition on a printed page contributes to reading; the use of gross motor activities to enhance pattern recognition has similarly not been researched. There are innumerable experimental studies attesting to the influence of adjusting levels of arousal and tension upon learning; however, making the division of the human personality into discrete mental and motor components is a somewhat precarious undertaking (Duffy 1962).

An atypical child's self-concept is, as is the normal child's image of himself, based to a large degree upon what he can do in rather obvious ways. The child's self-concept in turn influences the extent to which he will even attempt the new and unfamiliar tasks as well as those activities which he will select for his attention.

Perceptual-motor activities, if well planned and reasonably well sequenced, provide a helpful way for the teacher of physically and mentally handicapped children to enhance self-control, to improve performance in recreational and vocational tasks, and to manipulate components of the environment when attempting self-care skills. At the same time, perceptual-motor activities, if properly selected, provide an important channel through which children with difficulties in conceptualizing may be encouraged to better deal with their world.

BIBLIOGRAPHY

Ayres, A. Jean: Perceptual-Motor Dysfunction in Children. Monograph from the Greater Cincinnati District Ohio Occupational Therapy Association Conference, 1964, 1-23.

Bruner, Jerome S.: *Toward a Therapy of Instruction.* Cambridge, Massachusetts, Harvard, 1966.

Cratty, Bryant J.: The Perceptual-Motor Attributes of Mentally Retarded Children and Youth. Monograph, Mental Retardation Services Board, Los Angeles County, August 1966.

Cratty, Bryant J.: *Developmental Sequences of Perceptual-Motor Tasks, Movement Activities for Neurologically Handicapped and Retarded Children and Youth.* Freeport, Long Island, New York, Educational Activities, 1967a.

Cratty, Bryant J.: *Movement Behavior and Motor Learning.* 2nd ed. Philadelphia, Lea & F., 1967b.

Cratty, Bryant J.: *Social Dimensions of Physical Activity.* Englewood Cliffs, New Jersey, Prentice-Hall, 1967c.

Cratty, Bryant J.: *Perceptual-Motor Behavior and Educational Processes.* Springfield, Thomas, 1968.

Cratty, Bryant J.: *Active Learning.* Englewood Cliffs, New Jersey, Prentice-Hall, 1971.

Duffy, E.: *Activation and Behavior.* New York, Wiley, 1962.

Franklin, C.C.: Diversified Games and Activities of Low Organization for Mentally Retarded Children. Monograph, Southern Illinois University, Carbondale, Illinois.

Ilg, Francis L., and Ames, Louise Bates: *School Readiness.* New York, Harper, 1965.

Jacobson, Edmund: *Progressive Relaxation.* Chicago, U. of Chicago, 1938.

Kagan, Jerome: Personality, behavior and temperament. In Falkner, Frank (Ed.): *Human Development.* Philadelphia, Saunders, 1966.

MacCCoby, Eleanor E., Dowley, Edith M., and Hagen, John W.: Activity level and intellectual functioning in normal pre-school children. *Child Develop, 36:*761-769, 1965.

Mosston, Muska: *Teaching Physical Education: From Command to Discovery.* Columbus, Ohio, C. E. Merrill, 1966.

Semans, Sarah: Physical therapy for motor disorders resulting from brain damage. *Rehab Lit, 20:*4:99-110, 1959.

Chapter Eight

IMPROVING THE PHYSICAL FITNESS OF RETARDATES

Bryant J. Cratty

THE FINDINGS of several research studies confirm the fact that, as a group, retardates are less physically fit than are normal children. Although little effort has been made to thoroughly explore the causes of this deficiency, it has been speculated that retarded children often lack opportunities for vigorous physical activity, and even if these are available, the child may be reluctant to participate because of a lack of skill and/or self-confidence in vigorous games enjoyed by the more able normal child. With a decreased opportunity to participate in strenuous motor activities or the lack of inclination to do so, a child's physical capacities will not become fully developed.

When formulating a program for improving the fitness of retarded children, several guide lines should be kept in mind. Some of these principles are related to the nature of the development of improved cardiovascular and muscular efficiency, while other guide lines pertain to the physical and psychological makeup of retarded children and youth. The material which follows is organized into four sections. Initially, guiding principles are listed. These are followed by suggestions for equipment and facilities appropriate for physical programs for retarded children. The third section contains suggested fitness activities, including those intended to improve cardiovascular efficiency as well as those to improve muscular strength. The final portion of the chapter contains selected exercises, intended to improve strength and flexibility of various portions of the body. The material contained in this chapter is meant to provide general guide lines and suggested activities rather than a comprehensive compilation of all the possible games and exercises which might be employed for the improvement of physical vigor of retardates. The chapter bibliography contains references which should provide the reader with additional suggestions for physical activities appropriate for retarded children.

Program Guide Lines

The principles are as follows:

1. Any program of vigorous physical activities for retarded children should be preceded by a thorough physical examination. It is not unusual to find that within a group of retarded children, a number may have cardiovascular and/or structural abnormalities. For example, Benda (1960) points out that about 75 percent of children with Down's syndrome evidence concomitant cardiovascular problems including constricted aortas, leakage in the heart septum, and the like. If vigorous exercises are administered indiscriminately to groups of retarded children without a comprehensive medical evaluation of their performance capacities, it is possible that structural and/or physiological impairments could be aggravated.

2. To improve endurance or strength of an individual, some type of overload must be imposed upon his muscular and/or cardiorespiratory system. Passive exercises are not likely to improve strength, just as repetitive activities carried out well within the individual's capabilities are not likely to improve endurance.

3. Retarded children are not usually aware of the long-range objectives of muscular exercises. They are more susceptible to the immediate emotional content of the situation in which they are performing. Therefore, if it is to be expected that retarded children extend themselves while exercising, it is imperative to arrange incentives so that they are well motivated.

4. Fitness *games* are likely to elicit more interest on the part of retarded children than are the simple counting of exercises. Improving the ability of a retarded child to participate fully in a variety of games is likely to encourage him to overload his own systems, and is probably more effective than for an instructor to attempt to coerce him to maximum efforts without interjecting fun into the situation.

5. Strength and endurance activities are likely to improve the ability of a retarded child to think (to the extent to which he is encouraged to think) about the makeup of his exercise program. Keeping records of personal improvement, devising modifications of exercises, counting repetition, and similar intellectual activity on the part of retarded children should result in ancillary intellectual benefits from participation in vigorous physical efforts. To the limits of their understanding, retarded children should be informed of the nature of the muscular and physiological processes underlying their efforts. Learning the names of muscles and how muscles move bones, for example, should provide helpful adjuncts to a fitness program.

Equipment and Facilities

To expedite a fitness program for retarded children, special thought should be given to the type of equipment which might be used as well as to special facilities which might be required. Although most of the standard fitness apparatus (ropes, bars, gymnasium apparatus, etc.) appropriate for normal youngsters are also suitable for retarded children, certain modifications should be helpful when working with children having learning deficiencies.

Playground Markings

When working in a large area with retarded children having IQ's from 30 to 60, it may be desirable to provide special playground markings in order to afford them a comfortable "structure" within which to engage in exercises and in other developmental activities. In one of the Los Angeles schools for retarded children, I have found it helpful to employ a large grid made up of separate squares when working with large groups of trainable retardates.

The dimensions of this grid arrangement are as shown in Figure 8-1.

This general arrangement permits the children to acquire an idea of just where they should stand and at the same time, keeps children separated so that they will not contact each other when

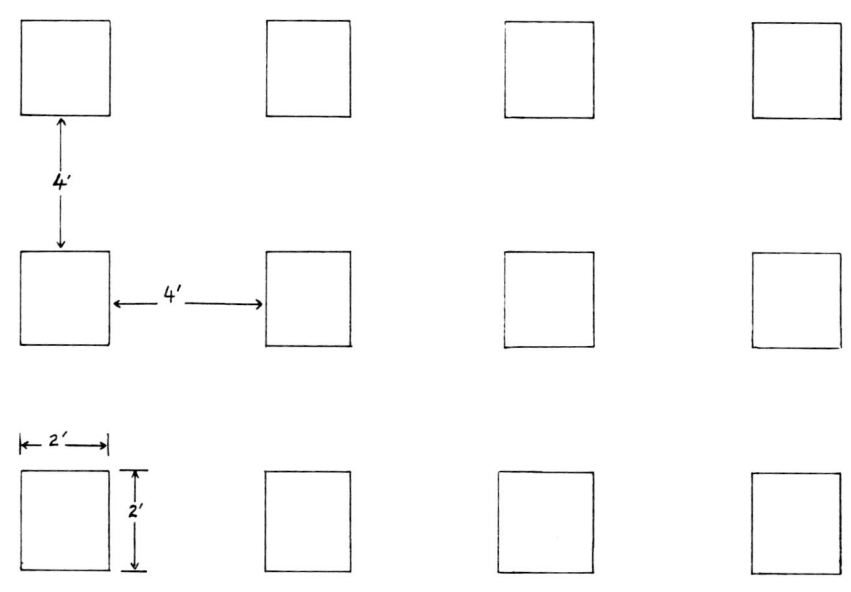

Improving the Physical Fitness of Retardates 341

Figure 8-1.

engaged in vigorous movements. These squares may be used to encourage the children to make decisions about their program ("How many ways can you jump in your square?") or perhaps to enhance left-right judgments ("Can you get into your square with your left foot first?"). The lines composing each square can be balanced upon in static positions ("Can you balance on one foot?") or at other times, the lines may be walked around as moving balance is practiced. The children may also jump from square to square, one at a time, playing follow-the-leader games or attempting to remember the series of movements engaged in by the previous child as he proceeded from square to square. If the squares contain numbers and/or letters (Fig. 8-2), the children may play games—running to numbers or letters called, jumping from square to square and calling the letter or numbers in the square landed in, etc.

Other playground markings which might be helpful include the markings shown in Figure 8-3 which are intended to provide exercise stations. Using this configuration, a child may perform a

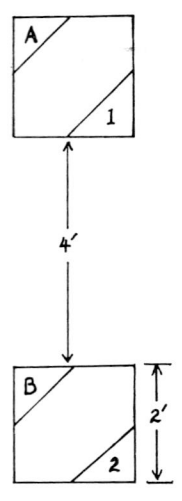

Figure 8-2.

different exercise at each station, proceeding from one to the other by jogging, walking, or skipping. This type of marking again affords retarded children a needed structure when performing exercises, and aids in the often encountered problem of controlling them as they engage in individualized activities. Additional vigor may be added to such a program by asking the child to increase by one repetition the number of exercises performed at each station as they proceed from one to the other. Records of improvement should be kept when engaged in this type of circuit training, which is designated to improve muscular fitness as well as endurance.

If funds and other conditions permit, more elaborate equipment may be constructed. Large obstacle courses are effective and motivating ways to improve the fitness both of retarded and normal children. Logs placed at various heights, when walked upon, aid in the development of leg power, balance, and agility (Fig. 8-4). Ropes suspended horizontally in groups of two or three, when traversed, require arm strength (Fig. 8-5). Wall boards, containing holes about 2 inches in diameter and 8 inches deep, may be climbed through the use of a dowel held in the

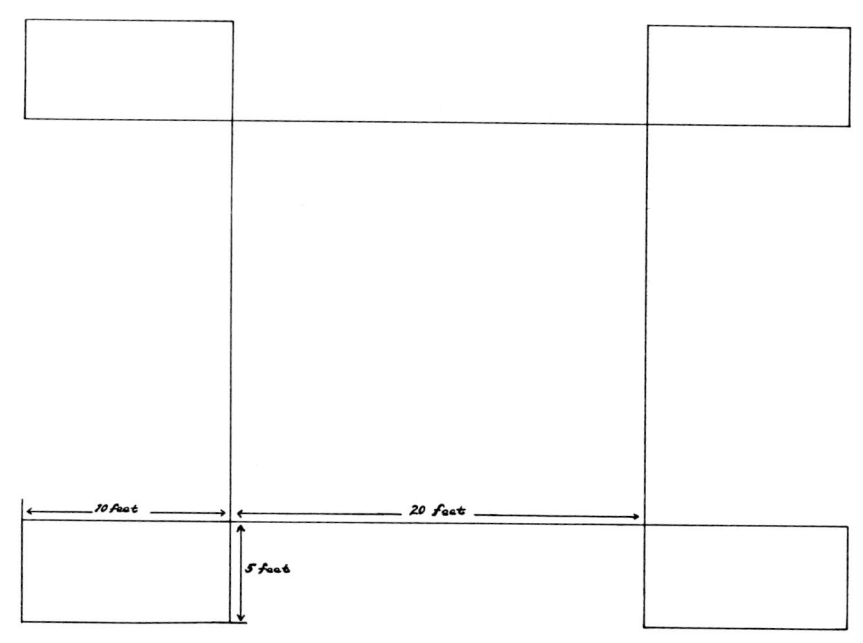

Improving the Physical Fitness of Retardates 343

Figure 8-3.

hands of children (Fig. 8-6). This activity requires marked effort by the shoulder-girdle muscles. Horizontal bars, adjustable to chest height, may be used to perform a modified pull-up (Fig. 8-7). Stepping under the bar and keeping the body stiff and feet on the ground, the child with shoulder-girdle weakness may improve by pulling himself up and down. Parallel bars may be also used for a modified pull-up activity if the child places his knees over the opposite bar.

Trampoline jumping has proved to be one of the most effective means of strengthening the trunk, back, and leg muscles of retarded children in our program at the University of California at Los Angeles (UCLA). All the antigravity muscles must work in unison as the child depresses the bed of the trampoline at the bottom of his descent. In order to gain maximum height on subsequent bounces and to avoid an uncomfortable "whiplash" effect, the children quickly learn that they must remain rigid as they

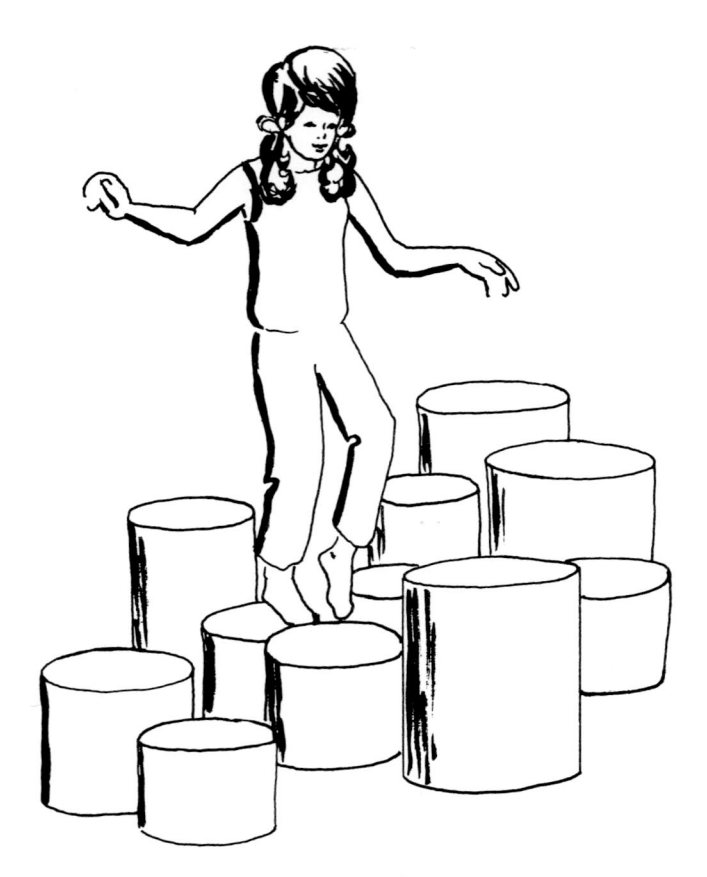

Figure 8-4.

touch the bed. Thus, while bouncing, the children are alternately exposed to vigorous static efforts by the larger muscles in the body, followed by rather complete relaxation of these same muscle groups as they reach the apex of each jump. It is believed that improvement of locomotor skills, balance, and agility has also been derived from engaging in this type of activity. If a trampoline is not available, some type of bounce board constructed of plywood or similar material will suffice.

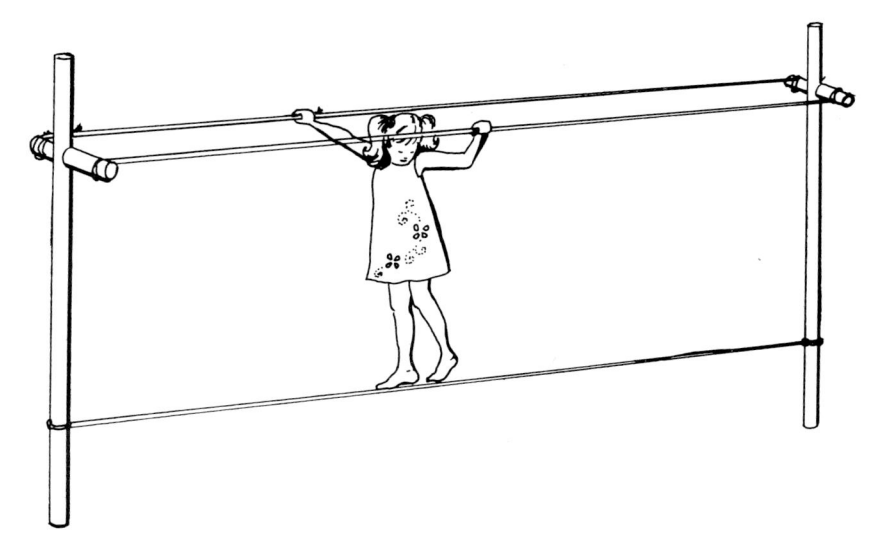

Figure 8-5.

Game Modifications to Promote Fitness

It is effective to modify the rules of the usual playground games prior to presenting them to retardates. Simplification of the rules should facilitate understanding and encourage increased participation. Games may be changed so that most of the children are interacting most of the time, thus preventing retarded children, whose attention spans are short, from forgetting where they are or what they are doing. At the same time, certain rule changes may result in more vigorous participation by retarded children. Examples of games in which helpful rule changes may be instituted are discussed below.

Base Games

Base games for retardates may be modified in several ways.
1. A fewer number of bases may be utilized; the runner, for example, may be required only to run to one base and then back home again before the fielders do something with the ball.

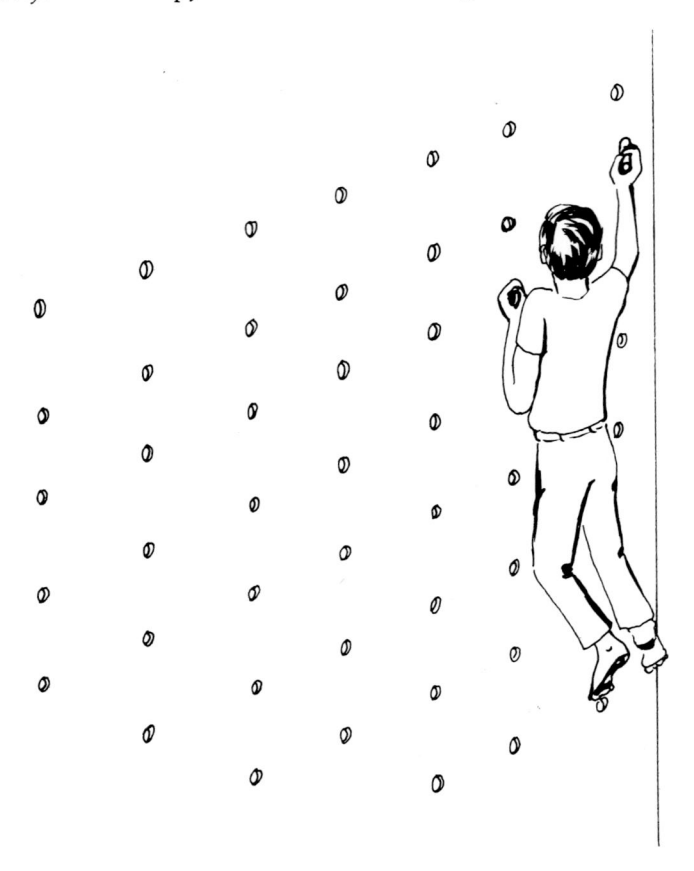

Figure 8-6.

2. The players may be first encouraged to explore the bases by walking around them, skipping around them, counting them, etc., without using a ball at all, prior to attempting more complicated games in which a ball is used.

3. The base runner may be required to run to a base away from the field of play, thus not confusing the fielders own movements as would normally occur (Fig. 8-8).

4. To encourage increased and constant participation by all the outfielders in base games with playground balls, all the fielders may be required to react to every ball hit or kicked to the out-

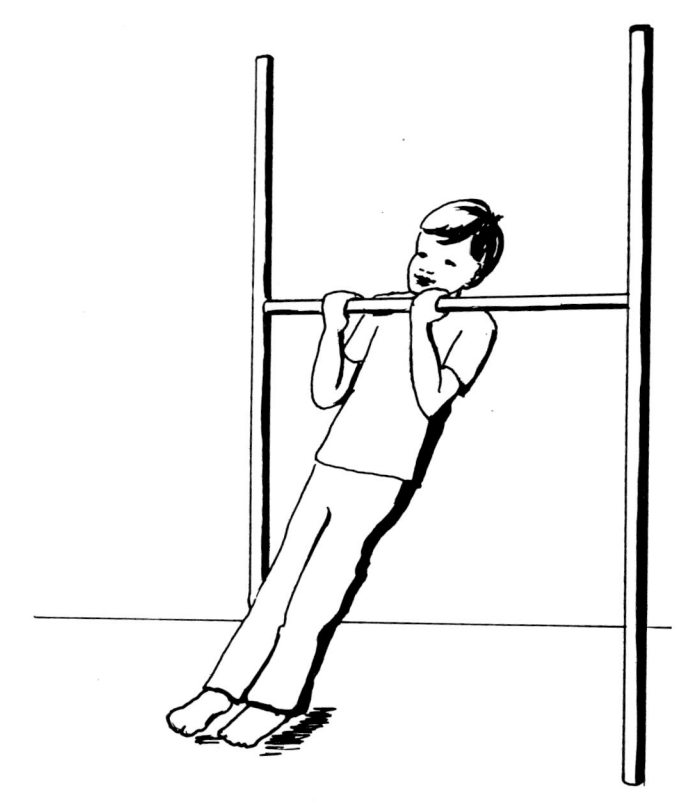

Figure 8-7.

field. For example, all fielders may be required to run and to quickly line up behind the fielder who first intercepts the ball. The ball may then be passed back from fielder to fielder with the last one in line yelling "stop" to terminate the efforts of the child striking the ball (who may be attempting to see how many bases he can circle before being told to stop). Using this type of activity, it is less likely that retarded children in the outfield will "lose contact" with the game situation than if their participation is required only intermittently as is usual in games of this nature.

Soccer

It is important that children deficient in skill learn how to move their feet with accuracy. For example, throwing efficiently

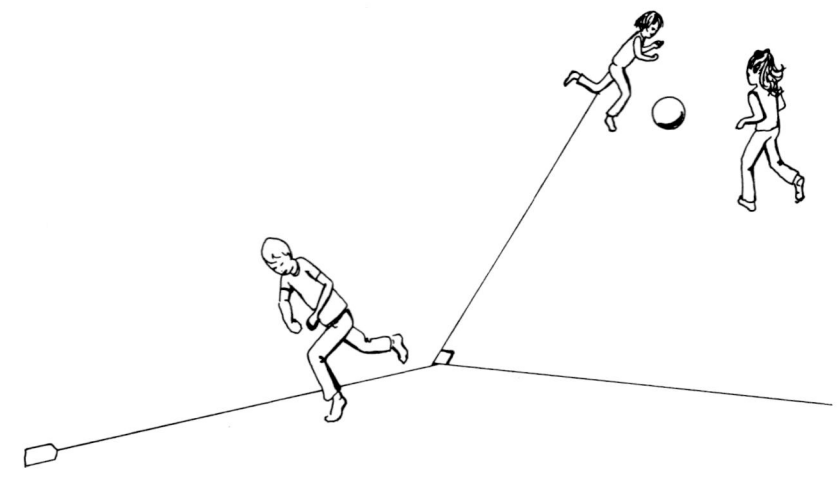

348 *Physical Therapy Services in the Developmental Disabilities*

Figure 8-8.

requires appropriate foot action as do most game skills. Various modified soccer games may be engaged in by retarded children to encourage increased locomotor agility, as well as to improve cardiovascular fitness. For example, three or four benches may be arranged in a square or triangle by placing them on their sides as shown in Figure 8-9. Using such an arrangement, each child can protect his own goal, while together they try to kick the ball through the other players' goals; winners are those having the least number of points scored against them. The same game may be made even simpler by having just two benches, two players, and two goals.

Suggested Exercises

Exercises carried out at the end of a physical education period for only a few minutes each day have resulted in significant improvement in the abdominal, back and shoulder-girdle strength of retardates participating in our program at UCLA. The four types of exercises we utilized are as described below:

1. Modified sit-up, keeping the knees bent so as to involve primarily the abdominal muscles, rather than the larger muscles of the legs (Fig. 8-10). This type of exercise can be made difficult

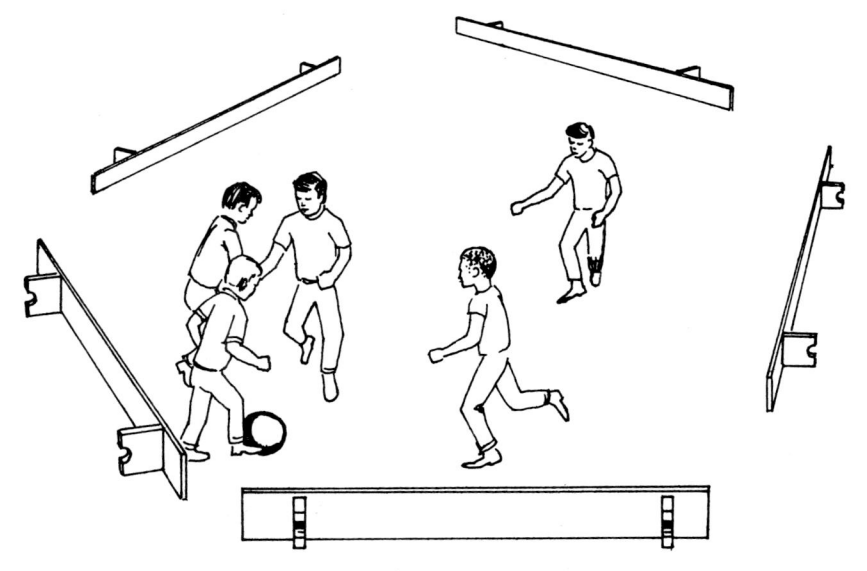

Figure 8-9.

by keeping the arms extended in back of the head, or slightly easier with the hands clasped behind the head. If the child has difficulty performing six to eight of these in this manner, he may be permitted to swing the arms forward and reach for his knees as he attempts to sit up.

2. Some type of pulling exercise is also engaged in, either the modified pull-ups described previously, or some type of rope climbing activity.

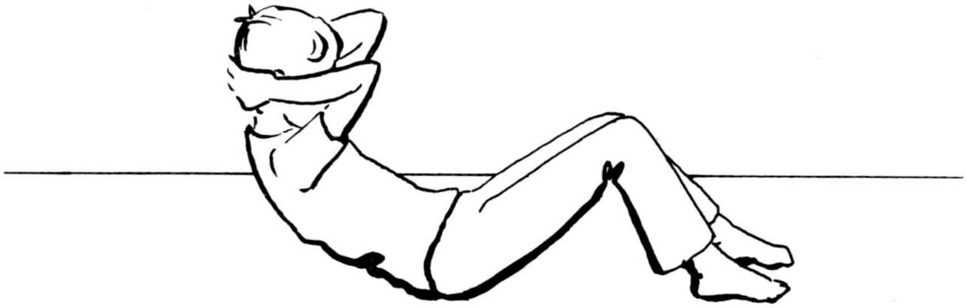

Figure 8-10.

3. Back-extensions are also performed to aid in the strengthening of the lower back. From a front-lying position and with the ankles held on the ground, the child is required to lift his shoulders and upper body off the ground by tightening his back, leg and hip muscles. This "up" position may be held for increased periods of time for more difficulty, or increased effort can be encouraged by asking the child to hold his arms to the side or over his head while holding this extended position (Fig. 8-11).

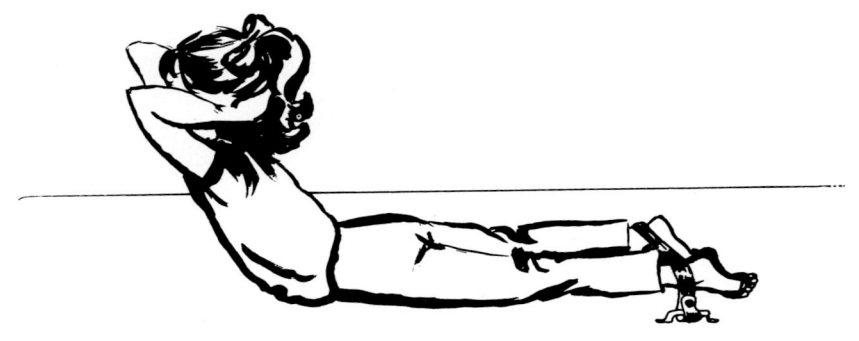

Figure 8-11.

4. Some type of pushing exercise is also engaged in, such as a modified push-up performed with the knees remaining on the ground. If the child is able, increased difficulty can be achieved by placing his feet on a box raised about a foot high.

Exercises intended to improve muscular flexibility should incorporate slow stretching movements, rather than the bouncing and stretching action normally seen. It has been found that the latter activity may cause undue muscle strain and impede the acquisition of muscular flexibility. Exercises to promote flexibility should concentrate upon the shoulder-girdle, trunk, hip, and legs, and be of a number of movements incorporating all the possible actions of the various larger joints of the body to their fullest range of motion without undue strain.

Summary

Programs to improve the fitness of retarded children should be preceded by thorough physical examinations for the participants. The content of the program may differ from that of normal children insofar as rule modifications for vigorous games may be needed and in that additional structure of space exercise may be required in the form of playground markings of various kinds.

To improve the fitness of retardates, they must be encouraged to participate vigorously in activities to enhance endurance and muscular efficiency. Thus, special consideration should be given to conditions which will result in maximum efforts of the children. Records of improvement should be kept so that they may see the results of their energy expenditures. Vigorous games are many times more interesting to them than simply performing exercises counted out by their instructor. Games in which every child is involved most of the time are more likely to enhance endurance, and at the same time, result in better attention to the game than would take place if a child's participation is required only sporadically.

A typical physical education period for retarded children should begin with general warm-up and stretching exercises, followed by the teaching of game skills and/or game participation. The period should be concluded by a few minutes of vigorous strength-producing exercises. Following such a program, there is sufficient evidence that significant gains may be expected in the physical fitness of retarded children.

BIBLIOGRAPHY

AAHPER–Kennedy Foundation: *Special Fitness Awards for the Mentally Retarded.* Washington, D.C., N.E.A.

Benda, Clemon E.: *The Child with Mongolism.* New York, Grune, 1960.

Blake, O., and Volp, Anne M.: *Lead-Up Games to Team Sports.* Englewood Cliffs, New Jersey, Prentice-Hall, 1964.

Cratty, Bryant J.: *Social Dimensions of Physical Activity.* Englewood Cliffs, New Jersey, Prentice-Hall, 1967a.

Cratty, Bryant J.: Strength, endurance plus flexibility equals fitness. In: *Developmental Sequences of Perceptual-Motor Tasks.* Freeport, Long Island, New York, Educational Activities, 1967b.

Cratty, Bryant J.: *Motor Activity and the Education of Retardates.* Philadelphia, Lea & F., 1969.

Cratty, Bryant J., and Sister Margaret Mary Martin: *Perceptual-Motor Ef-*

ficiency in Children, *The Measurement and Improvement of Movement Attributes.* Philadelphia, Lea & F., 1969.

Cratty, Bryant J.: *Active Learning.* Englewood Cliffs, New Jersey, Prentice-Hall, 1971.

DeVries, Herbert J.: Evaluation of static stretching procedures for the improvement of flexibility. *Res Quart Amer Ass Health Phys Educ, 33*:222-229, 1962.

Francis, R.J., and Rarick, G.L.: Motor Characteristics of the Mentally Retarded. U.S. Office of Education Cooperative Research Project #152, University of Wisconsin, September, 1967.

Hayden, Frank J.: Physical Fitness for the Mentally Retarded. Washington, D.C., Joseph P. Kennedy Foundation, 1964.

Howe, Clifford: A comparison of motor skills of mentally retarded and normal children. *J Except Child, 25-8*:352-354, April, 1959.

Johnson, G. Orville: A study of the social position of mentally handicapped children in the regular grades. *Amer J Ment Defic, 55*:69-89, 1950.

Wallis, E., and Logan, G.A.: *Exercise for Children.* Englewood Cliffs, New Jersey, Prentice-Hall, 1966.

SECTION THREE
Programs

Chapter Nine

PHYSICAL THERAPY IN A CHILDREN'S REHABILITATION CENTER

Nancy M. Fieber and Duane Kliewer

Significant progress is being made in meeting the educational, vocational, and health needs of the mentally retarded in the community. The special needs of the mentally retarded-physically handicapped are now being recognized. This chapter will describe the philosophy and organization of an outpatient physical therapy department and its role in a rehabilitation center serving children with handicaps. Suggestions are offered in keeping with the changing trends toward serving a broader scope of patients with developmental disabilities, increasing use of developmental and sensory-motor treatment approaches, better evaluation and management of the "whole child and his family," and necessary changes in the type of equipment and organization.

Traditionally, programs or clinics have been organized for special groups such as the cerebral-palsied, children's orthopedic, mentally retarded, or the "brain-injured." In some cases it has been difficult to tell which program was appropriate for a child with multiple handicaps, or which parent organization a parent should join. Such specialized programs result in the "left-outs"—the mentally retarded cerebral-palsied child left out of services for cerebral palsy; the cerebral-palsied child seen in a mental retardation clinic lacking adequate management of his motor problems; the child left out of a special education program because he cannot walk or is not toilet-trained.

The concept of a children's rehabilitation center for comprehensive diagnosis, treatment and service for the whole spectrum of developmental problems is emphasized increasingly in the literature. Such a center with its multidisciplinary team of specialists may serve to evaluate the whole child and his family, and provide guidance and treatment in a way that has not been possible in more limited clinics. The role of the pediatrician or pediatric neurologist as director of such a program is a trend in keeping with this broader scope. The basic team most frequently mentioned in mental retardation clinics has been the physician, psychologist, social worker, and public health nurse. Clinics for cerebral palsy and other neuromuscular disorders, with their remedial as well as diagnostic emphasis, have traditionally included physical, occupational, and speech therapists as members of their primary team. In a children's rehabilitation center, all of these must be represented.

The physical therapist's role in such a program is in assessment of various aspects of motor behavior, and in planning and implementing programs to guide and facilitate motor and perceptual development. In addition to providing direct treatment service, the therapist may provide consultative and indirect services through other disciplines. In planning assessment and service, the characteristics and needs of a variety of conditions must be considered.

WHO ARE THE DEVELOPMENTALLY DISABLED?

The children served in a children's rehabilitation center may include children with developmental delay, neuropathies such as cerebral palsy, myopathies such as muscular dystrophy of the Duchenne type, congenital anomalies such as meningomyelocele, and perceptual-motor handicaps. Sensory deficits such as visual or auditory impairment, behavioral manifestations such as hyperactivity or autism, seizures, and a variety of motor problems may also be seen.

Mental Retardation

Motor developmental delay, poor coordination, and poor physical fitness frequently accompany mental retardation. Hypotonia, hypermobility of joints, or congenital deformities may be present. Motor development in the child with general delay has been said to proceed along the same general continuums as in the normal, based on the maturation of the same underlying postural reflex mechanisms. Our observation of the motor development of children with delay at various ages has been that, in addition to the commonly recognized factors of sensory deprivation, parental rejection or overprotection, and lack of motivation, these children also exhibit substitutions or compensatory behavior which may contribute to further delay.

In some children not all aspects of the normal motor continuum will develop. For example, children with Down's anomaly, and others with hypotonia and hypermobility, may not use normal righting maneuvers between prone and sitting postures, but move between widely abducted legs. They may scoot in sitting rather than develop locomotion on hands and knees. Standing may be particularly delayed, and may be quite stiff with inability to squat down and stand up again. Orthopedic problems may develop as a result of low tone, hypermobility of joints, and faulty patterns of posture and weight-bearing. Incoordination in games and play may contribute to inability to interact socially with other children and to habitual failure patterns; possibly, it may influence motivation for learning (Cratty 1967, 1969). As the children grow older, motor incoordination may also handicap training for vocational skills and a place in the community.

Cerebral Palsy

The characteristics of children with cerebral palsy have been described in Chapter Three, Part I. They may exhibit delayed or uneven acquisition of the righting, protective, and equilibrium reactions basic to motor development, as well as retained primitive patterns of posture and movement. In addition, abnormal patterns of tonic reflex activity may interfere with or prevent the development of the normal patterns. Tone may be too low for postural fixation, too high for mobility, or may fluctuate. Deformities may develop as a result of stereotyped postures, persisting tonic reflex patterns, reinforcement of abnormal patterns by using them for functional purposes, and compensatory patterns. Some of these children will become ambulatory; others will be able to manage a wheelchair and assist in activities of daily living; some will require total care. Sensory handicaps, perceptual deficits or mental retardation may accompany the motor handicap.

Muscular Dystrophy

The child with progressive muscular dystrophy exhibits muscle weakness particularly of proximal muscles of shoulder-girdle and pelvic-girdle. Onset may be gradual; for example, as a preschooler the child may have difficulty getting up from the floor or climbing stairs. He develops compensatory patterns such as trunk sway, lordosis and backknee, and develops contractures from muscle imbalance, the pull of gravity and immobility. With progressive weakness he may lose the ability to ambulate, may manage some activities from a wheelchair, or may require maximum care. Although mental retardation or perceptual problems may be present in some of these children of the Duchenne type as a primary manifestation, deprivation may also contribute to secondary retardation (Cohen et al. 1968, Zellweger and Hanson 1967).

Meningomyelocele and Hydrocephalus

The child with meningomyelocele may have multiple deficits —orthopedic, neuromotor, sensory, bladder and bowel, and intellectual (Frederickson 1966). Spinal cord lesions may result in a variety of patterns of neurological impairment, such as paralysis, spinal spasticity and spinal reflexes, and the manifestations of upper motor neuron lesions superimposed (Stark and Baker 1967). In addition to congenital deformities of the feet and dislocation or subluxation of the hips, deformities may develop from unopposed active muscles, the pull of gravity, spasticity, and stereotyped postures.

The hydrocephalic child with very enlarged head and requiring special equipment and management in daily living may still be seen. Injuries and skin breakdown may be hazards with sensory deficit. Some of these children will become ambulatory with braces and crutches, others will lead wheelchair lives.

Sensory and Perceptual-Motor Disability

Sensory, sensory integrative and perceptual-motor deficits may accompany other handicaps of cerebral dysfunction or occur as the predominant disability. In addition to problems with sensory and motor differentiation, problems with development of body-image, motor planning or praxia, and visuomotor skills may occur which effect the development or training of motor skills and have been related to learning problems. Much work remains to fully understand the perceptual problems of the child with cerebral palsy, the child with mental retardation, or the child with minimal cerebral dysfunction and specific learning disabilities.

PHYSICAL THERAPY EVALUATION

The physical therapist carries out specific evaluation procedures as part of a coordinated assessment process and as a necessary prelude to the development of a total management program. Team evaluations should result in each discipline contributing its special knowledge in such ways that a concise picture of the whole child emerges. Only in this way can one avoid the danger of fragmentation inherent in multidisciplinary assessment. The physical therapist is responsible for assessing the total motor picture and should consider how it affects adaptive behavior, speech, and function both at home and school. While the occupational therapist is primarily responsible for adaptive skills, and the speech therapist for oral or respiratory functions, they cannot evaluate or treat adequately without also understanding the total motor picture.

Evaluation procedures should be broad enough to serve as a basis for some freedom in treatment technique. Generally, no one test procedure or form will serve the therapist's purpose of a thorough motor assessment. A flexible battery of tests is recommended, the therapist choosing whichever tests will provide the needed information. The emphasis in testing may vary according to the nature of the problems presented, with detailed assessment and objective scoring in one or more areas, and only brief comment or subjective observation in others.

The following outline may be used whether the child has developmental delay, cerebral palsy, muscular dystrophy, meningomyelocele, is perceptually handicapped, or has a combination of deficits:

1. Developmental and functional assessments.
2. Neurodevelopmental evaluation of postural reflex mechanisms and tone.
3. Evaluation of muscle strength.
4. Evaluation of musculoskeletal status in terms of range of motion, limb measurements, and postural deviations.
5. Evaluation of specific or integrative sensory functions.
6. Evaluation of perceptual-motor skills.

Developmental and Functional Assessments

Motor function should be correlated with normal development for age in all children with developmental handicaps. This may include gross and fine motor skills, adaptive skills and activities of daily living; it may be evaluated in detail or simply with developmental screening devices. As the child grows, activities of daily living tests may include brace management, crutch-walking skills, or wheelchair management.

Objective scoring is desirable and various scoring systems have been offered. Those which grade the quality of performance rather than simple pass-fail scoring may be of more value to a therapist. Scores for different aspects of motor function may be more meaningful than a single developmental quotient. Others will prefer describing a specific area in terms of age level. Therapists will find that tests measuring a continuum of presumably the same aspect of motor behavior (such as the development of prone antigravity function, sitting and prehension) are more useful in analyzing the causes of deficiencies, planning remedial measures and measuring progress than tests which group items of relatively unrelated motor behavior at the same age level with various weighting to each item. Therapists are referred to discussions of the general attributes of good tests (Stockmeyer 1965) and of specific tests (Semans 1965).

The developmental assessments described below may be useful in a children's rehabilitation center.

Screening Devices

A DEVELOPMENTAL SCREENING INVENTORY FOR INFANTS (Knobloch, Pasamanick and Sherard 1966). This Gesell-derived test may be useful both in screening for developmental deviations and as a "whole child" profile in the assessment of an infant with motor deviation. This test includes ages four weeks to 18 months, and scores each aspect of function (i.e. gross motor, fine motor, adaptive, language, and personal-social) in terms of maturity of age level. Items are scored as present, absent, or unknown, with separate columns for scoring observed and reported behavior. Therapists will find the items of visual coordination and attempted separation of fine motor and adaptive behavior useful. Test procedures are described in the form, and materials may be improvised within described guide lines.

THE DENVER DEVELOPMENTAL SCREENING TEST (Frankenberg and Dodds 1967). This test, derived from a number of developmental and intelligence tests, includes ages from birth to six years. Standardization with a normal age range of accomplishment is presented in graph form. Scoring is on a pass-fail basis, with division into gross motor, fine motor and adaptive, language, and personal-social behavior areas. A procedure manual and test kit are available with test forms. Along with its primary intended use in screening for developmental deviations, this test may serve to provide the therapist with a developmental profile of the whole child.

THE MOTOR DEVELOPMENTAL SCREENING EXAMINATION (Milani-Comparetti and Gidoni 1967a). This test is intended primarily as a rapid screening device for motor development in young children from birth to age five years. Functional motor achievements in terms of antigravity postural control is related to underlying reflex structures. A chart with the upper section describing spontaneous behavior involving postural control and active movement shows the continuums of development in several areas against an age scale or graph. The lower section graphs the disappearance of the primitive reflexes and appearance of righting, parachute, and tilting reactions as they relate to the spontaneous behavior above. These relationships are discussed by Milani-Comparetti and Gidoni in the original article (1967a). Adequate background and training is required in using this test. A careful reading of the original article is essential.

Motor Developmental Assessments

THE GESELL DEVELOPMENTAL SCHEDULES (Gesell 1940). This test measures motor development, adaptive behavior, language development, and personal-social behavior from four weeks to six years as described in the basic texts (Gesell 1940, Gesell and Amatruda 1954). Scoring arrives at a developmental quotient. A test kit and forms are available.

Gesell-derived motor development forms have been devised and used by many therapists to meet their own needs in recording motor skills and measuring progress (Johnson et al. 1951, Miller et al. 1955, Dallas Society 1963, Fields 1969, Willson 1969). A Gesell-derived motor developmental form might be a common assessment for all children seen by the physical therapy department in a children's rehabilitation center. Caution against arriving at a quotient when using only part of the original test in unstandardized form is suggested. Describing performance in terms of age level of success and range, as well as recording quality of performance is recommended. Further analysis by the therapist of musculoskeletal, neuromuscular, sensory and perceptual factors will be necessary in interpreting the child's performance and planning appropriate therapy measures.

THE ZAUSMER MOTOR DEVELOPMENT ASSESSMENT (Zausmer and Tower 1966). This test in preparation has been described as intended primarily for use by physical therapists as an assessment for cerebral palsy, but could be useful with other conditions affecting a child's motor development. Test items are grouped in separate units dealing with various aspects of motor behavior: head control, rolling over, crawling and creeping, kneeling, sitting, standing, walking and running; complex motor skills such as hopping, prehension and manipulation; complex manipulation skills and self-care; and play and sport skills. A rating scale for motor behavior has been presented (Zausmer 1964, 1966, 1968) with scoring considering several factors of motivation and quality of performance, and modified according to the age at which the function normally matures. While further testing or interpretation of the reasons for the child's performance would be necessary in planning treatment, this test should be helpful in objectively measuring progress for children who may not be able to perform motor milestones normally.

The Lincoln-Oseretsky Motor Development Scale (Sloan 1955). This test is designed to test motor abilities of children between ages six and fourteen years. It consists of 36 items involving a wide variety of motor skills such as finger dexterity, eye-hand coordination, and gross activities of arms, legs, and trunk arranged in approximate order of difficulty according to age. This adaptation of the original Oseretsky test does not claim to measure basic components of motor ability as did the original, but retains selected items which discriminate between performance of children at different ages and undoubtedly involves both maturational and learned factors. An objective scoring system relates total numerical score to percentile norms for boys and girls according to age. A manual and test kit are available.

It has been recommended that further standardization be done, and there is some question of reliability between different examiners. This test does not successfully exclude intelligence and perceptual factors in measuring motor coordination, and is not practical with many mentally retarded children. A current revision attempting to solve some of the above problems has been reported in progress, with a return to an attempt at qualitatively measuring basic areas of motor function at different age levels, and reducing intellectual, perceptual, cultural, and experiential influences (Stott 1966).

Therapists may find this test useful in relating a child's total score of motor abilities to what is expected for his age, but considerable further analysis of which items were failed and why would be necessary for use in remedial planning. The need continues for a test of basic motor abilities with continuums sensitive to neuromuscular dysfunction and covering a wide age range.

Functional Assessments

ACTIVITIES OF DAILY LIVING TEST (Buchwald 1952). This well-known functional test has served as the basis for many derivations useful in various settings. It includes evaluation of bed activities, hygiene or personal care, eating, dressing and undressing, hand skills, wheelchair activities, elevation activities and walking activities. It may be useful in its original form or adapted for use with young children by reference to Gesell scales for age level of activities. Traditionally used with physically handicapping conditions, the activities of daily living or adaptive profiles have also been utilized in assessment and management of the mentally retarded.

DAILY ACTIVITY INVENTORY AND PROGRESS RECORD FOR THOSE WITH ATYPICAL MOVEMENT (Brown 1950). This activities of daily living test was designed to check skills of children with a variety of motor or orthopedic problems. The 100 daily activities tested include bed activities, bathing and grooming, dressing and undressing, eating, management of wheelchair or appliances, standing and locomotion. With management of younger children, increasing developmental emphasis, and a trend toward less early bracing, an activities of daily living test might be modified to supplement developmental assessments and used primarily with older children who may require crutches, bracing, or wheelchairs.

THE PRESCHOOL FUNCTIONAL ACTIVITY TEST (Footh and Kogan 1963). This test was devised for measuring base lines and progress in cerebral-palsied children and is based on developmental scales and activities of daily living tests. The test consists of four sections: general motor development leading up to ambulation; wheelchair management; activities of daily living; and general activities or coordination in ambulatory skills. Objective scoring does not involve maturity levels or quotients, but arrives at a numerical score. Grading of general motor development is according to the quality of performance and amount of assistance necessary. A procedure manual with specific administration and scoring procedures has been prepared. This test has the advantages of objectively scoring improvement in a functional skill that may still fall short of independence. Further testing would be necessary in planning treatment.

Testing the Uncooperative Child

In testing an uncooperative or very retarded child or a child with hearing or visual defects, it may be difficult to use tests with specific procedures involved. In our experience a reasonable idea of the child's abilities according to developmental levels can be obtained through less formal testing. The stage may be set with toys and equipment that will invite the child to spontaneously show specific aspects of motor behavior.

Push and pull toys, dolls, blocks, cars and balls may stimulate spontaneous play. A ball in particular may provide the means of establishing some rapport between therapist and child and exploring imitative behavior as well as skills. The child may be placed on the stairs for observation of various aspects of balance, agility, foot preference and visual awareness. This may also give clues to his maturity level. A small chair and table with suitable toys on it may invite the child to demonstrate his maturity level in seating himself and manipulating objects. He may be placed on his back on the floor and his method of getting up observed. He may be placed in a squatting position and his independent balance and method of getting up observed. Balance, agility and motor planning may be observed in response to play equipment such as a jungle gym, slide or tricycle. Obstacle courses may be improvised and the child lured with a windup or friction toy or a ball.

Neurodevelopmental Evaluation of Postural Reflex Mechanisms and Tone

Evaluation of Muscle Tone

A detailed assessment of muscle tone will be indicated in a young child with a neuromotor deficit. More general observations or screening may be sufficient in assessing children with developmental delay and general low tone, or with minimal cerebral dysfunction. Evaluation of muscle tone in the child with cerebral palsy should explore patterns of distribution of hypertonus and the influence of various postures other than supine (Ch. 3). Assessment of tone by tests for capacity of muscle for lengthening and response to flapping of limb segments may also be useful in differentiating normal tone from hypertonus and hypotonus (Andrè-Thomas et al. 1960). In our experience in testing the child with possible minimal hypertonus, very rapid stretch from the shortened position of the muscle may elicit stretch reflex in the patterns of the tonic reflexes.

Evaluation of Postural Reflex Mechanisms or Background

Developmental assessment should be supplemented by evaluation of the basic postural reflex mechanisms underlying the motor developmental scales, the righting, protective, and equilibrium reactions as well as primitive mechanisms such as the grasp reflex or Moro reaction which may be retained in the child with developmental delay or cerebral palsy (Ch. 3; Milani-Comparetti and Gidoni 1967a,b, Andrè-Thomas et al. 1960). In children with developmental delay, the righting, protective, and equilibrium reactions are the building blocks for advancing the skills measured on the developmental scales. In working with the very young child with meningomyelocele, an understanding of the sequential acquisition of these reactions is useful in stimulating development and developing the necessary arm and trunk strength needed for later ambulation with crutches and the activities of daily living. With the cerebral-palsied child, the presence of abnormal patterns of posture and movement should be recorded with observation of interaction of normal and abnormal patterns (Ch. 3).

The following published tests may be useful in analyzing development of postural control and movement:

REFLEX TESTING CHART (Fiorentino 1963). This monograph describes testing of postural reflexes with specific test position, test stimulus, negative and positive reactions, and time of appearance and disappearance. Photographs of normal and abnormal responses illustrate each test. A reflex testing chart accompanying a motor development chart are presented. Therapists may find this text helpful in identifying disturbances of postural reflexes and reactions. The validity of the grouping of the reflexes according to levels of CNS integration, and timing of appearance and disappearance of various reactions may be questioned (Semans 1964).

CEREBRAL PALSY ASSESSMENT CHART OF BASIC MOTOR CONTROL (Semans et al. 1965). This test has been developed as a modification of the assessment chart developed by Karel Bobath and Berta Bobath (1958, 1960). Selected test postures show the nature and extent of the interference of abnormal posture and movements with the necessary postural control for various functional activities. Test procedures involve first passively placing the child in the test postures and observing interfering tension, contractures or structural deviations, secondly asking the child to maintain the test posture, and then observing the quality of the child's independent movement into the test posture. A numerical scoring system is used to grade each posture, making comparisons possible in specific areas as well as providing a total score. Both are useful as a guide in planning treatment procedures and measuring progress. Its administration, interpretation, and usefulness in planning treatment requires the necessary background and training in the Bobath approach to treatment of cerebral palsy. A more detailed assessment of interaction of maturing normal and abnormal patterns might be indicated in assessing the very young infant.

Testing of Synergies and Associated Reactions in Movement

Supplementary testing of upper extremity functioning may be useful in some children with cerebral palsy or with acquired central neuromotor deficits. We have found it helpful in analyzing the function of the hemiplegic upper extremity in particular. The evaluation of the combined or selective movements possible outside of the abnormal flexor and extensor synergies (Bobath 1959, 1960, 1965, Brunnstrom 1966) has been useful in planning, training and progressing toward more functional movement patterns. With the child who may not perform movements on command, the therapist may observe the combined motions and ability to reach, grasp, and release in different positions through play with the child.

The occurrence of associated reactions may be observed as the child performs fine or effortful activities with the uninvolved hand, in resisted effortful movement of the involved arm, and in spontaneous behavior when running about. The influence of tonic neck reflexes on these associated reactions may be explored by observing the child's spontaneous use of head rotation to facilitate effortful movement or by instructing the child to turn his head as he performs a movement (Walshe 1923). The effect of associated reactions of upper or lower extremities in effortful activity should be considered in planning treatment.

Postural Background and Other Disciplines

Observation of postural background should be related to those skills traditionally assessed by occupational and speech therapists. This is particularly important in the absence of these therapists. The influence of posture on visual fixation and pursuit, as well as manipulation, should be explored. As an example, certain children may be better able to visually follow and to manually exploit a toy when positioned in side-lying or over a bolster in prone than when in supine or propped sitting. Oral and respiratory mechanisms of feeding and prespeech should also be related to problems of postural control, tonic reflexes and primitive patterns in order to plan motor management with a continuity of treatment approach.

Evaluation of Muscle Strength

Assessment of muscle function by manual muscle testing is a familiar procedure to all physical therapists. Grading of muscle strength is based on the ability to move the part through its range against gravity or with gravity eliminated, and to hold the contraction against resistance (Daniels et al. 1946, Kendall and Kendall 1949).

Detailed assessment of muscle function and strength is an

important part of the evaluation in conditions such as muscular dystrophy or the myelodysplasias. In children with developmental delay general functional screening and assessment of trunk strength may be sufficient. When testing an uncooperative or very young child, the therapist may assess ability to move the part through its range or to stabilize by placing the child in various positions where active movement and postural fixation can be observed. For example, strength of posterior shoulder muscles may be appraised by inducing the child to reach up high with a toy, or to prop on his arms in prone. Lifting a toy may offer clues to ability to take resistance. Careful observation of use of play equipment can also offer clues as to muscle strength or specific weaknesses. In muscle testing of the infant, observing muscle function in the postural reflexes may be useful (Zausmer 1953, Andre-Thomas et al. 1960). For example, a young child with meningomyelocele may demonstrate active hip flexors and quadriceps as he is supported in supine suspension. His lack of hip extensors and hamstrings may show as he is supported in prone suspension and does not lift his legs in the Landau reaction.

Detailed muscle testing in cerebral palsy is not of first importance in evaluation of the motor deficit because this is a problem primarily of neuromuscular incoordination (Ch. 3.). It is important that the therapist evaluate the patterns of coordination in which a muscle group functions or does not function. Where antigravity tone or postural fixation is weak, this might be described in the context of the postural reactions or functional mechanisms involved. With the effect of long-term stereotyped postures and movement, secondary weakness may occur and this should be described.

Evaluation of Musculoskeletal Status in Terms of Range of Motion, Limb Measurements, and Postural Deviations

Range of motion and postural deviations may be measured and recorded in detail in some cases, and only briefly described in others. Hypermobility of joints should be recorded as well as limitations of range (Amer. Acad. Orthopaedic Surgeons 1965). Range of motion should be assessed routinely in conditions such as muscular dystrophy, myelodysplasias, or cerebral palsy.

Children with muscular dystrophy will be subject to development of contractures due to the pull of gravity, muscle imbalances, or immobility. The ambulatory child may typically have lordosis with hip flexor tightness or hamstring, backknee, and tight plantar flexors. Once he becomes nonambulatory and sits in a wheelchair, tightness of flexor muscles of hip and knee as well as plantar flexors may increase. The child with meningomyelocele may develop limitations of range due to stereotyped postures such as frog-legged posture in supine, unopposed active muscles such as hip flexors or ankle dorsiflexors, or spasticity in adduction. In cerebral palsy, persistent stereotyped postures, tonic reflexes and compensatory mechanisms may contribute to deformity. Evaluation and remedial measures should consider these causes as well as their peripheral results.

In assessing the child with developmental delay or the child with possible perceptual-motor handicaps, the therapist should routinely perform a rapid screening of joint range, posture, and limb length differences. In the child with developmental delay and low tone, hypermobility may contribute to problems with postural alignment in weight-bearing and further contribute to delayed acquisition of skills. The child with Down's anomaly, for example, may develop marked backknee, valgus of knees and feet, lordosis, and hip problems.

In our experience a number of children being assessed for perceptual-motor problems and possible specific learning disabilities have proved to have such postural problems as severely pronated feet, tightness of hip flexors or hamstrings and compensatory lordosis, leg length differences, and mild scoliosis. Interpretation of the child's performance in perceptual-motor tests is aided by consideration of these structural factors as well as assessment of muscle tone. Such information may also be contributory to identifying minimal cerebral palsy or minimal cerebral dysfunctions.

Evaluation of Specific and Integrative Sensory Functions

Physical therapists have traditionally performed various sensory tests for diagnostic purposes with conditions such as peripheral nerve injuries, spinal cord lesions, or cerebral vascular accidents. The possible relationships between sensory deficits and recovery of muscle function and practical functional use of hands and legs have been explored. With the awareness of the possible specific or integrative sensory deficits occurring in the syndromes of cerebral dysfunction and their possible contribution to perceptual problems, sensory testing should become more routine.

Primary sensations tested may include exteroceptive sensations such as touch, pain and temperature, and proprioceptive sensations such as kinesthesia and position sense. Cortical or integrative sensory functions may include tests for stereognosis, two-point discrimination, recognition of textures, graphaesthesia, and tactile localization. Useful references for sensory testing of children are Paine and Oppe (1966) and Denhoff (1967).

Brunnstrom (1966) has described gross testing for sensory loss in adult hemiplegia patients. Included are tests for passive motion sense of large and small joints of upper and lower limbs, fingertip recognition, and sole sensation. Similar methods may be useful in testing of some children, although not standardized according to age as are The Southern California Kinesthesia and Tactile Perception Tests by A. Jean Ayres (1966). This battery of six tests evaluates upper extremity somesthetic perception in children with norms established from four to eight years. Included are kinesthesia, manual form perception, finger identification, graphaesthesia, localization of tactile stimuli and double tactile stimuli perception. Procedures can be modified for testing children with neuromuscular dysfunction, but although verbal response is not required the child must be able to communicate in some fashion. This test may be useful in correlation of sensory deficit with motor deficit, or in evaluation of perceptual handicaps. Factor analysis studies have identified correlations with specific perceptual-motor syndrome clusters that may assist therapists in identifying and treating these deficits (Ayres 1965).

In testing the very young, retarded, or uncooperative child, gross testing of specific sensations such as temperature or pain are not difficult. Tactile awareness of parts of the body may be observed by touching the child with a wisp of cotton, touching him with an object or hiding it in his clothes. Responses may include such reactions as no awareness, awareness and activation without localization, ability to localize and bring hand to the spot, and tactile defensiveness, inappropriate anger or silliness. Such observations are helpful in understanding a child's problems with body image and praxia, his response to handling by a therapist, and in the training of motor skills. Observations of the way a child explores toys with "feeling" hands or the way his feet search for the rungs of the jungle gym offer some clues to integrative sensory functions.

Evaluation of Perceptual-Motor Skills

Although the validity of the various theories, tests and training of perceptual-motor functions needs further research, thorough evaluation of the child should include this area for better understanding of the individual child and for its contribution to better understanding of these problems in general. A physical therapist participating in testing children with possible perceptual-motor deficits should be familiar with the contributions of several disciplines—medicine, occupational therapy, education, and psychology, as well as physical therapy. An understanding of the theories, tests and remedial approaches of Ayres (1958, 1960, 1961, 1962, 1963, 1964, 1965, 1966, 1968), Knickerbocker (1966), Frostig (1961, 1964, 1969), Cratty (1966, 1967, 1969) and Kephart (1960, 1966) are recommended as basic preparation. These workers stress the importance of early sensorimotor learning in the later development of more complex perceptual and cognitive skills. They all relate the development of body scheme and body-image to the development of spatial and directional relationships. Various balance and agility skills and motor planning activities are included in both testing and training.

Gross Perceptual-Motor Tests

Tests useful in identifying gross perceptual-motor problems and as a basis for remedial planning are described.

SOUTHERN CALIFORNIA PERCEPTUAL-MOTOR TEST (Ayres 1968). This standardized test with norms for children four to eight years, includes sections testing imitation of postures, crossing the midline of the body, bilateral motor coordination, right-left discrimination, and standing balance. A manual and score sheets are available. This test is especially useful in identifying problems with integration of the two sides of the body. Except for the standing balance on one leg items, motor planning and coordination involve largely upper extremities and upper body, and physical therapists concerned with possible problems with gross perceptual-motor skills will need to test further.

THE CRATTY PERCEPTUAL-MOTOR TEST (Cratty 1966, 1969). This test was developed in studying the perceptual-motor attributes of mentally retarded children of school age, four to eleven years. Categories tested include body perception, gross agility, balance, locomotor agility, ball throwing and ball tracking at two levels of difficulty. Norms are offered for comparison of numerical scores with normal boys and girls, and children classified as trainable, educable, Down's anomaly, and educationally handicapped. This test is not difficult to administer, and is useful in identifying problems and planning motor training programs. Testing of the above attributes of motor skill and additional attributes of physical fitness and manual skills is also described by Cratty (1967). Performance is not scored objectively as tested in this manual, but is specifically related to suggested sequential remedial activities useful in a school or children's rehabilitation center program.

THE PURDUE PERCEPTUAL-MOTOR SURVEY (Kephart and Roach 1966). This standardized test for children six to nine years is intended as a test for perceptual-motor skills in those areas which Kephart has stressed as related to learning readiness (Kephart 1960). It includes items assessing balance and postural flexibility, body-image and differentiation, perceptual-motor match, ocular control and form perception. A numerical score is compared with norms. This is not meant as a test to identify specific motor disability or for use with known neuromuscular deficit. Intended for use by teachers as a basis for perceptual-motor testing and training in a special education setting, the test may also be useful for the therapist in working with school programs. We have found it useful in combination with other testing, particularly in regard to identification of laterality problems involved with crossing the midline and integration of the two sides.

A Psychoeducational Inventory of Basic Learning Abilities (Valett 1967). This evaluation and the accompanying remedial program include items in gross motor development, sensory-motor integration, perceptual-motor skills, language development, conceptual skills and social skills. Intended for use by educators, several sections would be of interest to a therapist working with a school program. This is not a standardized instrument, and relies on the examiner's judgment and experience in testing and interpretation.

Screening Tests for Minimal Motor Deficits and Learning Problems

The inclusion of gross and fine motor skills in screening tests for possible learning difficulties or minimal cerebral dysfunction has been explored. The Meeting Street School Screening Test (Denhoff et al. 1968, Hainsworth and Sigueland 1969) has been studied for its predictive value in identifying possible underachievers or school failures at first grade level. The following gross motor items were found to be significant: touching thumb to fingertips bilaterally, skipping, hopping on a line, and trunk strength in sitting from supine. Tests reflecting motor differentiation in terms of associated movements have been explored and found to be sensitive to maturation and to motor deficit (Abercrombie et al. 1964, Connolly and Stratton 1968). Tests involving distal alternate motion rate were found by DeHaven and co-workers (1969) to significantly differentiate children with minimal cerebral dysfunction from the normal.

General Suggestions

The physical therapist may supplement the tests of the physician, the teacher, the psychologist, or the occupational therapist with motor examination in more detail. Rather than merely scoring a child on the basis of performance in one-leg balance, balance beam tests, or hopping tests, the therapist may analyze further what underlying motor problem is to blame. In our experience, supplementing motor and perceptual-motor testing with evaluation of basic postural mechanisms, tone on passive manipulation, muscle strength, range of motion and structural deviations has been enlightening in a number of children referred for exploration of possible perceptual-motor problems.

No one test covers every aspect which might be explored in gross perceptual-motor skills. A narrative summary may describe results of objectively scored tests and specific areas of behavior such as static and dynamic balance, agility, gross and fine motor planning, laterality or integration of the two sides, body rhythms, and visual accuracy and tracking. The therapist should be prepared to test certain aspects of perceptual-motor behavior several ways. Increasingly we are seeing children who have received perceptual-motor training in too routinized and unvaried a training program based on test items in particular. They have developed ungeneralized splinter skills rather than the desired increased adaptability and generalization stressed by authorities such as Kephart (1960).

The problems and significance of various tests of handedness are not discussed in detail here. It is recommended that a therapist explore not only preferred use but skill and sensory differences in considering this problem. Usually these areas may be observed or recorded in the course of other testing.

Selection of Tests

The therapist should select those tests which seem most pertinent to the age or problems of the child to be assessed. With young children, a developmental assessment might be a common starting point. A functional or daily living test might be a common test where older children are seen. A nonambulatory child with developmental delay might first be tested by the Milani-Comparetti Developmental Test, or with a Gesell-derived form. He might also have a screening assessment of tone, structural deviations, and reactions to sensory stimuli.

An eleven-year-old child with muscular dystrophy would require a manual muscle test, measurement of range of motion, observation of gait and posture, and an activities of daily living test. A six-month-old cerebral-palsied child might be tested first with a Gesell-derived motor developmental scale, an assessment of tone, normal and abnormal postural-reflex patterns, and of range of motion and structured deviations. A developmental screening device may offer information about other aspects of behavior useful in planning management.

A nine-year-old child with possible perceptual-motor handicap and specific learning disability might be tested with a Gesell-derived scale, a gross perceptual-motor test, and a screening of tone, postural alignment, and range of motion. If sensory and fine motor testing is not available from an occupational therapist, screening or testing in detail should be done by the physical therapist.

The kind of complete evaluation suggested takes time to administer, interpret and prepare. Therapists under pressure for service or evaluation of many children may feel such an assessment is impossible, but only with thorough evaluation can a good general or individual program be planned. An initial evaluation of an hour or hour and a half will be adequate for planning and beginning treatment and preparing an initial report. Additional information can be added in subsequent visits modifying or supplementing initial findings, with evaluation being a continuous process. In a program where a child can be observed in a play group or preschool, the therapist can evaluate the child more gradually over a period of time.

THE TREATMENT PROGRAM
Setting Goals

The general goals of physical therapy in the syndromes of cerebral dysfunction and other handicaps interfering with motor development are to assist the child in developing his motor and perceptual potential, to prevent or control deformity, to help the family in daily care and management, and to provide the child with as many sensorimotor experiences of normal childhood as possible in preparation for living and learning. The term treatment is used for its dynamic remedial implications in the management of the child and need not be associated with cure.

Adequate assessment will provide the basis for forming specific therapy goals for the individual child. Goals should be presented in terms of short-term and long-term expectations. Examples are as follows:

1. In a young child with developmental delay and frogged legs, a long-term goal of achieving weight-bearing in standing may involve a short-term goal such as facilitation of the chain reaction of extension in prone in order to fix the hips in extension.

2. In an infant with hemiplegia, preparation for balance, functional use of the hand, and prevention of deformity may involve facilitation of protective extension of the arm as a short-term goal.

3. In a child with meningomyelocele and unopposed hip flexors, early instruction of the mother in prevention of hip flexion deformity by prone positioning and passive motion may assist in reaching a long-term goal of independent crutch-walking with the hips forward.

When prognosis may be uncertain, as in the very young child with cerebral palsy, long-term goals may be open-end initially and evolve with time. Reevaluation at specific intervals should assess progress and the goals themselves. With setting of goals, interpretation of these to the parents, and consideration of a number of factors, an appropriate program may be planned.

Types of Programs

The treatment program involves the general organization of physical therapy services and the manner in which needs of an individual child and family are met. Several factors are considered to determine whether services are organized on a group or individual basis, administered by therapist or parent, or include home visits. The types of patients served by the department, the age span, and what other services for handicapped children are available in the area will influence the general program. A center serving a local community only will plan services differently from one serving a large area. The social-economic groups served and the practical aspects of transportation and costs should be considered. The approach to treatment itself may influence the organization of the program. The best use of trained professional personnel, providing care for the most children possible is a necessity.

Several terms may be used to describe different types of therapy programs. An *active treatment program* refers to regular scheduling such as a twice weekly or daily plan in which the therapist administers treatment to the child. Parent instructions should support such a plan, emphasizing the parents' role in long-term care of the child. In some instances parents may be instructed in specific treatment techniques, while in others they may be instructed in supportive *remedial management*. Active treatment should not continue indefinitely but be used at specific times in the child's long-term management such as initially when diagnosis or prognosis is being explored and foundations of parent-training are being laid, during times of change, steady progress, or regression, or at points in development where the therapist's skill is particularly needed.

Remedial management might be used to describe therapy programs where family, school, and nursing personnel are instructed periodically in therapeutic handling and positioning of the child in daily care and play. Remedial management is something more than a *maintenance program* which is limited to range of motion exercises, mobility activities such as assisted locomotion or use of standing and locomotor equipment, or physical education activities. Specific therapeutic handling and positioning may be designed to encourage developmental progress in specific areas and avoid reinforcement of abnormal postural patterns or deformity-producing postures.

Developmental guidance programs with periodic reassessment and suggestions to parents in developmental stimulation may meet the needs of several types of situations—for example, the child with mental retardation and motor delay, the young child with signs of possible specific learning disabilities or perceptual handicaps, the child with cerebral palsy who has made good progress with early treatment and presents a "hidden handicap." The dilemma of how to offer early remedial services to the infant with suspected cerebral palsy may be solved with a developmental guidance program during ongoing assessment and diagnosis.

Role of Physical Therapy at Different Ages

A physical therapy program must meet the changing needs and priorities of the child at different ages. Several phases may be involved in a child's long-term management program, with physical therapy playing different roles in each (Denhoff 1960, Ellis 1967).

Infancy

Increasing interest in early diagnosis, treatment, and education for the very young child with mental retardation or physical handicaps places the highest priority on provision of services for this age group. At the same time, sensory-motor development may have the highest priority in early management of the infant.

Recent approaches to treatment of neuromotor deficits have increasingly emphasized developmental concepts and use of sensory input to influence motor output. (Chs. 3, 4, and 5) Facilitation of active postural reactions or movements is possible without intelligent cooperation or effort by the child, making possible dynamic treatment of very young or retarded children who could not cooperate in more traditional therapeutic exercise regimens (Ch. 3; Bobath 1967).

THE INFANT WITH DEVELOPMENTAL DELAY. The physical therapist in a children's rehabilitation center or public health program may play a key role in specific developmental guidance and stimulation for mentally retarded children with developmental delay during infancy, helping the child to reach his best motor and perceptual potential, and assisting the parents in their insight and acceptance of the child's handicap (Nunley 1967, Ames 1966).

There has been relatively little work done exploring motor training for the retarded child at an early age, although great strides have been made in providing motor training for older children. Programs of developmental stimulation have been quite general. The child has been helped to walk by helping him walk, or to sit by propping him in sitting, with little recognition of the necessary sequence of prerequisites for these milestones. Parents have wanted to help their child develop as well as he can, but without specific guidance they may not have understood activities appropriate for his level and may have expected too much or too little of their child. The therapist may interpret and demonstrate to the parents the type of play and handling that will stimulate the needed prerequisites for the next developmental milestones. Faulty patterns of posture and weight-bearing may be controlled before they lead to more serious orthopedic problems.

Parent instruction may be scheduled as periodic developmental guidance individually or in small groups. In some instances, more frequent scheduling such as once weekly may be indicated for a period. A comprehensive developmental guidance program ideally requires close cooperation between disciplines, with joint assessment or instruction by physical therapist and occupational therapist or public health nurse at intervals.

The following case history is an example of a developmental guidance program for an infant with developmental delay.

Case Summary: Greg, a 9½-month-old child with Down's anomaly, was referred to the physical therapy department for evaluation of motor status as part of general clinic evaluation. Psychological testing showed mental retardation in the moderate range. Physical therapy assessment included the Milani-Comparetti examination, a Gesell-derived motor scale, and assessment of range of motion and postural alignment.

Findings: At 9½ months gross motor development was at approximately the four-months level, or less. Greg had head lag as pulled to sit and although he could roll to prone he had difficulty freeing his arms forward. In prone his head was raised intermittently to 60° and he supported on his forearms, but hips were frogged in flexion-abduction. He could not travel on his stomach or assume all fours. In horizontal suspension, extensor tone was also inadequate as was protective extension or parachute reaction. Placed to sit he was completely flexed forward and tended to slide or slump in the high chair. Held to stand, he was non-weight-bearing and had no downward parachute reaction of the legs. Reach, grasp and exploitation of toys were more advanced, although he avoided bilateral play requiring shoulder-girdle fixation. Joints were hypermobile and muscle tone low.

Greg showed early compensatory behavior which could contribute to further delay. Although he could support on his forearms in prone and reach for a toy, he would immediately roll to his side to exploit it rather than sustaining antigravity extension in prone and practicing that very necessary level of motor behavior. He could manage a one-

Physical Therapy in a Children's Rehabilitation Center 381

handed toy, such as a small rattle, in supine and might play briefly with it in that position, but for bilateral exploitation of a toy demanding two hands, he would roll to his side to play.

He had the advantage of loving parents who wanted to help him attain his best potential. They had questions about daily management and toys at his level of function. A developmental guidance program in physical and occupational therapy with joint scheduling was recommended, to be coordinated with the public health nurse at intervals. As the family lived a distance from the center, an interval of two to three months was planned.

Goals and Activities: Greg's current developmental level was interpreted for his parents in terms of what basic postural mechanisms were then developing or would next develop, which were slow, and how they related to functional skills. They were shown ways in the handling of daily care and play to stimulate him to practice prone skills at his level, encouraging lifting the head, supporting and weight shift on his arms and the chain reaction of extension to the hips. These activities were interpreted as preparation for upright posture in sitting and standing. Ventral righting of the head and trunk was demonstrated in lap play and in picking him up.

To attain rolling, Greg needed better segmental righting reactions as well as better prone extension. Stimulation of protective extension forward in sitting was explained as preparation for beginning independent balance. Preparation for weight-bearing on the feet was demonstrated holding Greg to sit astride his daddy's leg on the floor with weight shift over the feet, and assisting him to stand up. The parents asked if use of an infant walker would be helpful in getting Greg to walk. The therapist explained that at that time Greg needed to accomplish certain prerequisites first in prone extension and flexible weight-bearing, and that being placed in standing without these might contribute to knee and foot alignment problems.

Toys were shown the parents by the occupational therapist which might invite two-handed manipulation, visual pursuit and fixation, and sensory awareness. Tongue protrusion was noted, but Greg enjoyed making lip sounds and was babbling. Sensory stimulation for awareness of lips and tongue was begun.

Subsequent visits with the therapists followed Greg as he developed. Later problems with stiff total extension patterns in getting to stand and in stance were overcome, and flexible weight-bearing achieved. A tendency to move between sitting and all fours with one leg extended and abducted, a possible contributor to joint alignment problems, was overcome with the encouragement of good rotation patterns. When Greg began spending time on his feet in cruising, pronation of the feet was noted, and corrective shoes were prescribed by the orthopedic consultant. Progression to solid foods and self-feeding were guided by the occupational therapist, and stimulating toys were demonstrated. Beginning body-image concepts and imitative behavior were encouraged. Problems with diet and toilet training readiness were discussed with the public health nurse. Guidance with early language stimulation was given by the speech therapist.

Periodic social service interviews with Greg's parents revealed they had developed realistic understanding of his condition and expectations for the future. They were delighted with his accomplishments as he grew and satisfied that they were helping him reach his potential. When Greg was three-years-old he entered a special education nursery school program in his community. Suggestions were sent by the therapists to this program regarding sensory and perceptual-motor training and a once-yearly reevaluation was planned.

THE INFANT WITH MENINGOMYELOCELE AND HYDROCEPHALUS. The physical therapist's role has broadened from emphasis on ambulation training for the child with meningomyelocele to include early management in infancy. Physical therapy consisting of positioning, splinting, and range of motion exercises for prevention of deformity should begin shortly after birth while the child is still under treatment in the hospital (Kinsman 1966, Ames 1966).

On discharge, the family should be taught these measures and follow them at regular intervals. Range of motion exercises should be taught with careful attention to any tendency toward subluxation to dislocation of the hips. Guidance should be given in positioning the infant in daily care both for prevention of deformity and encouragement of development.

Prone positioning to encourage development of active antigravity extension patterns and to counteract hip flexion is recommended. If the posterior defect is closed, the child may be positioned in supine on a thick foam rubber pad with a cut-out area. In time he may be placed in an infant seat to encourage development of his use of hands and enable him to see what is going on around him. Side-lying should involve precautions for abduction of the upper leg.

The family may be taught handling techniques for facilitation of the normal maturing postural mechanisms in the course of daily care and play—that is, the appropriate righting, protective and equilibrium reactions underlying functional development (Ch. 3). This approach, with control or inhibition of abnormal posture and movement when spasticity is present, is similar to that of cerebral palsy except for the added possibilities of peripheral paralysis and spasm. Where no spasticity or upper motor neuron involvement is present the child may be kept as close as possible to the normal sequence of development and provided active exercise of upper extremities and trunk as preparation for later functional training.

The child should be brought into a standing position as close to the normal age as possible for optimum timing of learning functions in standing as well as needs for weight-bearing according to Shurtleff (1966). Bracing or special standing equipment such as a prone-stander may be used (Hueter and Blossom 1967). In the child with hydrocephalus and spasticity, consideration should also be given to the developmental level of readiness, adequacy of head control and the state of abnormal posture and movement patterns.

The medical and physical problems of these children may dominate their early management. The need for attention to other kinds of stimulation and learning should be considered in a comprehensive plan.

THE INFANT WITH MYOPATHY. The child with muscular dystrophy may not be diagnosed and referred as a young infant, but other myopathies, some of which may be progressive, may be seen in a children's rehabilitation center. Successive motor assessment may aid in the determination of changing status. Helping parents in positioning and handling the child to encourage function and avoid deformities may be accomplished with periodic instruction.

THE INFANT WITH CEREBRAL PALSY. Physical therapy for the child with cerebral palsy should begin as early as possible, preferably in the first year. A dynamic developmental approach begun at that time may have the best prognosis for establishing normal sensorimotor patterns, preventing deformity, and helping the child reach his best developmental potential (Ch. 3; Kong 1966, Bobath 1967, Blumenthal 1958, Derham 1967).

The early developmental treatment of the infant is best achieved by parent instruction in a home program with regular supervision by the physical therapist. Scheduling may vary from an active treatment plan of once or twice weekly to once or twice monthly, according to the problems presented by the child, the need of the mother for instruction or support, and practical problems of getting into the center. A period of active treatment with intensive parent instruction is ideal to prepare for a good home program.

It is recommended that a therapist with special training in the area of child development, preferably in the neurodevelopmental techniques, be the key person dealing with the total developmental stimulation of the infant with cerebral palsy so that the treatment of the child is not fragmented (Jones 1969). A "whole child" approach is desirable, since continuity of treatment approach is necessary in all aspects of the child's management. Early attention to respiratory coordination and feeding problems involving jaw control, sucking and swallowing, or spoon-feeding of solids should be managed in the context of the therapist's evaluation of the total motor picture and treatment plan (Ch. 6).

Sensory stimulation should be controlled so that abnormal posture and movement is not reinforced. Placement of visual stimuli such as crib mobiles and mirrors may be specific according to the positioning needs of the child. Visual pursuit may need to be encouraged with special techniques controlling posture so that the child can pursue but does not reinforce tonic reflex activity when he does so. The therapist will explore auditory stimuli that do not cause a startle reaction. The child should be assisted to exploit toys without reinforcing associated reactions. When the child is seen by several therapists, close coordination of activities is necessary.

Developmental treatment approaches for infants with developmental handicaps may be translated into the handling of daily care and play to a great extent, and demanding exercise routines need not be imposed on the family. Although home visits are desirable at intervals, the pressure of staff time may make them infrequent or impossible. The therapist, therefore, must take great care to find out how the family lives, to know the infant's schedule and habits, to deal with normal infant toys and furniture insofar as possible, and to apply and teach treatment principles accordingly.

The Preschool-age Child

As the child approaches two to three years of age, prenursery school training, language, self-help activities, and the need for group experiences have increasing priorities. The child may now require physical, occupational, and speech therapy as well as attend a nursery school program. Communication between the various therapists and the teacher is necessary to avoid conflicting treatment efforts.

The need for group experiences may be met in physical therapy or joint therapy groupings of children with similar therapy needs. These may supplement and support individual treatment or instruction where they are needed. They may be helpful in preparing for participation in a nursery school program. Group activities should be planned for the benefit of the children, rather than as a means of solving pressure for service.

THE PRESCHOOL CHILD WITH DEVELOPMENTAL DELAY. As they reach the preschool stage of development, some children with marked motor delay who are not ambulatory may need a period of active treatment to achieve ambulation. Others will have achieved ambulation but still lack many functional motor skills such as sitting directly on a chair, squatting or picking up a toy from the floor, climbing stairs safely, or stepping up a curb or step without rail or assistance. Because a child cannot ride a tricycle or climb the play equipment he may begin to avoid or fail in the gross motor play and exploration activities important in physical fitness, perceptual development, and in social adjustment. If a therapeutic nursery school is not available, these children may benefit by a home developmental guidance program stressing opportunity for continued development of balance and agility and perceptual-motor skills. Guidance in choice of play equipment and structured play activities can combine learning with fun.

Case Summary: Karen was three years old at the time of her assessment by the Meyer Children's Rehabilitation Institute. She was found to be mildly retarded, but particularly delayed in social-emotional and motor development. No specific neuromotor disability was diagnosed. Physical therapy included assessment on a Gesell-derived scale, the Milani-Comparetti examination, evaluation of range of motion and postural deviations, and some screening of perceptual-motor aspects.

Findings: Karen was able to creep on all fours, to rotate between sitting and all fours, to pull to stand and cruise around the furniture. She walked with both hands held, but did not try to stand alone or get up from midfloor. She had great difficulty standing up from a squat, equilibrium reactions were poor in stance, and she lacked trunk-hip stability. Protective extension was not developed backward in sitting, and she could not accommodate to disruption very well without using her hands for props. Muscle tone was low and joints hypermobile; for instance, a tendency to backknee and pronation of the feet was noted, especially on the left.

Karen was very fearful, especially of movement in space. She did not know the parts of her body, imitate movement or follow verbal instructions regarding movement. She did not localize tactile stimuli well. Attention span was brief and tolerance for structure poor. The occupational therapist reported that dressing skills were particularly delayed because of poor body-image development and inability to balance with both hands free.

It was recommended that Karen enter the nursery school program and be placed on an active twice weekly physical therapy program for a period of three or four months. Plans were made to include Karen's mother at regular intervals, an important consideration for children attending a daily program of nursery school. An orthopedic evaluation was recommended. Corrective shoes and a short-leg brace were prescribed for the left ankle.

Goals and Activities: Long-term goals established for Karen were to achieve ambulation and practical functional skills needed for daily living, to enable her to learn to use play equipment important for social as well as perceptual-motor development, and to develop awareness of her body and its movements.

Short-term goals and activities for Karen were to develop flexible weight-bearing and standing up from a squat, to go forward on her hands to plantigrade and be assisted to come to stand, to develop protective extension backward in sitting, to achieve better trunk-hip stability in prone, kneeling, and standing, and to stimulate equilibrium reactions in sitting and standing.

Encouragement of walking, gradually lessening direct assistance, began with pushing a small chair or weighted doll buggy. Instruction of her nursery school teacher and aids enabled carry-over of therapeutic goals to the nursery setting. Karen soon progressed to walking with one hand held or a light touch on the shoulders. Direct contact was reduced by having her hold a stiff doll's arm with therapist or teacher holding the other, and finally holding a floppy rag doll between them. Karen began getting up from midfloor and walking alone in about three months, and began enjoying trying the play equipment and the stairs. At that time a recommendation was made that the active plan be extended an additional three months to get her started with ambulatory skills and continued stress of perceptual-motor development.

It was very interesting to note that climbing the jungle gym was very difficult, and raising and lowering her weight on a flexed leg was still difficult. She could not organize arms and legs, and appeared to have no ability to "feel" with her leg and foot for a rung. As she reached the top of the jungle gym she could not get into position to go down the slide. On the stairs she had great difficulty seeing or feeling the edges, and tended to slide, trip, and skip stairs rather than step down. Karen's program increasingly stressed body awareness, motor planning, sensory reinforcement, and coordinating vision with movement.

At the end of the next three months period she had mastered stairs with a rail and was trying a low step with no rail. She had learned to ride a tricycle with rubber loop fasteners for her feet on the pedals, and to sit on a chair without climbing on. She played games such as carrying a pail and squatting to pick up a trail of poker chips and followed colorful yarn through obstacle courses. She was beginning to respond in games involving body awareness and imitation of movement. Although she had improved generally in visual attention and judgments it was felt she still needed work in this area. It was recommended that active treatment be discontinued and that needs for continued functional and perceptual-motor training could be met in the nursery school group program conducted by the therapists with the teachers.

THE PRESCHOOL CHILD WITH MENINGOMYELOCELE AND HYDROCEPHALUS. The child with meningomyelocele who is a potential crutch-walker will require an active treatment plan as he prepares for ambulation in parallel bars and with crutches. Parallel bars at home should be constructed when possible. A child who is too young to follow instructions for crutch balancing exercises may learn to shift weight and raise a controlled crutch as he hits a large ball or the child-size punch-a-clown. Needs for trunk and upper extremity strengthening may be met in mat activities appropriate for the child's age. Play equipment may meet his physical and social needs; for example, there are various vehicles which a child can propel with his arms.

The therapist may guide the family in choice of chairs for home, nursery school, or transportation. Modified chairs or special head supports may be devised for the child with an enlarged head. Continued caution regarding skin care is needed as the child moves in his environment. The child's needs for group experience, nursery school training, and attention to development as a whole are just as important as in the child with developmental delay or cerebral palsy.

THE PRESCHOOL CHILD WITH CEREBRAL PALSY. With early treatment of the very young child with cerebral palsy, the motor handicap may be hidden or minimal by the time the child reaches two to three years of age. Such children should have periodic retesting by the clinic during the preschool years for potential learning problems. The physical therapist may assess perceptual-motor development, watch any minimal structural problems, and offer the parents developmental guidance.

Other children with moderate handicaps may be on active treatment plans emphasizing prerequisite developmental needs or the achievement of ambulation. Instruction of the parents in carry-over of therapy goals to the home may involve planning special equipment such as modified chairs and tables, standing tables, parallel bars, or wheelchairs. The therapist should attempt to utilize and modify normal children's furniture if at all possible, and not forget to suggest suitable play equipment. A chair seat for a wagon or sled, or swing set or tricycle modifications may assist in providing more normal play experiences. When the child has orthopedic surgery and wears casts for a period, the therapist should assist the parents in devising ways to position and manage the child.

The severely mentally and physically handicapped child with cerebral palsy should have a trial period of active treatment if at all possible, to explore potential for any improvement, satisfy concerns that all has been done, and prepare families for long-term care. They should then be followed periodically for remedial management for the purpose of maintaining mobility, encouraging functioning at their level, and assisting the family with daily care problems. Guiding the parents in choice or construction of equipment that may assist in sitting, transporting, bathing, and feeding can be of help as the child grows. Structuring simple passive movements and a variety of positions throughout the day may combat deformity. Sensory stimulation with appropriate auditory, tactile, and visual stimulation at the child's level should be demonstrated. Assistance with feeding problems may be most important of all. A coordinated plan with the occupational therapist and public health nurse is suggested, with home calls at intervals for instruction and support of the parents. Where a day care program is available, instruction of the staff in remedial management and appropriate stimulation should be done.

THE PHYSICAL THERAPIST'S ROLE IN THE NURSERY SCHOOL PROGRAM. The nursery school program in a developmental center is the ideal setting for observation and evaluation of the child by the physical therapist, and for carry-over and translation of therapy goals. The therapist should demonstrate techniques of handling to assist or control movement and posture for children on therapy programs.

Teachers should be instructed to avoid keeping the physically handicapped nonambulatory child in a chair the entire time so as to avoid immobility and flexor deformities. He may be positioned in prone over a support or in side-lying to play, be allowed to move on the floor if he is able, and to stand in a standing table if indicated. Sitting postures to be avoided or encouraged should be demonstrated. The teacher should be informed what to expect and what to allow the child to do, what to assist the child to do, and what not to press the child to do. The therapist should assist with modification of play equipment and suggest suitable furniture.

In a small program, the therapists may be closely knit into the nursery school program, and may work with an individual child in the school setting. In a larger program it may be more practical to assign a therapist to the nursery school at specific times for the purpose of assisting the nursery school staff with the management of the physically handicapped children. A physical therapy carry-over sheet for each child (Chart 9-I) may be helpful to the teachers who must in turn supervise aides and volunteers. In our experience, a carry-over program in the nursery school has been of great value. A child resistant to changing habits may cooperate in a group setting when the teacher, finding her sitting back between her heels, says "No, Betty, that is not a good way to sit. We are sitting with our legs in front."

The physical therapist may work with the nursery school teacher, the occupational and speech therapists in assessing the general functional level of the nursery group in motor and per-

CHART 9-I

MEYER CHILDREN'S REHABILITATION INSTITUTE
PHYSICAL THERAPY CARRY-OVER SHEET
POSTURE AND LOCOMOTION IN THE NURSERY SCHOOL

Purpose: Encourage Functional Skills and Maintain mobility.
Instructions: Circle activities child should be encouraged or expected to do, or those not desired.

Locomotion

Travel: Carry child____ Rolling____ Tummy crawling____ Creeping all fours____ Cruise furniture____

Comments:

Walk with Assistance: Do not walk____ Two hands____ One hand____ Hands on shoulders____ Push chair____

Comments:

Standing Table Yes____ No____ Comments:

Sitting

Chair Needs: *Armless Chair* ____ Armchair ____ C.P. Chair ____ *Wheelchair* ____
Trunktie ____ Footstool ____ Abd. Block ____ Trunktie ____
Abd. Block ____ Trunktie ____
Trunktie ____

Getting to Chair, Child Should: Pull up and sit alone____; Pull to stand but have help to turn and sit____; Pull to kneel before lifting____; Be lifted____.

Encouragement of Sitting Development on Bench: (Story time, etc.)
A. Assistance or close supervision____. B. Needs hands balance____.
C. Reach for toy____.

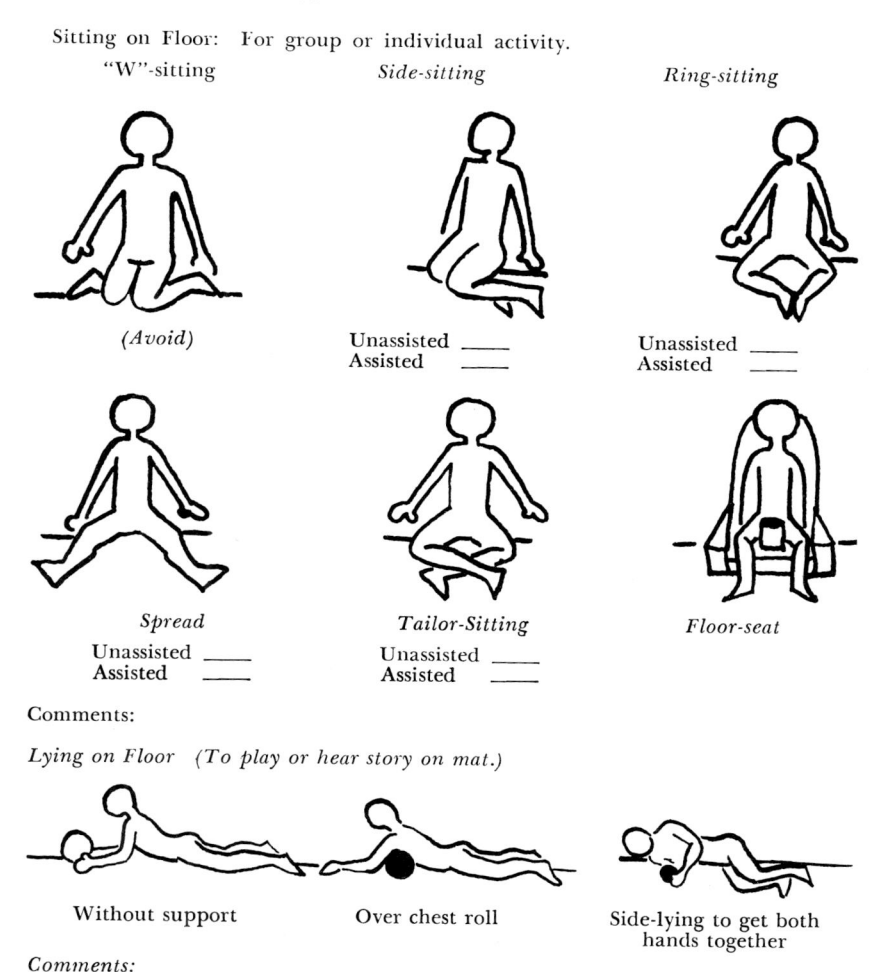

Physical Therapy in a Children's Rehabilitation Center 391

Sitting on Floor: For group or individual activity.

"W"-sitting — (Avoid)

Side-sitting — Unassisted ____ Assisted ____

Ring-sitting — Unassisted ____ Assisted ____

Spread — Unassisted ____ Assisted ____

Tailor-Sitting — Unassisted ____ Assisted ____

Floor-seat

Comments:

Lying on Floor (To play or hear story on mat.)

Without support

Over chest roll

Side-lying to get both hands together

Comments:

---

ceptual-motor skills. In some settings a complete team assessment will be available for each child; in others, not all children will be assessed by all departments. A simplified motor scale in age graph form may assist the school staff to assess their groups as a basis for understanding and planning needed perceptual-motor activities (Chart 9-II). Group functional motor and perceptual-motor activities may be demonstrated by the therapist with empha-

CHART 9-II

MEYER CHILDREN'S REHABILITATION INSTITUTE
GROSS MOTOR SKILLS

Name: B.D.

Skill			15 mos	18 mos
Sitting	Sits supported in chair or needs special chair.	Sits indep. on floor, legs in front.	Faces/climbs on chair. Safe armless chair.	Seats self directly on small chair (backs).
Getting to stand	Gets to sit, to all fours, or pulls to kneel.	Pulls to stand by furniture.	Gets up from midfloor—turns to hands and feet.	
Standing balance	Balances erect on knees—no hands.	Stands alone briefly.		
Agility skills and walking		Walks with hands held.	Walks independent.	Runs stiffly.
Stairs			Creeps up.	Walks up hand held. Creeps down.
Play equipment				Pull and push toys.

NOT CORRELATED WITH

Body-image and motor planning	Knows parts of face, hands, feet.	Identifies body parts generally. 3 yrs	Knows body surfaces front, back, sides.	Imitates simple movement.

Instruction: Record in red ink date child observed to perform function described.
Record progressions when they occur.

Comments:

sis on interpreting the level of the children and prerequisites needed for advancement. We have found written lesson plans helpful to the school staff. These are reinforced and translated by the teachers into many situations, and also posted for the information of the parents.

21 mos	2 yrs	3 yrs	4 yrs	5 yrs
		Gets up with partial turn to one side.		Gets up directly. No rotation.
Squats to play.	Picks up toy from floor.	Stands one leg momentarily.	Stands one leg 4-8 sec	Stands one leg indefinitely.
	Jumps down—one foot leading.	Jumps down feet together.	Hops a few feet. Gallops.	Skips alternately.
Up with rail. Down hand held.	Up and down alone holds rail. Both feet to step.	Walks up and down—no hands. Alt. feet up.	Alternates feet both up and down.	
Rides astride toys.	Climbs ladder and goes down slide.	Pedals and steers trike well.	Catches tossed ball, elbows bent.	
AGE GRAPH ABOVE				
Relates body surfaces to objects.	Relates body surfaces to directional movement.	Imitates motor sequences.	Can do motor sequences on verbal command.	

The School Age Child

The younger physically handicapped child of school age may still be continuing to progress and benefit by active treatment; others may require periods of active treatment following surgical procedures. Eventually, however, progress may level off, and the emphasis of therapy shifts toward continuing physical care, maintenance of mobility and function, recreation, and physical education (Ellis 1967).

THE SCHOOL AGE CHILD WITH MENINGOMYELOCELE. Some children with meningomyelocele will be achieving independent ambulation with crutches and braces and require intensive gait training. At this age, group mat work may provide stimulation and motivation. Children may assist each other with the use of weights and pulleys or in leading the group in the mat routine. Wheelchair management and activities of daily living should be stressed for the nonambulatory children. Continuing parent instruction should emphasize prevention of deformity, care of the skin, and how to teach self-care of bowel and bladder functions to the child when possible.

THE SCHOOL AGE CHILD WITH CEREBRAL PALSY. The younger nonambulatory children with cerebral palsy may still benefit by work stressing head control or sitting, moving between postures, assisted ambulation, or use of their upper extremities in self-care or school-related activities. Some will be achieving independent ambulation. Parents must be trained to understand and assume the responsibility for long-term needs for maintaining mobility and preventing deformity. Semans (1966) has emphasized the importance also of teaching the child with cerebral palsy self-control and responsibility in maintaining mobility, alignment and appearance. The need for continuing supervision and physical activity as the child approaches adolescence is stressed to counteract the common development of obesity and deterioration at that time (Ellis 1967).

THE SCHOOL AGE CHILD WITH MUSCULAR DYSTROPHY. Although onset may occur during the preschool years, typically the child with muscular dystrophy is referred for physical therapy at school age. Any active treatment plan should emphasize from the beginning the instruction of the parents in a daily routine of deformity prevention (Gucker 1964). Early emphasis on positioning to avoid the influence of hip and knee flexion in sleeping as well as in sitting may involve the use of splinting if necessary. Range of motion exercises should be instituted early to prevent contractures in the typical lumbodorsal fascia, hip flexors, hamstrings and plantar flexors. If contractures are beginning, stretching may be important in preventing the loss of ambulation (Gucker 1964).

Also needed are active and assistive exercises emphasizing trunk, shoulder-girdle, hip extensors and abductors, knee extensors, and ankle dorsiflexors. Pool therapy, if available, may provide active exercise for even the very weakened child. When ambulation is threatened by increasing deformity, orthopedic procedures will involve early mobilization and ambulation. In the nonambulatory phase, the wheelchair patient may benefit by assistive upper extremity devices such as overhead suspension or ball-bearing feeders. Management at home may be assisted by use of lifts or other special equipment.

THE SCHOOL. A child requiring special physical facilities or continued physical therapy may attend a special school where this is provided. Although the educational program has the highest priority in the school setting, the special school for the physically handicapped should be organized to meet their physical needs, requiring something more than wheelchairs and ramps. A carefully controlled regimen of positioning throughout the school day and opportunity for mobility should be planned, especially if the child is nonambulatory and relegated to a wheelchair. Use of appropriate wheelchairs, special cerebral palsy chairs, and desk or tray modifications should be supervised by the therapist for control of posture and to enable the child to benefit from the learning experiences of the classroom.

It is important, however, that nonambulatory or assisted-ambulatory children with cerebral palsy, muscular dystrophy, or meningomyelocele not sit all day in school. Classroom work may be done with the child positioned in prone-lying over bolsters on floor mats, on orthopedic carts, or standing in a standing table. The opportunity to move about on the floor at certain periods is desirable for mobility. The therapist should inform the teacher and others handling the child what to expect the child to do, which postures to avoid, and how opportunities for mobility can be provided without disruption of the classroom's primary purpose. This can be accomplished with cooperative planning between therapists, teachers, and administrators, and realistic consideration of means to carry out such a program, such as volunteers or aides to assist in the physical management of the children.

The need for physical activity and recreation may also be met in modified sports activities and wheelchair games devised in physical therapy or physical education. The therapist should assist and encourage community sponsored opportunities for recreation and camping as well.

Many ambulatory children will enter a normal school setting where there is no physical therapy supervision. Any necessary information about a child's special needs or limitations should be made known to the school by the therapist and referring physician. Regular scheduled therapy may no longer be indicated for most of these children, but checkups at regular intervals should be planned for parent and child instruction in any necessary maintenance activities.

The need for physical fitness or perceptual-motor training in special education programs for the mentally retarded will be met by remedial physical education programs in many schools. Therapists may serve in a consultant role to schools organizing or promoting such programs in cooperation with other health professions and educators (Nunley 1965). Where the need exists, perceptual-motor training programs may be conducted in the children's rehabilitation center.

Programming for the Child with Perceptual-Motor Disability

All disciplines involved with testing or training a child with developmental problems need to be concerned with the development of perceptual-motor skills and to be aware of the various sensory and perceptual problems that may occur. Perceptual training is not a separate aspect of the child's management to be dealt with at a specific time by a specific discipline but should be made a part of occupational therapy, speech therapy, physical therapy, and education.

Early Perceptual-Motor Training

The physical therapist, in dealing with specific neuromuscular deficits, must understand other problems which may exist, including apraxia, integrative sensory deficits such as astereognosis, and inability to understand verbal instructions. The therapist must base choice of techniques on an understanding of the whole child, and not see him solely as a neuromuscular problem. In achieving a particular level of accomplishment such as moving about on the floor by rolling, crawling, or creeping, a child must also learn to solve spatial problems of near, far, around, under, and through and be provided with appropriate visual and sensory stimuli within his range. Toys may be suspended over the floor or attached to furniture in order to elicit spontaneous efforts to erect on arms, to reach, and to pursue.

Motor training should involve toys, play, and games which can provide meaning, purpose, perceptual experiences, and satisfaction in achievement for the child (Ayres 1960, 1966; Morgenstern 1968). Ayres stresses that goal-directed movement with its associated feedback is necessary for development of the ability to motor plan or apraxia. Children who may not be able to see the purpose of the therapist's objectives of improved motor function may have this need met in constructive and creative play.

The preschool years are important in the development of a variety of fine discrimination and perceptual-motor skills. At this age games and play should be planned for the home or nursery school providing sensory input, enhancing the development of body-image, teaching conscious motor planning and awareness of the body in space, direction, and time. These are especially needed for the child with a visual deficit (Turner and Siegel 1969). Experience involving visual judgments, pursuit, and attention are also needed (Kephart 1960, Radler and Kephart 1960, Frostig 1964, 1968, Knickerbocker 1966, Ayres 1958, 1960, Cratty 1967).

The importance of structuring movement activities to help the child gain in impulse control and extending attention is stressed by Cratty (1967). Motor activities in a group setting, if not carefully structured, can result in the opposite effect—exciting the child who tends to hyperactivity.

Programs for the School Age Child with Perceptual-Motor Disabilities

In addition to incorporating sensory and perceptual training in the treatment program for cerebral palsy, in the developmental guidance program for the mentally retarded child with motor delay and in the preschool programs, the physical therapist may participate in perceptual-motor training for school age children with specific perceptual handicaps and related learning disabilities. Although the problems of this group of children are increasingly receiving the attention of educators with remedial programs incorporated in the school setting, a need may exist in many areas for supplementary programs in a children's center.

Perceptual-motor-training classes may be conducted one day a week after school with grouping based on ages and characteristics of dysfunction. Such classes are ideally a joint project of physical therapy and occupational therapy with the close cooperation of the psychologist. Small groups of four to six can be managed by two or three professionals. When several children require individual control or assistance, additional help from aids may be needed. General plans should be based on thorough testing by each department. The concepts of Kephart, Frostig, Cratty, and Ayres may be consulted for remedial activities to fit the needs of the individual and group.

The first half hour may be devoted to gross perceptual-motor activities planned by the physical therapist, the second half hour to finer skills planned by the occupational therapist. With the therapists working together for both periods, a clearer understanding of the child's problems is possible. It is suggested that a notebook be kept for each class, and specific lesson plans be prepared for each week with observations on performance recorded. In conjunction with class lesson plans, home carry-over instruction sheets should be prepared and discussed with the parents. The child's teacher should be informed of the program, invited to visit, and supplied with appropriate worksheets by the occupational therapist.

Some children living a distance from the children's center may be placed on a home program with material also provided to their school. A report by the psychologist and therapists summarizing the child's evaluation should be sent to the teacher with specific suggestions for remedial training. In a school situation, teachers may be helped in preparing lesson plans for group perceptual-motor programs with a progression of activities by references to several sources (Vallet 1967, Hacket 1967, Cratty 1967, Frostig 1969). A home program workbook for parents may be devised with progressions of suggested activities and sample lesson plans.

It is important to emphasize to parents, teachers, and therapists the need to vary and challenge the child's ability in skills, working for improved generalization and not mere splinter skills. It is also important to stress the need to *teach* perceptual-motor integration and transfer of learning to these children—not just to provide sensory stimulation and gross motor activities and expect transfer to occur (Cratty 1967).

Case History: Bobby
Perceptual-Motor Training Program for Child
with Minimal Cerebral Dysfunction

Chief Complaint: Bobby was referred to the Meyer Children's Rehabilitation Institute at six years eleven months by his family pediatrician because of difficulties in first grade. His teacher reported major difficulties in reading, with possible visual perceptual and auditory memory deficits and poor coordination. She complained of poor concentration and described him as hyperactive. He wandered around the classroom aimlessly, disturbed the class, and was a loner on the playground. She reported he was becoming isolated, and appeared defiant and disobedient.

Social Service Interview: Bobby was the third of four children of educated professional parents. There appeared to be some difficulties in parent-child relationships, inconsistency combining over-criticalness with indulgence. Though the father spent little time with his family he expressed a responsible attitude with eagerness to cooperate, but some denial of Bobby's problems was shown by his mother.

History and Physical Examination: Bobby apparently had a normal prenatal, delivery, and neonatal course and development was apparently normal until the present complaints. He had suffered a fall at three years and was hospitalized and treated for concussion but no sequelae had been noted at the time. The neurological examination was within normal limits except for indications of difficulties with fine motor coordination, integrative sensory functions, and balance on one leg. The EEG was normal.

Psychological Testing: This included the Stanford-Binet, Form L-M; Bender Visual-Motor Gestalt Test; Frostig Developmental Test of Visual Perception; and the Vineland. Bobby scored within the average range of intelligence with an IQ of 95; however, there was considerable discrepancy between verbal and visual-motor functions. Test evidence supported a diagnosis of minimal cerebral dysfunction affecting visual-motor coordination and figure ground discrimination, as well as being productive of perseverative and rigid behavior. Bobby appeared to have poor self-concept, and expressed resentment towards his environment.

Speech and Hearing: Hearing and speech and language development were within normal limits, but difficulties were noted in auditory memory and in expressing thoughts through gesture.

Although diagnosis was possible on the basis of the above examinations, detailed assessment by the full team was done as a basis for remedial planning specific to his needs.

Occupational Therapy: Tests used were the Ayres Southern California Perceptual-Motor Test, the Southern California Kinesthesia and Tactile Perception Tests, the Ayres Space Test, and the Southern California Figure-Ground Visual Perception Test. Results showed difficulties with gross and fine motor planning and bilateral coordination tasks or activities which required crossing the midline with one extremity. He was right-handed and sighted with his right eye. Right-left discrimination was not established. Sensory deficits were noted in kinesthesia, stereognosis, and tactile localization. In addition to visual figure-ground difficulties, he had poor control of tracking across the midline. Grasp of a pencil was very tense, and he wrote very small, tending to break off pencil points.

Physical Therapy: Tests used were the Cratty Perceptual-Motor Test, the Purdue Perceptual-Motor Scale, evaluation of trunk strength, muscle tone, postural and structural deviations. Findings supported the observations of the occupational therapist. In addition, although Bobby gave the impression of good gross motor agility because he moved so much, it was found that both static and dynamic balance and agility skills such as hopping and skipping were all below age level. He had poor trunk strength, and ball skills were very poor.

Difficulty with motor planning involving sequencing was noted on either visual or auditory clues, but particularly the latter. He had trouble inhibiting unwanted movement and often exhibited tension in attempt at control. No abnormality of muscle tone on passive manipulation or structural deviations were noted. Impulsiveness was marked with poor ability to sustain attention or to try his best to finish a task. Sensitivity to failure was noted, and avoidance of tasks with silliness.

Diagnosis: A diagnosis of minimal cerebral dysfunction with average intelligence, and adjustment reactions associated with learning deficits was made.

Recommendations: A broad approach to remediation was stressed.
1. School program adapted to his handicap. As no special classroom for perceptually handicapped children was available, a regular classroom in an ungraded setting with remedial reading program was recommended.
2. Perceptual-motor training class once weekly at the Meyer Children's Rehabilitation Institute conducted by the occupational and physical therapists.
3. Further psychological evaluation regarding Bobby's personality dynamics and family counseling.

A trial basis of a stimulant drug was instituted by his family pediatrician. Significant improvement in behavior was noted, but impulsiveness and short attention span remained problems. Over the summer he began work with the remedial reading specialist, attended the perceptual-motor training class, and was seen by the psychologist. Bobby's father took more time for regular outings with Bobby for swimming and fishing, and included other boys his age.

The perceptual-motor class included four children, both boys and girls. The first half hour was devoted to gross motor activities with the following emphasis for Bobby:
1. Improved trunk strength and physical fitness.
2. Balance and agility skills in combination with visual attention and accuracy.
3. Body perception: awareness of feeling of movement—timing, force, rhythms; increasing control of inhibition of unwanted movement; and right-left discrimination.
4. Motor planning involving coordination of the two sides, crossing the midline, sequencing, "thinking and movement" and "creative movement," and strengthening responses to auditory clues in particular.
5. Ball skills—catching, throwing, bouncing; game sequences.

6. Increasing impulse control and extending attention were programmed into many tasks, as were success and fun.

The second half hour was devoted to fine motor activities emphasizing the following:
1. Visual-perceptual skills (figure-ground, form perception, position in space, etc.).
2. Eye-hand coordination, visual tracking, and prewriting work. The Frostig worksheets were included in these activities.
3. Sensory discrimination.

Reevaluation was planned at six month intervals. Attendance was regular, and home lesson plans were carried out. These also served the purpose of helping his parents understand the nature of his problems. When school began in the fall, Bob was placed in an ungraded setting, with special remedial classes and tutoring outside the classroom. No special remedial physical education was available so he continued in the perceptual-motor group. Reports were sent to his school, his teacher visited the class, and suggestions and worksheets were provided. Simple techniques were demonstrated such as covering all but one row of a worksheet, reinforcing verbal instructions with demonstration and manual assistance, and pre-writing work with the recommendations of teaching him longhand.

One Year Follow-up Report: Bobby was now eight years old. His teacher reported he was making progress at school with his remedial reading and in general behavior. The therapists reported improving motor planning, awareness and control of movement, but he still scored below the age level on these and in sensory tests for stereognosis, kinesthesia, and tactile localization. Body rhythms though improved were still difficult, as were motor planning sequences. He had improved scores in balance and agility skills but these were below age level. Right-left discrimination was fairly good in his own frame of reference but not in translation to another person or object in space.

The Frostig test scores had improved: fine eye-hand coordination had improved but was still below age level; figure-ground discrimination, form constancy, position in space and spatial relationships were all at age or above. Ball skills were improved if impulse control was good. It was found that Bob's self-control was best when the task was adequately challenging and demanded more self-control. In games, bouncing a ball in place or against the wall, Bob and the ball were all over the place, out of control. He did better when he had to stay in a prescribed circle on the floor and used target circles on the wall demanding accuracy, or when he had to continue bouncing the ball while going from standing to kneeling and up again with a beanbag balanced on his head. Lesson planning for the therapists was really challenging because success was also very important.

It was recommended at the staff conference to continue the program. Program emphasis continued to stress motor planning and sensory discrimination, gross and fine coordination emphasizing the relationships of the two sides of the body, directionality or transfer of right-left concepts outside his own frame of reference, pre-sports skills, and impulse control. Over the summer Bobby also continued work with his reading, but had plenty of time for fun. He showed marked improvement in sports skills and participated with his father in Little League, where he was reportedly one of the better players on his winning team!

Second Year Report: Bob was now nine years of age. His school reported good progress in reading, with continued remedial work recommended. He was a happy boy, had friends, and his parents felt Bob was a different boy in all circumstances. He still had periods when impulse control was difficult and required some isolation for reduction of distractions in the classroom to assist attention. His pediatrician was exploring reduction of medication. The therapists reported improvement in all areas. Retesting showed motor planning and bilateral integration within normal limits for age. Balance and agility skills, and ball skills were at or above age norms. Right-left discrimination was generally at age, but continued to require reinforcement. Fine coordination and sensory testing of kinesthesia, stereognosis, and tactile localization were all at age. Fine rhythmic coordination skills such as writing had improved, but he still tended to segment when copying geometric designs.

It was felt that Bob's needs could now be met by his school program with areas needing reinforcement suggested to his parents and the school. It was recommended that he participate in structured organized sports activities over the summer. He was dismissed from the perceptual-motor training group, with reevaluation or assistance available at the request of parents or school.

This boy's history and progress emphasize several important principles as listed below:

1. Multidisciplinary team assessment for defining the problems of the child in detail as basis for specific remediation particular to his needs, rather than fitting the child to a prescribed program.

2. Remedial approach on a broad front—medication, manage-

ment of emotional and family problems, appropriate school program with remedial reading, and the perceptual-motor training.

3. Cooperation between parents, school and the children's center.

A Good Home Program

The long-term physical therapy of the physically handicapped child is a joint therapist-parent responsibility, and a good home program should be an important goal in every child's management. The role of the therapist as a teacher with the family and child in an outpatient facility is stressed rather than administration of treatment in the traditional sense (Ellis 1963, 1967, Semans 1966). The adequacy of the home program will be much more influential in the child's progress or lack of it than treatment by the therapist. The needs of the specific family and child should determine the relative amounts of treatment and instruction and the interval for regular therapist support.

The physical therapist and other disciplines concerned with the care of the child should plan any home instruction program with realistic consideration of what is possible in the particular home, and with recognition for the importance of other things in the life of the child and family. Parents subjected to intensive treatment regimens that interfere with daily life and do not allow the child to be a child, may become exhausted and disappointed with their child's failure to show corresponding improvement. This may result in further shopping around or feelings of inadequacy, guilt, and rejection. At the opposite extreme are the many parents who have been to clinics and specialists without getting specific help in the care of their child. Most parents want and need to be able to help their child themselves. We have had the experience that with adequate instructions and support, many parents can carry out home programs beautifully. At the same time, there are those parents who cannot and should not be involved in direct treatment of their own child.

Home instructions should be interpreted to the parents through specific short-term goals, and the means to achieve them demonstrated with specific techniques or activities. Treatment should be translated into daily life in terms of what the child does all day, and the equipment and toys the child may use at home. Use or modification of normal infant or children's furniture is recommended whenever possible.

Finnie describes practical management of the child with cerebral palsy in carrying out bathing, toilet training, dressing, feeding, and at play (Finnie 1968). A parent well trained in translating the child's treatment into activities of daily life does not need to provide a specific amount of treatment time or number of repetitions, but will see to it that the child is treated even on those days when "not a thing gets done!" The ways the mother positioned the child for play, the way she dressed him, held him on her lap, and picked him up and carried him all may involve indirect treatment. The therapist should be sensitive to those families that need more routinized structured programs, however, and be careful not to overburden them. Some instruction of any members of the family or even sitters who may take care of the child for significant amounts of time should be done if possible.

Written instructions prepared for an individual child and family will be well worth the preparation time in terms of establishing a good home program. They are absolutely essential with those who cannot be seen frequently. It may be necessary to revise techniques or correct a parent's interpretation of instructions. The written program or summary of goals gives the parents a good starting point and reinforces them when confronted with well-meant advice by relatives and friends.

The provision of resident accommodations for parents and children, including siblings if necessary, is recommended for a center serving a large area (Ellis 1963). Even when the family lives a long distance from the center, this will make it possible to carry out adequate evaluation, parent instruction and periodic follow-up visits. Staff may observe the daily care problems and explore methods of helping the family with the management of a severely handicapped child. Several days attendance in a diagnostic nursery school group where staff may observe the child may assist in evaluation.

In addition to specific instructions prepared by the therapist, the physical therapist or center staff as a whole should explore parent-oriented materials distributed by various associations dealing with specific aspects of dysfunction such as The Easter Seal Parent Series, United Cerebral Palsy, the National Association for Retarded Children, the National Association for Brain-Injured Children and the Association for Children with Learning Disabilities (see Bibliography for addresses). Parent group discussions and educational programs with presentations by various team members and guest speakers may contribute to general understanding of their child's problems.

Coordination Between Services

Achieving the goal of whole child management means carrying the team concept further than usual to avoid fragmentation of the child's program. Coordination and cooperation between services is relatively simple and easy to organize if roles are clearly defined. More challenging is whole child management with adequate communication and planned overlap of treatment techniques. Egland (1966), in encouraging interdisciplinary cooperation, suggests that new interdepartmental cooperation courses may have to be designed in clinical and educational centers to reach interdisciplinary understanding and assistance.

Coordination with Occupational Therapy

Close coordination and agreement in treatment principles are particularly important between physical and occupational therapists. In our experience, several arrangements for cooperation have proved rewarding to the therapists and the children. Combined evaluation and treatment or instruction are helpful in bringing about immediate understanding and communication on the problems of the child, establishing goals, and determining each therapist's part in parent instruction. These have been especially useful in children with perceptual-motor disorders, the severely multiply handicapped child, the family from a long distance on a home program, and with infants.

Readiness of either discipline to understand something of the other's scope and to bridge the gap till follow-up is arranged is valuable in a large program where patients are not routinely seen by all members of the team. For example the occupational therapist evaluating a child finds he is a spastic hemiplegic in need of general motor management by the physical therapist. The occupational therapist may instruct the mother in some work in protective extension until physical therapy can be arranged. As another example, suppose the physical therapist, who screens in daily living skills in evaluating a mentally retarded child, finds the child ready for feeding himself with certain modified utensils and instructs the parent on how to go about teaching this until an appointment can be made in occupational therapy. In a program with less pressure on staff time, immediate consultation should be arranged; but, if a delay is likely, the child should be helped. This kind of overlap is especially needed where there is a physical therapist and no occupational therapist.

Coordination with Speech Therapy

Physical therapy and speech therapy have obvious overlap with each other and with occupational therapy in evaluation of feeding functions and motor control of the speech mechanisms in the child with cerebral palsy (Ch. 6). It is recommended that the speech therapist plan some joint work periods with both physical and occupational therapy for a unified motor approach and to learn how to take advantage of situations when tone is more normal and better speech functions possible (Crickmay 1966). Physical and occupational therapy are also ideal situations for carry-over of the speech therapist's goals.

Coordination with the Psychologist

The psychologist in a children's rehabilitation center may contribute to management of the whole child through evaluation and counseling and in working with the therapists in perceptual-motor training, developmental stimulation of infants, behavior management and the use of reinforcement.

The physical therapist's use of reward or reinforcement through a sense of accomplishment and social approval are not new. The use of a more specific reward system in operant conditioning has been explored in behavior management and training of daily living skills with severely retarded children (Breland 1965). Its use in motor training is beginning to be explored by physical therapists (Trotter and Inman 1968, Rice et al. 1968, Foss 1966).

Coordination with Nursing Services

The physical therapist will find coordination with the public health nurse valuable in supporting the therapy program (Holtgrew 1964, Wolff 1964, Curfman and Arnold 1967, Haynes 1967, Barnard 1968). The nurse may be invited to attend parent instruction sessions to have treatment goals interpreted, to observe the specific treatment techniques, and to be informed of equipment or toys recommended. The nurse may support the family in their efforts, assist in obtaining or devising equipment or toys, share the responsibility, and communicate essential information to the management team. In this role the nurse is not actually carrying out physical therapy treatment, but is important to a successful treatment program.

Some cases may require delegation of specific physical therapy treatment on a regular basis to the nurse, when neither parent or therapist treatment is possible (for example, in a home program where the mother is ill or working). Physical therapy program planning, instruction, and follow-up is supervised by the physical therapist. The parents should not be left out but whenever possible should be included in the instruction sessions, with the goal for both therapist and nurse being to encourage the parents' responsibility and participation. Una Haynes (1962, 1965), in describing the nurse's role in home management of cerebral palsy, points out that physical therapy services are not able to meet the demand or need, and that such services have not been as available for the severely handicapped as for the child with a better prognosis. She describes home management programs conducted by the public health nurse with physical or occupational therapy consultation.

It is our belief that physical therapy treatment should be specific and under the supervision of an adequately trained therapist. It is recommended, however, that therapists coordinate and work with the public health nurse in extending services and meeting the needs of the child and family. In our experience these have been satisfying working relationships with mutual respect and rewarding benefit to the children involved.

The Schedule and Service

Several approaches are suggested in solving the problems of pressure for service in order to use staff time to best advantage. Good parent training programs have been described. The training of physical therapy aides for specific delegated treatment of children may be necessary in many programs where the emphasis is on active treatment and children are in daily attendance.

Patient priorities can be established. Blocks of time can be designated for specific patient groups or purposes such as daily patients, group work, parent instruction programs, infant programs, developmental guidance, perceptual-motor training programs, or for out-of-town rechecks. Blocking the time should be coordinated with other services involved. With the establishment of priorities, some children may be assigned to a rotation list for a specific block of time, so that some instruction is provided until their program needs can be met.

Organization of Space and Equipment

The organization of space and equipment for outpatient services in a children's rehabilitation center physical therapy department must be considered in terms of the same criteria determining program needs, such as age span and types of patients served. Suggestions have previously been given for a program emphasizing the role of the therapist as a teacher to the family, the child, related disciplines and students. The setting for a developmental and whole child approach to treatment will bear little resemblance to the traditional physical therapy department but will be equipped and decorated so as to invite children to play and learn.

Space

The convenient availability of the therapy departments to each other for coordination of services and joint therapy is recommended in planning new facilities. A physical therapy department should also be planned for flexibility, allowing rearrangement to meet changing needs. Large rooms without permanent partitions may be divided only by equipment, or may be partitioned for a quiet area or infant area. Easily folded back partitions with adequate soundproofing would be ideal. A flexible organization of space enables the therapists to work separately for parent instruction, together in group work, or to move around with the child during treatment.

We have found the concept of instruction areas practical. These are used primarily to instruct the mother. Other people involved in regular care of the child (personnel from day care or preschool programs, public health nurses, and students) may observe. An observation room with one-way window is useful at times; however, discussing and interpreting to the observer is usually necessary.

Instruction areas are patterned after typical nursery school space organization. A doll play, playing-house area has a children's table and chairs, dishes, doll beds, and vanity. Donations of several talking dolls and clothes have been popular. The therapist may work with standing reactions as a little girl "powders her nose" or a little boy "shaves" at the vanity. Another instruction area includes a collection of building blocks, cars, and tractors at a kneeling table and mat area.

The needs for an infant area include typical infant furniture such as swings, jumpers, rocking seats, as well as crib and high chair. Infant toys that provide visual, auditory and tactile stimuli, and infant feeding equipment are kept in this area. It is desirable to separate this area from the general area because of crying babies at times, and to keep toys and equipment clean. The infant area might well be cooperatively used with the occupational therapist, the speech therapist, and the psychologist.

A large area is equipped with gross motor play equipment for use in treatment and developmental guidance. This area includes an adjustable jungle gym and slide, barrel on rack, box, rocking boat, rocking horse, folding tunnel, scooter boards, tricycles and other vehicles, walking beams and balance boards, balls, beanbags, hoops, and jump ropes. A trampoline, inflated jumping tire, or old mattresses are desirable for a number of perceptual-motor activities. The gross motor play area may be used also by the other therapists and the nursery school and ideally might be located conveniently for use of all.

These areas have toys and equipment out in view inviting the child to play. Bright figures are on the walls, and various geometric shapes, stepping stones, and lines on the floor. An area with reduced stimuli for the distractible or hyperactive child is also needed.

Equipment

We have enjoyed using toys in treatment. A therapist may find many uses for the life-size plastic punch-a-clown in working with the child in standing. Learning to stand up in extension-abduction-external rotation can be fun astride an animal instead of a bolster. Prone work over a bolster can be done with the child's hands in the sandbox. Building a tower with large blocks can involve many "squats up and down." Shoulder-girdle fixation in prone work over the bolster can be obtained with a stick for a xylophone in each hand. Toys or balloons suspended at various heights from the ceiling or old curtain bars invite the child to reach up as the therapist works on prone or creeping balance. Therapists are referred to several sources for suggestions of use of toys in treatment (Rogers and Thomas 1949, Frantzen 1957, Logan 1957).

Adjustable parallel bars, mirrors, stairs, and ramp are necessary and may be separated in a gait training area or placed about the instruction areas or gross motor play area. Fewer treatment tables and more mat areas are appropriate to a children's program since more functional work is done on the floor. Folding mats may be more convenient than those which are hung on the wall.

With the treatment of younger patients, we are finding that simple modifications of normal children's equipment and furniture are often possible. Examples of typical modifications or special equipment should be available for demonstration to parents, such as several types of small chairs with abduction blocks, straps, or attached footstools, sit-astride type chairs, floor seats, and standing tables. Examples of small wheelchairs with various modifications make it possible to try these before expensive equipment is ordered. An adjustable jackknife cerebral palsy chair should be available for exploring of position and angle with some severely involved children. Although we do not recommend walkers for use in training most young cerebral palsied children, some may be needed for older severely involved or retarded children and other types of patients. The usual assortment of crutches, splinting media, bandages, straps and webbing, foam rubber and goniometers are needed in a children's department.

Many departments will not require hydrotherapy rooms, unless the program involves management of the hurt and sick child, or postoperative cases. This area should be separated from the rest of the department with the necessary tiled floors and walls. A therapeutic pool, while valuable for treatment of patients such as children with muscular dystrophy, or those recovering from acute paralytic disease, will find its use for recreational purposes increasingly important. Facilities should be planned for dressing facilities adequate for wheelchair patients, and a ramp or equipment to lift patients in and out of the pool. In a department using electrodiagnostic and therapeutic equipment, it is suggested that this be stored as a safety factor away from the children's area.

Conclusion

The management of children who are physically handicapped, mentally retarded, or who have other developmental disabilities is one of the most challenging and rewarding areas of physical therapy. The therapist is challenged to bring his education, training, imagination, and special knowledge of motor function and dysfunction to a wider scope of problems. His role in assessment and planning of treatment, and as a teacher is emphasized. All disciplines are challenged to learn from each other and to work together for better prevention, evaluation, and remedial management of the child with handicaps.

BIBLIOGRAPHY

Abercrombie, M.L.J., Lindon, R.S., and Tyson, M.C.: Associated movements in normal and physically handicapped children. *Develop Med Child Neurol, 6:*573, 1964.

Amer. Acad. Orth. Surgeons: "Joint Motion," Method of Measuring and Recording. 1965. 29E. Madison St., Chicago, Ill. 60602.

Ames, Mary D.: Mental retardation and the child with C.N.S. deficit. *J Amer Phys Ther Ass, 46:*444, 1966.

Andrè-Thomas, Saint-Anne Dargassies, and Chesni, Y.: *The Neurological Examination of the Infant.* Little Club Clinics in Developmental Medicine, No. 1. The Spastics Society. London, Heinemann, 1960.

Association for Children with Learning Disabilities (ACLD), Director of Services, 3739 S. Delaware Place, Tulsa, Oklahoma 74105.

Ayres, A. Jean: The visual-motor function. *Amer J Occup Ther, 12:*130, 1958.

Ayres, A. Jean: Occupational therapy for motor disorders resulting from impairment of the central nervous system. *Rehab Lit, 21:*302, 1960.

Ayres, A. Jean: Development of the body scheme in children. *Amer J Occup Ther, 15:*99, 1961.

Ayres, A. Jean: Ayres Space Test. Western Psychological Services, Los Angeles, 1962.

Ayres, A. Jean: The development of perceptual-motor abilities: A theoretical basis for treatment of dysfunction. *Amer J Occup Ther, 17:*221, 1963.

Ayres, A. Jean: Perceptual-Motor Dysfunction in Children. Monograph from the Greater Cincinnati District Ohio Occupational Therapy Association, Cincinnati, Ohio, 1964.

Ayres, A. Jean: Tactile functions, their relation to hyperactive and perceptual-motor behavior. *Amer J Occup Ther, 17:*6, 1964.

Ayres, A. Jean: The Southern California Motor Accuracy Test. Western Psychological Services, Los Angeles, 1964.

Ayres, A. Jean: Patterns of perceptual-motor dysfunction in children: A factor analytic study. *Percept Motor Skills, 20:*335, 1965.

Ayres, A. Jean: Interrelation of perception, function, and treatment. *Phys Ther, 46:*741, 1966.

Ayres, A. Jean: The Southern California Kinesthesia and Tactile Perception Tests. Western Psychological Services, Los Angeles, 1966.

Ayres, A. Jean: The Southern California Figure-Ground Visual Perception Test. Western Psychological Services, Los Angeles, 1966.

Ayres, A. Jean: Southern California Perceptual-Motor Test. Western Psychological Services, Los Angeles, 1968.

Barnard, Kathryn: Teaching the retarded child is a family affair. *Amer J Nurs, 68:*305, 1968.

Blumenthal, Edna, and Banham, Katherine, M.: A cerebral palsied infant under treatment. *Phys Ther Rev, 38:*323, 1958.

Bobath, Berta: Observations on adult hemiplegia and suggestions for treatment. *Physiotherapy, 45:*279, 1959; *46:*5, 1960.

Bobath, Berta: The very early treatment of cerebral palsy. *Develop Med Child Neurol, 9:*373, 1967.

Bobath, Berta, and Bobath, Karel: An assessment of the motor handicap of children with cerebral palsy and of their response to treatment. *Occup Ther J, 21:*19, 1958.

Bobath, Karel: The long term results of treatment. In *Child Neurology and Cerebral Palsy*. Little Club Clinics in Developmental Medicine, No. 2. The Spastics Society. London, Heinemann, 1960.

Bobath, Karel: The prevention of mental retardation in patients with cerebral palsy. *Acta Paedopsychiat, 30:*141, 1963.

Bobath, Berta, and Cotton, Estu: A patient with residual hemiplegia. *J Amer Phys Ther Ass, 45:*849, 1965.

Breland, Marion: Foundation of teaching by positive reinforcements (Ch. 7), and Application of method, (Ch. 8). In Bensberg, Gerald J. (Ed.): *Teaching the Mentally Retarded, A Handbook for Ward Personnel*. Atlanta, Southern Regional Education Board, 1965.

Brown, Mary Eleanor: Daily activity inventories of cerebral palsy children in experimental classes. *Phys Ther Rev, 30:*415, 1950.

Brunnstrom, Signe: Motor testing procedures in hemiplegia, based on sequential recovery stages. *Phys Ther, 46:*357, 1966.

Buchwald, Edith: Activities of daily living testing. In *Physical Rehabilitation for Daily Living*. New York, McGraw, 1952.

Cohen, Herbert J., Molnar, Gabriella E., and Taft, Lawrence, T.: The genetic relationship of progressive muscular dystrophy (Duchenne type) and mental retardation. *Develop Med Child Neurol, 10:*754, 1968.

Connolly, Kevin J., and Stratton, Peter: Developmental changes in associated movements. *Develop Med Child Neurol, 10:*44, 1968.

Cratty, Bryant J.: The Perceptual-Motor Attributes of Mentally Retarded Children and Youth. Monograph, Mental Retardation Services Board of Los Angeles County, 1966.

Cratty, Bryant J.: *Developmental Sequences of Perceptual-Motor Tasks*. Freeport, Long Island, New York, Educational Activities, 1967.

Cratty, Bryant J.: *Motor Activity and the Education of Retardates*. Philadelphia, Lea & F., 1969.

Crickmay, Marie C.: *Speech Therapy and the Bobath Approach to Cerebral Palsy*. Springfield, Thomas, 1966.

Curfman, H.G., and Arnold, C.B.: A homebound therapy program for severely retarded children. *Children, 14:*63, 1967.

Dallas Society for Crippled Children: The Dallas Motor Development Test, 1963.

Daniels, Lucille, Williams, Marian, and Worthingham, Catherine: *Muscle*

Testing, Techniques of Manual Examination. Philadelphia, Saunders, 1946.

DeHaven, George E., Mordock, John B., and LoyKovich, J.M.: Evaluation of Coordination Deficits in Children with Minimal Cerebral Dysfunction. *Phys Ther,* 153-161, 1969.

Denhoff, Eric: *Cerebral Palsy—The Preschool years: Diagnosis, Treatment and Planning.* A Monograph in Russ, J.D. (Ed.): American Lectures in Cerebral Palsy. Springfield, Thomas, 1967.

Denhoff, Eric, and Langdon, M.: Cerebral dysfunction, a treatment program for young children. *Clin Pediat, 5:*332, 1966.

Denhoff, Eric, and Robinault, Isabel P.: *Cerebral Palsy and Related Disorders, a Developmental Approach to Dysfunction.* New York, McGraw, 1960.

Denhoff, Eric, Sigueland, Marian L., Komich, M. Patricia, and Hainsworth, Peter K.: Developmental and predictive characteristics of items from the Meeting Street School Screening Test. *Develop Med Child Neurol, 10:* 220, 1968.

Derham, R.J.: The early management of cerebral palsy. *Develop Med Child Neurol, 9:*30, 1967.

Easter Seal Parent Series, National Society for Crippled Children and Adults, 2023 W. Ogden Avenue, Chicago, Illinois 60612.

Egland, George O.: Physical therapy, occupational therapy, and speech therapy. *Phys Ther, 46:*1116, 1966.

Ellis, Errington: The indications for residential treatment of cerebral palsy in the early years of life. *Develop Med Child Neurol, 5:*32, 1963.

Ellis, Errington: How long should treatment be continued? *Develop Med Child Neurol, 9:*47, 1967.

Fields, Ruby D.: Physical abilities of the mentally retarded child. *Phys Ther, 49:*38, 1969.

Finnie, Nancie R.: *Handling the Young Cerebral Palsied Child at Home.* London, Heinemann, 1968.

Fiorentino, Mary R.: *Reflex Testing Methods for Evaluating C.N.S. Development.* Springfield, Thomas, 1963.

Footh, Wilma K., and Kogan, K.L.: Measuring effectiveness of physical therapy in the treatment of cerebral palsy. *J Amer Phys Ther Ass, 43:* 867, 1963.

Foss, B.M.: Operant conditioning in the control of movements. *Develop Med Child Neurol, 8:*339, 1966.

Frankenberg, W.K., and Dodds, J.B.: Denver Developmental Screening Test. *J Pediat, 71:*181, 1967.

Frantzen, June: Toys—The Tools of Children. National Society for Crippled Children and Adults, 1957.

Fredrickson, Dorothy: The Child with hydrocephalus or myelomeningocele.

I. Initial and continuing physical therapy evaluation. *Phys Ther, 46:*606, 1966.

Frostig, M.: *Move, Grow, Learn Program.* Chicago, Follett, 1969.

Frostig, M., and Horne, D.: *Teacher's Guide—The Frostig Program for the Development of Visual Perception.* Chicago, Follett, 1964.

Frostig, M., Lefever, W., and Whittlesey: *The Marianne Frostig Developmental Test of Visual Perception.* Consulting Psychologists Press, 3rd ed., Palo Alto, California, 1961.

Gesell Developmental Schedules. The Psychological Corporation, New York.

Gesell, Arnold: *The First Five Years of Life.* New York, Harper Bros., 1940.

Gesell, Arnold, and Amatruda, C.S.: *Developmental Diagnosis.* New York, Paul B. Hoeber, 1954.

Gucker, Thomas: The orthopedic management of progressive muscular dystrophy. *Phys Ther, 44:*243, 1964.

Hackett, Layne, and Jenson, Robert G.: *A Guide to Movement Exploration.* Palo Alto, California, Peek, 1967.

Hainsworth, Peter K., and Sigueland, M.L.: *Early Identification of Children with Learning Disabilities: The Meeting Street School Screening Test, Meeting Street School, Providence, Rhode Island.* Published by Crippled Children and Adults of Rhode Island, Inc., 1969.

Haynes, Una: Role of the nurse in programs for patients with cerebral palsy and related disorders. *Amer Nurses Assoc,* 1962. Reprinted by United Cerebral Palsy Association, Inc., New York.

Haynes, Una: Nursing Needs of Infants with Cerebral Palsy or related Neurological Disorders. Paper presented at Annual Meeting of American Academy of Cerebral Palsy, December, 1965. Reprinted by United Cerebral Palsy Association, Inc., New York.

Haynes, Una: A Developmental Approach to Casefinding, with Special Reference to Cerebral Palsy, Mental Retardation, and Related Disorders. Washington, D.C., U.S. Department of Health, Education, and Welfare, Children's Bureau Publication #449, 1967.

Holtgrew, Marion M.: A Guide for Public Health Nurses Working with Mentally Retarded Children. Washington, D.C., U.S. Department of Health, Education, and Welfare, Children's Bureau Publication, 1964.

Hueter, Anne, and Blossom, Bonnie: A prone-stander. *Phys Ther, 47:* 386, 1967.

Johnson, M.K., Zuck, F.N., and Wingate, K.: Measurement of motor handicap in children with neuromuscular disorders such as cerebral palsy. *J Bone Joint Surg, 33A:*698, 1951.

Jones, Margaret: Practical Aspects of the Diagnosis, Prognosis and Management of the Cerebral-Palsied Child. Instructional Course, American Academy of Cerebral Palsy, Las Vegas, Nevada, December 3, 1969.

Kendall, H.O., and Kendall, F.M.P.: *Muscles, Testing and Function.* Baltimore, Williams & Wilkins, 1949.

Kephart, Newell C.: *The Slow-Learner in the Classroom.* Columbus, C.E. Merrill, 1960.

Kephart, Newell C., and Roach, Eugene G.: *Purdue Perceptual-Motor Survey.* Columbus, C.E. Merrill, 1966.

Kinsman, Deborah: The child with hydrocephalus or myelomeningocele. Part II. Comprehensive physical therapy program. *Phys Ther, 46:*611, 1966.

Knickerbocker, Barbara: Programming Units Related to the Five Syndromes of Perceptual-Motor Dysfunction. Proceedings of Occupational Therapy Seminar on Perceptual Motor Dysfunction, Evaluation and Training. Madison, Wisconsin, June, 1966.

Knobloch, Hilda, Pasamanick, B., and Sherard, E.S.: A developmental screening inventory for infants. *Pediatrics, 38:*Part 2, Dec., 1966. Available from Division of Child Development, Department of Pediatrics, Childrens' Hospital, Columbus, Ohio.

Kong, Elisabeth: Very early treatment of cerebral palsy. *Develop Med Child Neurol, 8:*198, 1966.

The Little Club Memorandum on Terminology and Classification of Cerebral Palsy, *Cereb Palsy Bull, 1:*27, 1959.

Logan, J.A.: There is more to toys than meets the eye, as seen by the physical therapist. Reprinted from *Crippled Child,* October, 1957, and distributed by National Society for Crippled Children and Adults, Chicago, Illinois.

Milani-Comparetti, A., and Gidoni, E.A.: Routine developmental examination in normal and retarded children. *Develop Med Child Neurol, 9:*631, 1967a.

Milani-Comparetti, A., and Gidoni, E.A.: Pattern analysis of motor development and its disorders. *Develop Med Child Neurol, 9:*625, 1967b.

Miller, A.S., Stewart, M.D., Murphy, M.A., and Jantzen, A.C.: An evaluation method for cerebral-palsied *Amer J Occup Ther, 9:* May-June, 1955.

Minear, W.L.: A classification of cerebral palsy. *Pediatrics, 18:*841, 1956.

Morgenstern, F.S.: Psychological handicaps in the play of handicapped children. *Develop Med Child Neurol, 10:*115, 1968.

National Association for Retarded Children, Inc., 386 Park Avenue, South, New York, New York.

New York Association for Brain Injured Children, 305 Broadway, New York, New York.

Nunley, Rachel L.: The physical therapist at home with the mentally retarded. *Phys Ther, 47:*926, 1967.

Paine, R.S., and Oppe, T.E.: *Neurological Examination of Children.* Little Club Clinics in Developmental Medicine, No. 20/21. The Spastics Society. London, Heinemann, 1966.

Radler, D.H., and Kephart, Newell: *Success Through Play.* New York, Harper, 1960.

Rice, Harold K., McDaniel, Martha W., and Denney, Sarah L.: Operant conditioning techniques for use in the physical rehabilitation of the multiply handicapped retarded patient. *Phys Ther, 48:*342, 1968.

Rogers, Gladys G., and Thomas, Leah: Toys, games, and apparatus for children with cerebral palsy. *Phys Ther Rev, 29:*1, 1949.

Semans, Sarah: Book review of *Reflex Testing Methods for Evaluating C.N.S. Development* by Mary R. Fiorentino, Springfield, Thomas, *Phys Ther, 44:*404, 1964.

Semans, Sarah: Specific tests and evaluation tools for the child with C.N.S. deficit. *J Amer Phys Ther Ass, 45:*456, 1965.

Semans, Sarah: Principles of treatment in cerebral palsy. *Phys Ther, 46:*715, 1966.

Semans, Sarah, Phillips, Rosalyn, Romanoli, Madeline, Miller, Ruth, and Skillen, Mary: Cerebral palsy assessment chart of basic motor control. *J Amer Phys Ther Ass, 45:*463, 1965.

Shapiro, Alexander: Provisions of special facilities for ineducable spastics. *Cereb Palsy Bull, 3:*573, 1961.

Shurtleff, David B.: Timing of learning in the meningomyelocele patient. *Phys Ther, 46:*137, 1966.

Sloan, William: The Lincoln-Oseretsky Motor Development Scale. *Genet Psychol Monog, 51:183, 1955.* Available from C. H. Stoelting Company, Chicago.

Stark, Gordon, D., and Baker, Geoffrey C.W.: The neurological involvement of the lower limbs in myelomeningocele. *Develop Med Child Neurol, 9:*732, 1967.

Stockmeyer, Shirley: A pattern for evaluation in the assessment of motor performance. *J Amer Phys Ther Ass, 45:*453, 1965.

Stott, D.H.: A general test of motor impairment for children. *Develop Med Child Neurol, 8:*523, 1966.

Trotter, Ann B., and Inman, Douglas A.: The use of positive reinforcement in physical therapy. *Phys Ther, 48:*347, 1968.

Turner, M., and Siegel, I.M.: Physical therapy for the blind child. *Phys Ther, 49:*1357, 1969.

United Cerebral Palsy Associations, Inc., 321 W. 44th St., New York, New York 10036.

Valett, Robert E.: A psychoeducational inventory of basic learning abilities. In: *The Remediation of Learning Disabilities, A Handbook of Psychoeducational Resource Programs.* Palo Alto, California, Fearon, 1967.

Walshe, F.M.R.: On certain tonic or postural reflexes in hemiplegia with special reference to so-called associated movements. *Brain, 46:*1, 1923.

Willson, M. Ann: Use of a developmental inventory as a chart of progress. *Phys Ther, 49:*19, 1969.

Wolff, Ilse S.: Nursing Role in Counseling Parents of Mentally Retarded

Children. Washington, Department of Health, Education, and Welfare, Children's Bureau, 1964.

Zausmer, Elizabeth: Evaluation of strength and motor development in infants. *Phys Ther Rev, 33:*November-December, 1953.

Zausmer, Elizabeth: The evaluation of motor development in children. *J Amer Phys Ther Ass, 44:*247, 1964.

Zausmer, Elizabeth: Motor Evaluation in Cerebral Palsy. Instructional Course, American Academy of Cerebral Palsy, Miami Beach, Florida, December 11, 1968.

Zausmer, Elizabeth, and Tower, Gail: A quotient for the evaluation of motor development. *Phys Ther, 46:*725, 1966.

Zellweger, Hans, and Hanson, James W.: Psychometric studies in muscular dystrophy. Type IIIa. (Duchenne). *Develop Med Child Neurol, 9:*576, 1967.

Chapter Ten

PHYSICAL THERAPY IN RESIDENTIAL FACILITIES

Carol Ethun Williams

Introduction

THIS CHAPTER WILL DEAL with the special problems faced by the physical therapist in planning and carrying out a physical therapy program within a residential facility for the mentally retarded. Although the specific treatment approaches are determined largely by the conditions existing in the individual patient, the therapist working under the conditions imposed by the average residential setting must make certain adjustments and compromises in order to provide optimal care to the patients needing physical therapy. It will rarely be possible for the therapist to personally provide all the individual treatment indicated on an ideal basis. This means that most physical therapists, although trained in providing treatment directly to the patient, must readjust their own thinking towards the role of teacher and supervisor for allied personnel (i.e. nurses, physical therapy aides, child care technicians, and other patient care attendants).

Development and refinement of procedures, techniques, and theorems are, and must be, continuous processes within all medical and allied professional specialties. Although still a relatively new profession, physical therapy is faced with a situation the resolution of which will affect the future development of the profession. There simply are not enough trained physical therapists to meet the increasing demand for services. New knowledge, better technical skills, greater understanding, and increased awareness have all contributed to the growth of the profession. Physical therapists are contributing to the direct care of patients with a multitude of disabilities, and are receiving referrals from a host of medical specialists. Consider also the fact that patients are treated at both ends of the age spectrum. It is not possible to recruit, train, and mobilize enough physical therapists to meet the current need for direct professional services, especially within residential facilities for the mentally retarded. The most workable solution at present is the extension of services through supportive personnel. This fact must be kept in mind when planning a physical therapy department within an institution for the mentally retarded.

Basic to the successful introduction of a new program will be first, a good understanding on the part of the physical therapist of the real functional operation of the patient care system, particularly at the ward level, and second, adequate support from the institutional power structure. The therapist would do well to first spend sufficient time on the wards to become fully acquainted with the hour by hour routines and problems of the ward personnel. With this background, realistic planning can be started. This planning process should involve the key administrative personnel from the superintendent or medical director to the chief nurse and ward supervisors. This helps to enlist their support and can provide the physical therapist with many helpful ideas which will smooth the actual implementation of the program.

The general philosophy of institutional personnel may present a challenge to the therapist trying to introduce and develop a new physical therapy program. Although most attendants will be concerned about and dedicated to their residents, in some institutions prolonged exposure to essentially a maintenance approach of "keep them clean and fed" may slow the acceptance of a truly therapeutic regimen. Here, the therapist who is a good student of human psychology may succeed through skillful use of various motivating approaches. A "special project" in which only one ward is chosen for intensive training and demonstration often arouses interest throughout the institution. It is particularly helpful if the administration or the personnel system provides for salary increases for those attendants who qualify as a result of such special training. Special insignia can be awarded to attendants who successfully complete the training course, and other inducements can be used to arouse interest in learning and applying these new skills.

Administration of the Physical Therapy Department

The philosophy and stated objective of the physical therapy department should be prepared by the chief physical therapist or physical therapy administrator and should reflect the overall purposes or objectives of the residential center. This philosophy will give direction to the physical therapy program. The chief physical therapist is responsible for planning and developing the physical therapy program and for coordinating it with the total interdisciplinary program of the residential facility. The chief therapist should have a position of equal authority with other department heads and should participate in the formulation and implementation of general goals and policies relating to the organization and operation of the center. Physical therapists should participate in all committees dealing directly with patient care.

It is the responsibility of the chief therapist to plan, organize, and direct the physical therapy program, supervise the personnel, both staff and voluntary, and coordinate the activities of the department with other patient care programs. Further responsibilities include the review and evaluation of the departmental programs, preparation of budgets including moneys related to staff and equipment, and recruitment of personnel. The physical therapy administrator is also responsible for training all personnel involved in the application of physiotherapeutic procedures. He should participate in health education programs provided for all professional and supportive personnel employed by the institution, as well as those programs directed toward community education.

Program Planning

The accumulation and interpretation of certain data is essential to early program planning in residential facilities. This should include a detailed survey of the resident population, overall institutional programs and personnel, and other resources in the community.

Resident Population

Each resident should have a gross assessment of his motor status with a correlation between actual level of motor development and the expected level for normal children within comparable age groups.* There should be an assessment of physical fitness, including such factors as strength, endurance, coordination and posture. Structural deformities must be evaluated in terms of possibilities for correction, surgical intervention, and need for appliances, as well as consideration of prophylactic measures where progressive conditions exist.

This type of resident survey leads quite naturally to the development of a functional profile in which significant data about individual residents can be categorized in appropriate groups giving an overall picture of the institution population. Each department, or special interest group, can develop its own functional profile according to those data which hold special significance. The functional profile developed by the physical therapy department would contain information regarding age and sex, diagnosis or significant history including behavioral characteristics, level of mental retardation, skills in activities of daily living, and general awareness of environment. Items within this functional profile will tend to fall into logical grouping which in turn will serve as criteria in the development of priorities. For instance, age and diagnosis will tend to correlate in that many of the conditions associated with institutionalized children do not lead to longevity (e.g., myelomeningocele with hydrocephalus, many chromosomal anomalies, and gross congenital cranial anomalies).

Very young children may present congenital structural deformities, but few will present the acquired deformities frequently seen in older residents. In general, lower levels of retardation correlate with poor degrees of physical fitness. The wearing of orthopedic appliances tends to correlate with the necessity for surgical procedures. Certain diagnostic characteristics have positive correlation with both the wearing of orthopedic appliances

---

*A variety of child development tests and forms are available and physical therapists should be aware of their content. See Chapter Nine.

and the necessity for surgical procedures; examples include the congenital clubfoot deformities and the myelomeningoceles.

The completed functional profile should contain the information which will best aid in the development of a physical therapy program designed to accommodate those residents who can most appropriately benefit from physical therapy. If the functional profile shows that the majority of the residents are young, moderately retarded children with low developmental quotients and few orthopedic appliances and/or surgical procedures, the program designed will be one in which the stimulation of major developmental motor milestones are stressed. A primarily geriatric population will require services appropriate for the conditions common to old age—arthritis, hip fractures and certain degenerative conditions. When the profile shows a high incidence of severe and profound levels of retardation, the plans must consider, as a minimum, a program for maintenance of the functional level and correction or prevention of deformities. Moderately retarded individuals requiring postsurgical care must have attention given to functional activities and improvement of physical fitness. The mildly retarded will generally require only those physical therapy services normally needed by nonretarded individuals.

Priorities must be considered also during this planning stage. Here again, functional profiles can help in selecting those children for whom physical therapy would have maximum benefit. Children whose hydrocephalus has not been arrested and those with severe cranial congenital anomalies may not be the most appropriate candidates for physical therapy. Other congenital anomalies may respond to appropriate physiotherapeutic, prosthetic or orthopedic procedures. However, where the level of mental retardation is severe and/or profound, the ability to manipulate appliances in a functional manner may not be possible.

All children with cerebral palsy should be closely evaluated in terms of their suitability for physical therapy. Referring again to the functional profile, the data regarding age, level of retardation, structural deformities, appliances and surgical procedures will contribute to the placement of this individual on a priority list. One must not consider priority as an all or none factor. Cases presented for physical therapy immediately following surgery should be given a high priority for the *direct* services of a registered physical therapist. An infant with cerebral palsy should be given priority for treatment by the physical therapist with consultation to the ward personnel so that proper steps are taken to insure appropriate handling and management of this child in the ward setting. Three- to seven-year-old children who are nonambulant but present no specific neurologic or orthopedic handicaps must be given priority for group therapy programs designed to stimulate lags in motor development. A 15-year-old child who is sluggish, obese, and walks with stooped shoulders must be given priority for a physical fitness program. The priorities then are not so much to determine who does and who does not receive physical therapy but rather to determine the nature of the physical therapy, and by whom the physical therapy procedures are administered.

Personnel and Programs

Program planning, as described above, must consider the nature and extent of the handicap, whether it is static or progressive, which therapeutic or prophylactic measures are indicated, and which department is best equipped to provide the service required. Time is a very expensive commodity, and we are well aware of the critical shortage of trained technical and professional personnel. Therefore, it is imperative that skilled people utilize their time in performing those tasks directly related to their special skills. Time spent in planning means that patients will receive the attention of the person best qualified to meet their particular needs, and also that highly trained persons will be performing only those tasks which require their particular skills.

COTTAGE AND WARD PROGRAMS. Most institutions are divided into nonambulant, semiambulant and ambulant wards or cottages. There generally is also a further division by age and/or functional level. These divisions of resident population make it convenient for attendant personnel to provide special programs of care and training for the residents under their supervision. Time studies (at Central Wisconsin Colony and Training School in

1963) of cottage and ward personnel have shown that time which could have been devoted to direct patient care was being spent on performing janitorial, clerical, and other housekeeping tasks. Administrators must bear in mind the actual amount of time available for ward personnel to perform special program activities before any decision to add these activities to their work schedule is made. Other considerations are the selection of special activities, the capabilities of the attendants, time available for training, and personnel available for supervision.

Special activities appropriate for inclusion in cottage and ward programs include the following examples:

1. Daily physical fitness exercises. Type and duration of these exercises should be selected and graded according to the age and motorial status of each group of residents. The session should begin with general flexibility exercises such as reaching, bending, and twisting. These might be followed by stretching and coordination exercises such as toe touching or windmilling. Following these, a group of endurance or strengthening exercises should be considered such as push-ups, sit-ups, or endurance running.

2. Practice periods for activities being stressed in various therapeutic settings. As teachers assign homework which is to be done on an extracurricular basis, therapists frequently assign special exercises which are to be carried out away from the physical or occupational therapy department. Activities leading to the major developmental milestones can be practiced on the ward or in the cottage setting. Youngsters can be guided in rolling and creeping activities. Crutch-walking can be supervised and encouraged by ward personnel. Cottage attendants who have been given adequate instruction can supervise residents during balance, endurance, and functional activities.

3. Activities of daily living (ADL). Feeding, dressing, and grooming activities may be initiated by special therapists, but follow-through on the ward is essential to the successful acquisition of these skills by the resident. This is particularly true where special appliances are necesssary. The application and removal of braces, splints, and other appliances should be carried out by the

resident on the ward with proper supervision and considered as an activity of daily living.

4. Behavior modification. There are a variety of ways in which these programs have been set up, but each is similar in that a criteria for behavior is established and the resident is rewarded when he exhibits behavior appropriate to the criterion. If the reward is significantly meaningful to the resident, he eventually alters his behavior to meet the established criteria in order to receive the reward. Further detail on these techniques is not within this purview, and is already available in the literature (Rice 1968, Trotter and Inman 1968, Watson 1968, Bensberg et al. 1965, Girardeau and Spradlin 1964).

NURSING SERVICES. Many activities now performed by physical therapists were once considered part of basic nursing care. These include such treatments as ultraviolet and infrared light treatments, massage, and range of motion exercises. Institutions which employ a sufficient number of nurses or supervised nurses aides can utilize these individuals for administering these treatments. In some institutions aide personnel are instructed by the physical therapist in the techniques of passive exercises as a routine part of their in-service training. This means that appropriate residents can be given a passive range of motion on a routine basis with a minimum of professional time expended. Progression of gross physical deformities is minimized and significant deviations are brought to the attention of the ward physician.

It is important that registered nurses, practical nurses and nurses aides develop a holistic attitude regarding the nature of the infant or young child with multiple handicaps. The infant with a severe physical handicap is unable to experiment with his own body and to explore his surroundings. Because of his inability to move, he is unable to establish a proper relationship between himself and distance, size, and space. He may be in a posture of generalized flexion with a closed hand and therefore has no experience of size, shape, and texture. It is the experience of moving that allows a normal child to learn to judge distances and space properly. He has had many opportunities for trial and error in attempting to grasp before he could reach, and in bumping into things because of a mistaken impression of either distance or size. In addition to being bound in primitive and pathological postures (such as the posture of the asymmetrical tonic neck reflex), the child is unable to gain a concept of "self" in the usual manner by sucking his thumb, scratching his tummy, pulling his ears, or playing with his toes.

It becomes the task of the people who provide his routine daily care to compensate for this lack of sensorimotor experience. Nursing service personnel must, however, have a firm understanding of normal child development, both in terms of gross behavior such as rolling, creeping, standing, and walking, and also in terms of the maturation of the primitive reflex behavior exemplified by the gradual appearance and/or disappearance of certain automatic postural and adaptive reactions.

A detailed account is not necessary at this time, but the following summary of development is presented: (1) the gradual acquisition of head control, leading to the performance and perfection of other adaptive reactions, and (2) the acquisition of fine motor skills, which is possible because of the modifications of the child's primitive and total reflex-like patterns of movements and is due to the increasing factor of inhibition (Bobath 1962).

Head control and equilibrium reactions are absent in a newborn baby. Whether in the prone or the supine position, the newborn shows a predominance of flexor tone which is symmetrical in distribution. The neck-righting reaction is present but all others are absent. As the nurse passively turns the head of the newborn to one side, a rotation movement of the whole body is initiated and the child turns to his side. Further turning of the head leads to a continued movement of the body in rotation and the child will ultimately turn from the prone position to the supine position and vice versa.

Between the fourth and sixth week, the baby begins to raise his head while lying in the prone position. This is due to the appearance and gradual increase in strength of the labyrinthine-righting reactions acting on the head. It is not until the sixth month that the child is able to lift his head while lying in a supine position. With elevation of the head and beginning development of head control comes the gradual development of extensor tone throughout the body. It is this extensor tone which ultimately enables the child to maintain his position against gravity. Equally important is the fact that head control gives the child independence over visual exploration of his environment. Extensor tone develops gradually in a cephalocaudal direction. The neck and spine begin to extend first and are followed by the shoulders and hips, arms and legs; ultimately, the hands and fingers open.

At about six months the equilibrium reactions appear in the prone and supine positions and continue to develop later in kneeling, sitting, standing, and walking. The acquisition of extensor tone in the arms and hands and the development of equilibrium reactions coincide as the upper extremities are used for support of the body in crawling and a little later in creeping. Further development of the equilibrium reactions leads to the ability to maintain balance in kneeling and later in standing and walking, thus emancipating the arm and hand for manipulation of objects.

It is this evolution of righting and equilibrium reactions just described which gives the child the normal postural background upon which all motor activities accomplished by the child will take place. An infant child moves and reacts in total primitive reflex-like patterns. Coinciding with the development of a proper postural background, a gradual modification of these total reflex patterns is taking place. The grasp reflex in which the fingers, hand, and elbow grasp in a total movement of flexion gradually is modified. The arms extend, the hands open, and the fingers can move independently, whether the other parts of the extremity are in flexion or in a state of rest. In other words, the child now has the ability to grasp an object and to release it regardless of whether the arm is in a state of motion or rest, and whether it is flexed or extended. It is not until the fourteenth to fifteenth month that the child is able to pick up small objects between the thumb and forefinger. The acquisition of these fine motor skills is dependent upon and in direct proportion to the developing degree of inhibition—the ability to suppress all but the desired part of any intended movement. Inhibition is a characteristic of maturation which results in the breaking up of total movement patterns and allows for a variety of precise and fine movements (Bobath 1962).

The nurses and aides must be thoroughly familiar with these concepts of child development in order to approach the handling of the multihandicapped child in that manner which will (1) inhibit the abnormal postural reflex activity, thereby normalizing the muscle tone, and (2) facilitate normal postural reactions in their proper developmental sequence with progression to the learning of normal movements and skills (Bobath 1962). (See Ch. 3.) Of prime importance—and this must be conveyed to nursing service personnel—is the fact that all handling of the child has a definite effect on his eventual acquisition of sensorimotor skills. Voluntary and involuntary motion, normal and abnormal motion occur in patterns. These patterns are developed as a direct response to the daily handling of an infant or child when he is being carried, dressed, bathed, picked up or put down. The child learns to protect himself as he develops righting and equilibrium reflexes. As he uses his basic patterns to cooperate (or to resist) and later to perform his own voluntary activities, he builds up a stockpile of movement patterns for use in later life. Unless nursing service personnel are taught to handle the neurologically handicapped child properly, his supply of movement patterns will be limited and abnormal.

The keynote to management is handling and positioning. Any child, with or without physical handicap, has a multitude of needs which require the personal contact of another individual. He must be fed, bathed, dressed, and fondled. He is moved from crib to chair, and from chair to floor. Each time he is picked up he should be given the opportunity to reach for the hands which must be offered to him, and whether he responds or not, his arms can be brought away from his body into extension and shoulder protraction. In this way he is provided with an opportunity to respond to the normal stimulus (the offered hands); with proper handling, the abnormal patterns of retraction are overcome. Carrying the child presents another opportunity to break the abnormal total extension pattern. It is simple and pleasant to carry a child with his legs straddling the crest of the aide's pelvis and his arms hugging her neck (Fig. 10-1). This avoids a total extension pattern and properly influences the child's arm, neck, spine, and legs. "Handling," then, refers to any manipulation of the child's body for any purpose whatsoever, and any change in his position or location which requires the personal contact of another individual (Ethun 1966).

When consideration is given to the general concepts regarding the care, management, and development of a multihandicapped child on a practical day to day basis, a formal series of exercises is not necessary. It is far better to give nursing service personnel sound knowledge and concepts that they can use, reuse and modify from patient to patient. It is recognized, however, that many

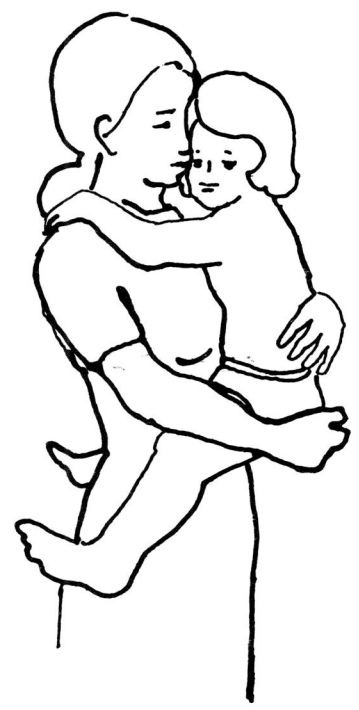

Figure 10-1. This position for carrying an infant or a small child prevents shoulder retraction and hip adduction.

432 *Physical Therapy Services in the Developmental Disabilities*

children with severe spasticity or tension athetosis are difficult to handle when first approached. The warming-up exercise illustrated (Fig. 10-2) will generally lead to a loosening up or relaxation

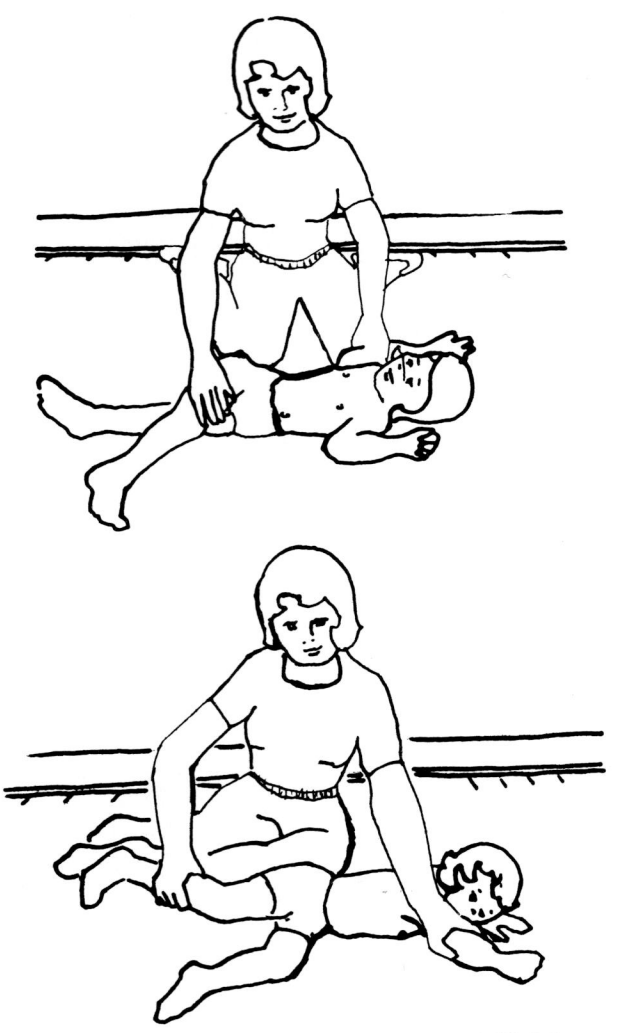

Figure 10-2. "Warming-up exercise." *Top,* with the child lying on his side, the shoulder-girdle is moved into retraction with simultaneous protraction of the pelvic-girdle. *Bottom,* the process is then reversed. This should be done three or four times on each side.

of this type of child. With the child on his side, the shoulder-girdle is moved into retraction with simultaneous protraction of the pelvic-girdle. The maneuver is then reversed and the hip is moved into retraction with simultaneous protraction of the shoulder. This process should be repeated three or four times on each side. This maneuver results in a rotation movement through the body axis and leads to the breaking up of the abnormal postural reflexes. The child can now be moved into one of a variety of positions depending upon the activity in which he is to be engaged. It is of the utmost importance that his position be varied frequently during the day and that the positions be appropriate for the activity intended. Frequent alteration of the child's position increases his supply of sensorimotor patterns while the risk of deformities is diminished.

It is frequently said that the perfect sitting posture is one in which the spine is extended, the hips and knees are flexed to 90°, the legs are perpendicular to the floor and the feet are supported in a neutral position. It must be remembered, however, that a child who is restrained in a special chair for extended periods, no matter how "perfect" his posture, is in real danger of developing flexion contractions of the hips, knees, and ankles. Furthermore, control of his posture is being obtained by mechanical means and he is deprived of the opportunity to learn control of his own posture. This postural control must be allowed to develop as a result of natural processes. That is not to say that special chairs such as the relaxation chair and adapted equipment do not have a place in a residential institution. Rather it is to emphasize that special equipment is designed or adapted for a special purpose: to improve function and to provide environmental stimulation. These items should be used for brief periods of time during which a child is practicing those activities for which the use of the chair was intended. For most children (unless special adapted equipment is necessary for function), the floor, a low stool or an ordinary chair, perhaps with some minor adjustments, will be better for the child and will give him a chance to move or use his hands in a functional way.

Several illustrations are presented depicting the use of the bolster (Figs. 10-3–10-5, 10-10). Positioned on the floor or on a mat, the bolster provides support in side-sitting, prone-lying, and kneeling for the infant, toddler, and severely handicapped youth. The bolster may be constructed by covering the central spool from a commercial carpet roll with foam rubber. The diameter desired will determine the quantity of foam rubber necessary. After the foam rubber is taped in place around the carpet spool, the entire bolster is covered with a water resistant fabric or plastic. It is suggested that a bolster with a diameter of 10 to 12 inches can be used with a greater variety of children; however, if several are to be made, they may be as small as 6 inches or as large as 18 inches in diameter.

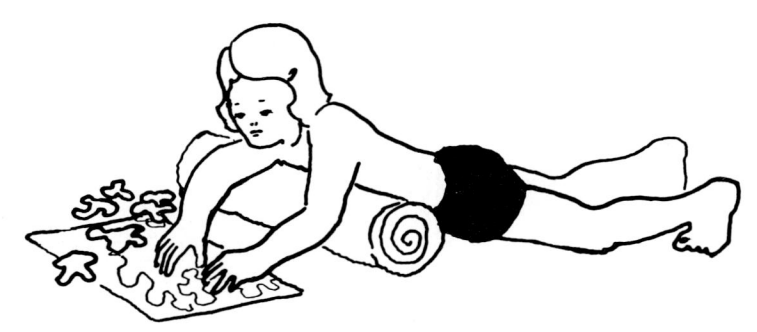

Figure 10.3. (See legend for Fig. 10-4.)

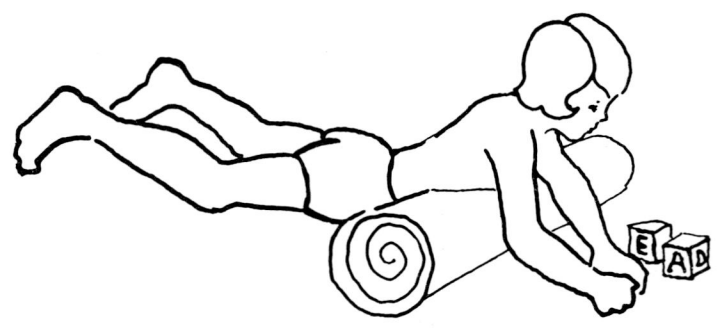

Figure 10-4. The size of the bolster can be varied to make this position suitable for the small infant and the teenager or adult handicapped to any degree of severity. It is particularly helpful when head control and upper extremity function are limited. (Also see Figure 10-5.)

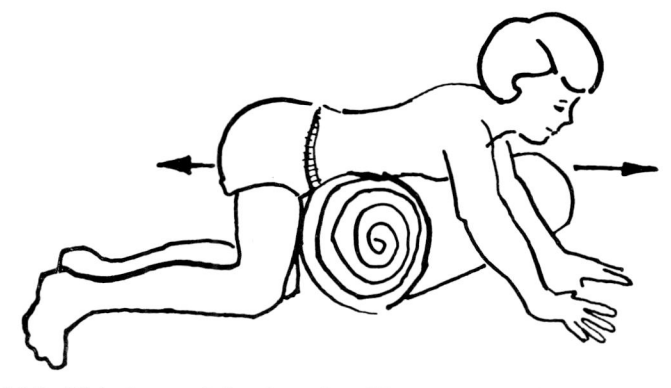

Figure 10-5. This form of "rock and roll" prevents deformities by encouraging weight-bearing on hands and knees, and also facilitates creeping.

To carry the discussion on concepts of proper management further, it should be pointed out that the *first thing* to teach the nurse and aide is to be observant—to distinguish the abnormal movement patterns from the normal ones. It is also necessary that they have an understanding of the underlying causes of the acquisition of deformities. Putting these two ideas—observation and understanding—together, the aide has the information necessary to handle a child in a manner that will both inhibit the pathological patterns and encourage or facilitate the normal patterns. Figure 10-6 illustrates that sitting position which is frequently easier for the multihandicapped child to independently assume. This position gives the child a wide base of sitting support between his feet. Because of the inherent predisposition of handicapped children to lower extremity adduction—internal rotation—compensatory flexion deformity, *this position should be avoided*. Figures 10-7–10-13 are presented as alternate choices for positioning throughout the day.

Young children and infants are frequently bathed and dressed while lying in a supine position. This position will tend to stimulate extensor tone as well as exacerbate those pathological reflexes which are extensor in nature. For this reason dressing, bathing, and feeding should be done with the child in a sitting position as soon as possible. It might also be pointed out that in the

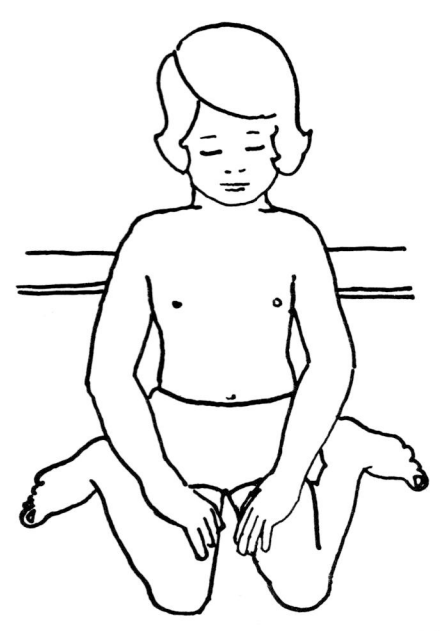

436 *Physical Therapy Services in the Developmental Disabilities*

Figure 10-6. This is frequently the first position in which a handicapped child can sit unsupported. However, it *should be avoided* because of the inherent predisposition to lower extremity flexion-adduction internal rotation deformity.

sitting position, the child is better able to assist with the activity; if he has not progressed that far, at least he can make visual contact and follow the progress of the activity. In Figure 10-14, note the position of the attendant's forearm holding the baby's shoulder in protraction, thus placing his hands in a position of function for grasping those objects placed before him.

EDUCATION. Two-way communication between teachers and physical therapists is the best way to assure that proper attention is given to the sensorimotor training of the mentally retarded. We have long aimed for an understanding between educators and therapists as to what each is attempting to accomplish so that current program goals might be reinforced on a mutual basis. Recent years have brought about an even closer communication between

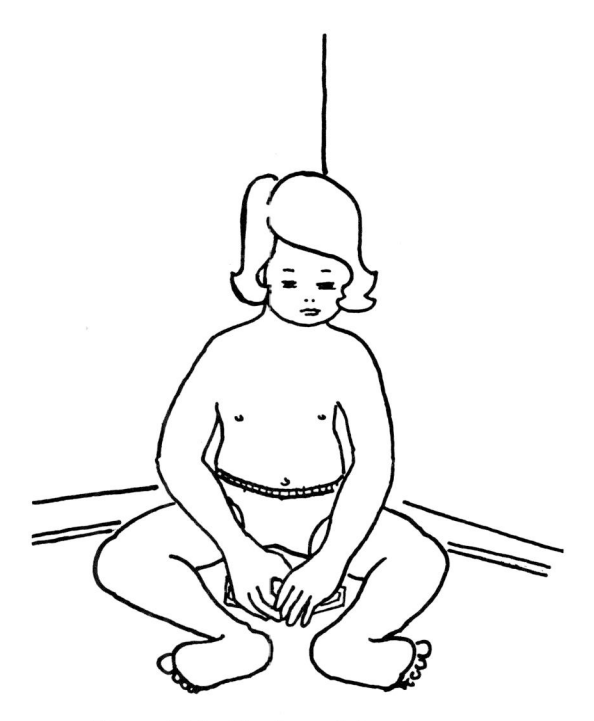

Figure 10-7. (See legend for Fig. 10-8.)

these two groups, resulting in the development of techniques which can be conducted with equal proficiency by teachers and therapists. Whether referred to simply as "movement activities" (Ch. 7), "educational rhythmics" (Robins and Robins 1963, 1966), or classified under a multitude of labels from musical gymnastics to trampoline therapy, these techniques all contain elements of motor, intellectual, and sensory training. The rationale may vary, depending upon the expositor. Various relationships between these three elements are cited from simple cause and effect to complex theorems espoused in multisyllabic professional jargon. The significant fact remains that given these three elements upon which to build a therapeutic program, a variety of technicians, with a slight change in approach to their clients, can supplement

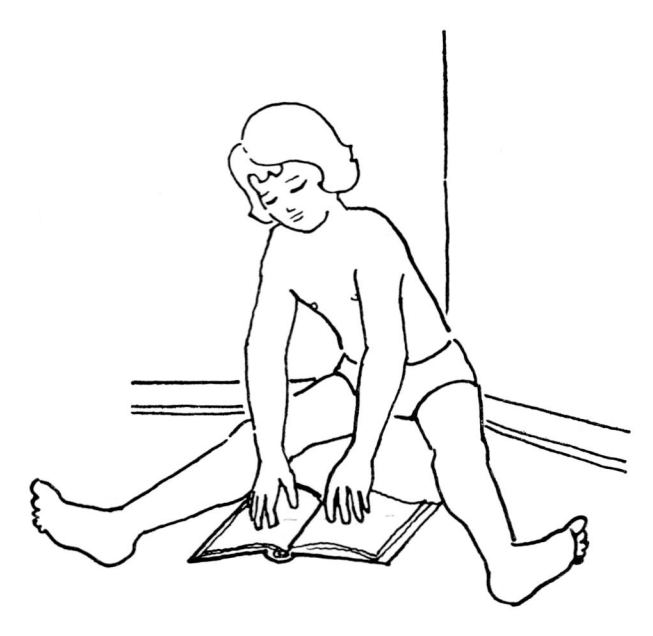

Figure 10-8. The child's back should be straight. If he needs additional support, he can be placed against a wall or in a corner instead of the center of the room. Parents should be encouraged to modify the basic postures shown in these illustrations to fit the capabilities or limitations of their child. They should be urged to have the child assume, or be placed in, as many different positions as possible throughout the day.

their program and the programs of other departments and provide more stimulating experiences for the residents.

RECREATION. Leisure time activities provide first and foremost an opportunity for the residents of an institution for the mentally retarded to have fun. Retarded children start out life several steps behind other children, and despite many giant steps now being made, never quite catch up. This means that a retarded child cannot pass up any opportunity for learning and for growing. The *fun* of a recreation program should not be replaced by the sometimes heavy business of learning, but should always be supplemented with elements of physical, social, and sensory training.

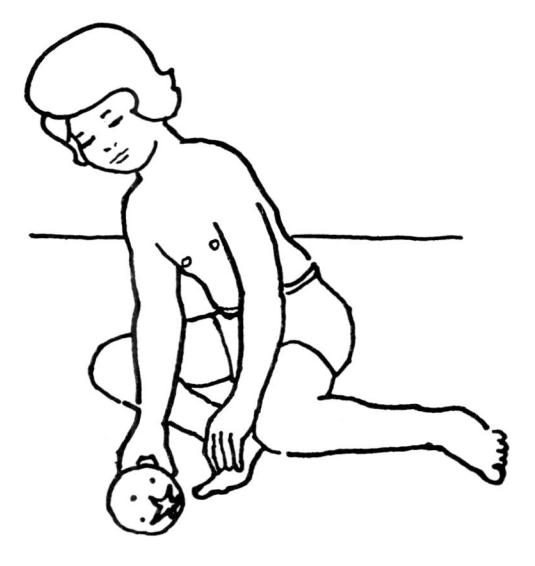

Figure 10-9. (See legend for Fig. 10-10.)

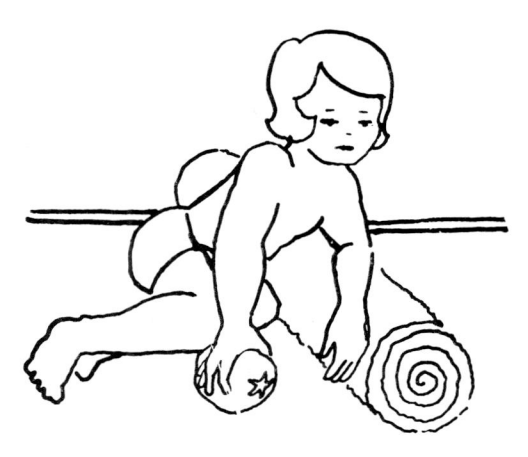

Figure 10-10. Careful attention must be given to alternating the direction in which the child sits.

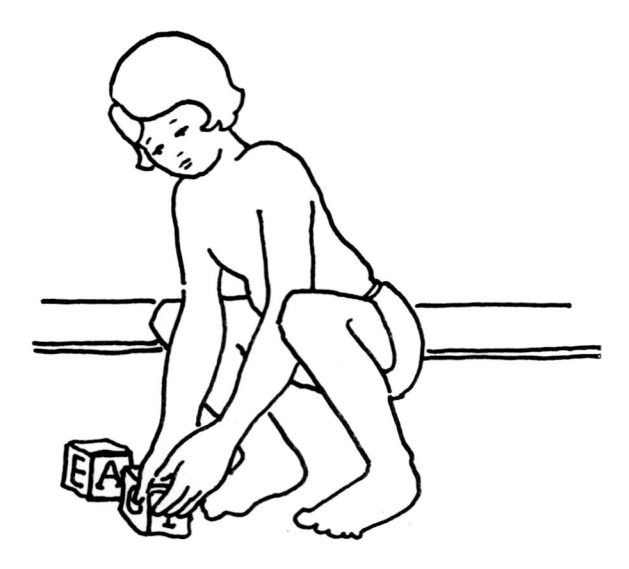

Figure 10-11. The heels should be on the floor as much as possible.

Also to be considered is the fact that much of the work in the physical therapy department, and most especially for the mentally retarded, is exceedingly repetitious and can become exceedingly dull without special effort. It behooves the physical therapist to approach the recreation specialist for means of providing fun and variation to specific activities without sacrificing their therapeutic value.

It is just as logical for a recreator to request the training of a resident in a specific functional activity in order to include him in certain recreational programs. If more of this type of interprofessional collaboration were going on in our institutions, we would hear fewer complaints about communication gaps and going at cross purposes. There are many activities, such as the educational rhythmics mentioned above, which are common to both therapists and recreators. Swimming, for example, is both fun and therapeutic. The swimming pool is also a good place for postsurgical gait training. Bicycling (tricycling for youngsters) is a tradi-

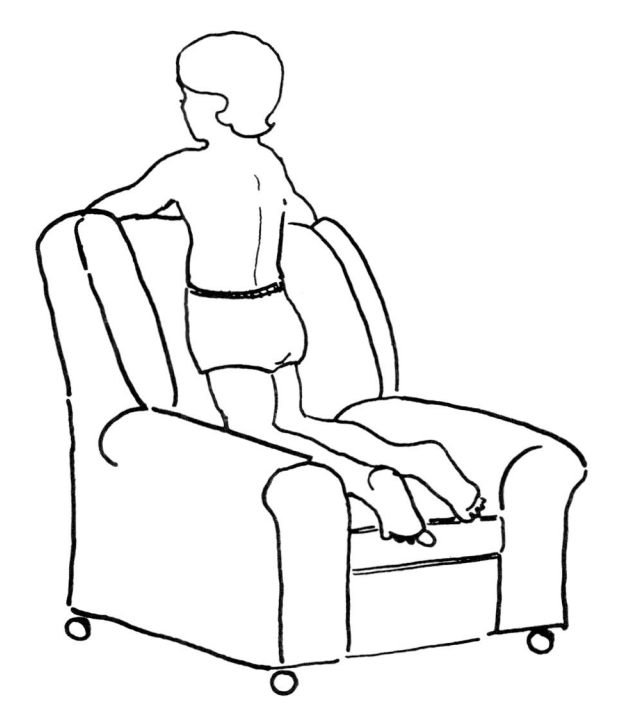

Figure 10-12. This is a good position for watching television.

tional part of physical therapy. Having mastered the techniques, a "bike hike" is fun. It may be that institutional administrators will have to make a strong catalytic contribution to the interprofessional relationships before we will see much change. The very best time to do this is when both programs are in the planning stage.

OTHER PROGRAMS. It is not necessary to elaborate on all of the departments generally found in residential facilities. The principle involved is to find either concepts or techniques which are common to two or more departments and to build an approach to patient care which is based on these commonalities. Some will be even more closely allied than those above, such as the relationship between occupational therapy and physical therapy. Interest in

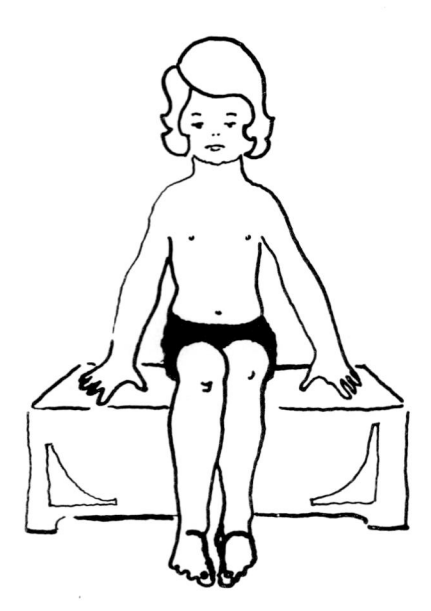

Figure 10-13. Careful attention to the height of the bench will assure that the feet are flat on the floor.

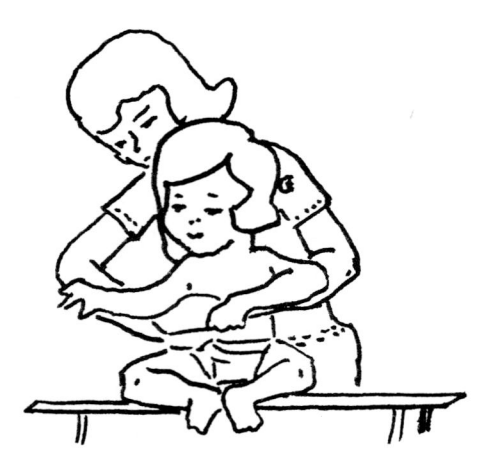

Figure 10-14. Bathing, dressing and feeding should be done in the sitting position as early as possible. Note shoulder is held in protraction.

physical fitness is a common tie between physical educators and physical therapists. Of particular importance is that these commonalities are found and considered early, and that administrative policy is such that interdepartmental approaches to resident care are treated with respect, approval, and recognition.

Survey of Community Resources

It is not necessary to dwell upon the variety of community resources commonly available to residential institutions in general. Those community agencies which may have a specific contribution toward the development of a physical therapy department, however, should be mentioned. Administratively, these extrainstitutional factors should be considered during the planning stages so that policies can be dealt with and patterns for interagency activities established. The state and local affiliates of the following agencies should be approached regarding their possible participation in the program: United Cerebral Palsy Association, Inc., Association for Retarded Children, National Foundation—March of Dimes, and the Society for Crippled Children and Adults. Participation of these agencies with various institutional programs has taken many forms. In New York State, the physical therapist employed by the state United Cerebral Palsy Association is actively engaged in the in-service training programs for employees in the residential facilities for the mentally retarded. United Cerebral Palsy of Wisconsin, Inc., has provided extensive physical therapy equipment for the state institutions and has paid for advanced training for many of the professional employees. In other areas, the Association for Retarded Children has provided financial support for training programs and direct consultation for developing institutional services. The National Foundation and the Easter Seal Society each has on their national staff a registered physical therapist who is available for consultation.

The availability of medical services in the community will have a direct effect on the physical therapy program. It must be determined whether orthopedic consultation is most feasible outside the institution on a fee-for-service basis, or whether a physician should be retained "on call" or on a regularly scheduled day of consultation, perhaps, a full-time institutional surgeon may be employed. The availability of commercial brace and appliance shops must be considered as well as the feasibility of forming an institutional brace shop. Financial arrangements and administrative protocol must be established for necessary surgery, appliances, and equipment. State Crippled Children's Services may become involved with the financial aspects of these problems. In some states, this agency may become more directly involved with patient care by providing individual home care or supervision to patients awaiting admission or recently returned from institutional care.

The Physical Therapy Department

Although repeatedly stated throughout this chapter, it is worthy of emphasis that many institutionalized individuals can benefit from the attention of the physical therapist although not all will require his direct service. Already discussed are those activities related to physical therapy but administered by other personnel. The following section will describe those activities directly related to the function of the physical therapist and the physical therapy department. It follows throughout this section that many children will receive specialized treatment by a qualified therapist while others will be attended to by trained physical therapy assistants or specially trained volunteers.

Specific Problems

Children who are slow to develop motor skills, even though complicating physical handicaps, if present, are relatively minimal, require the attention, but not the direct service, of a physical therapist. We recognize that most mentally retarded children are slow to pass from one stage of motor development to the next, and that many retardates fail to develop beyond a very rudimentary level. Studies are being considered to record graphically this deviation from the normal developmental sequence and to determine the possibilities of causal factors. We know, for instance, that most patients with Down's syndrome pass through all stages of motor development but spend a longer time at each individual stage, thus requiring a longer period of time for acquisition of motor skills (Koch 1963).

Developmentally retarded children under the age of six years can be treated in groups of approximately 16 by trained nonprofessional personnel in a structured situation geared to stimulate the development of gross motor skills. Supervision and instruction of the volunteers and therapy assistants, as well as direction of the program, is provided by the registered physical therapist. At the Central Wisconsin Colony and Training School, Madison, this type of "group therapy program" has been conducted since 1961 and generally has 40 to 50 children enrolled. Each child is given a motor skills achievement test which forms the basis for his specific program of developmental stimulation. Written directions are given to the nonprofessional workers just as home instructions are given to parents. In addition to this ongoing program of instructions on a per patient basis, each therapy assistant and volunteer is given an orientation to the basic principles of physical therapy including general comments on pathology, anatomy, kinesiology, and child development. Specific techniques are demonstrated and explained, and the importance of safety measures, body mechanics, and professional ethics is stressed.

Children with inadequate head control, such as those with minimal to moderate hydrocephalus, are placed in the prone position over a bolster. Later they will progress to sitting on the floor in a corner, and still later, against the flat wall. With further development of head and trunk control, they will progress to the crawler or infant walker for experience with locomotion. Further head and trunk control is developed along with experience in weight-bearing as the child is placed in the standing box (Fig. 10-15). The amount of control offered can be varied according to adaptive inserts placed within the box. With further improvement in balance and control he will graduate to the standing table, and at about the same time he will move to the small orthopedic walker. Weight-bearing, balance, motivation, and locomotion are known prerequisites to ambulation. In addition to these structured activities, each child is given a period of time for free play during which he is encouraged to move about the room, roll-

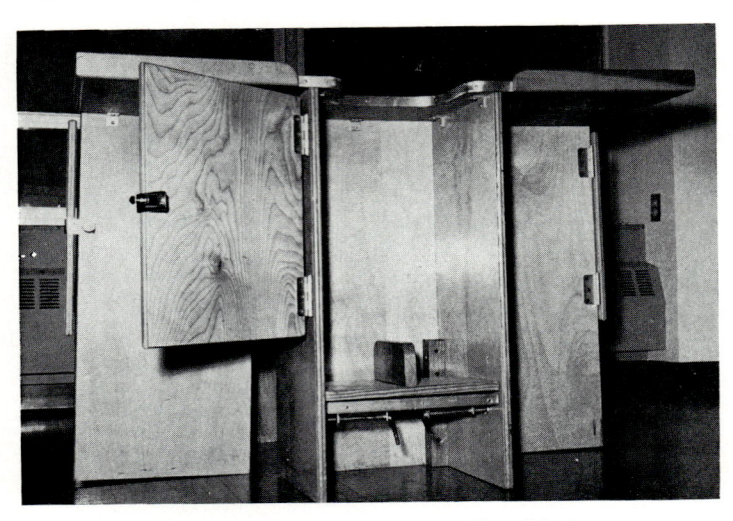

446 *Physical Therapy Services in the Developmental Disabilities*

Figure 10-15. Standing box. Note adjustable inserts.

ing, creeping, or crawling at will. Appropriate toys and games are provided for motivation. There will of course be variations for individual children, but in general the regimen just described is the format followed for most children in the group therapy program. Whether the child has Down's syndrome or phenylketonuria or one of the many chromosomal or metabolic disorders, as long as no major orthopedic or neurologic handicap is evident he is appropriate for this group therapy program.

The group therapy program for young children with an uncomplicated motor retardation can be summarized as follows: a combination of activities combining such factors as locomotion, weight-bearing, control or balance, and motivation are utilized in stages of progression according to the child's developing abilities and eventually resulting in independent ambulation. Equipment designed with these factors in mind is used by trained nonprofessional personnel under the supervision and direction of a registered physical therapist.

Young ambulatory children with balance or coordination problems can also be treated in groups. At first, emphasis is placed on gross motor coordination; elements of fine sensorimotor coordination can be added after the group has gained more control over gross body movements. To add fun and interest to the exercises, they can be conducted as games and can be given appropriate names according to the age of the group. The following exercises were developed from similar exercise programs described by the Bobaths (1967) and by Robins and Robins (1966).

1. Rock and roll. In kneeling and in standing, the child is gently pushed back and forth between two people in both the lateral and the AP plane.

2. Walking the plank. The children walk between two strips of tape which are placed on the floor approximately 10 inches apart. Later they will walk along a 10-inch plank which is elevated about 4 inches from the floor. Still later they will walk along a 2" x 4" similarly elevated.

3. Marching to music. High step marching, with strict rhythm and reciprocal arm swing. May be combined with "follow-the-leader" or "walking the plank."

4. Up and down, in and out. First, reciprocal flexion and extension of legs; then reciprocal abduction and adduction of legs; then a combination, while one leg flexes the other abducts, and reverse. This is done with the children lying in a supine position.

5. Monkey see—monkey do. The therapist (volunteer or aide) and children stand facing each other with matching colored objects in the hand of the same side (mirror image; e.g. green flag in child's left hand and therapist's right hand, red flag in child's right hand and therapist's left hand). The children then follow the movement initiated by the therapist, matching color for color, with a constant rhythm. This can also be done with children in wheelchairs.

Children with meningomyelocele should be seen very early by the physical therapist. Even while other orthopedic deformities are being corrected, and providing hydrocephalus is minimal, the therapist can be directing efforts to stimulate the development of head and trunk control and sitting balance. When this is accomplished, the child is ready to be included in a small group of similarly handicapped children. Prior to the time braces are ordered and the children are engaged in gait training, they will participate in preambulation activities. These exercises are designed to develop upper extremity strength and trunk control and to encourage locomotion. Bilateral independent use of the arms is essential and rolling a large ball from person to person is a good first step. Most of these children will never walk without the use of crutches; therefore, it is imperative that the upper extremities and shoulders have superior muscle strength. Large blocks, 4 x 4 x 6 inches, can be used to elevate the trunk and legs as the children move about while sitting on the floor. The maneuver is identical to that required for crutch-walking, elbow extension and shoulder depression.

A race among several children will add interest to the exercise. As confidence improves, sawed off or "shorty" crutches may be substituted for the large blocks. The children's game of wheel barrowing is also a good exercise, and it too can be executed in the form of a race. Repeated physical and psychological evaluation will help the physician determine when the child has obtained sufficient maturity and is ready for bracing. Institution aides will require thorough instruction in proper methods for applying, removing and caring for braces, and the physical therapist should be prepared to continually reinforce this instruction. Because these children all have a tendency toward skin ulcerations which tend to heal slowly once allowed to develop, extreme care must be taken to gradually build up the patient's tolerance to wearing braces. For the same reason, tolerance for standing is acquired in a graded manner.

Facilities and Equipment

The physical therapy department in a residential facility should be considered as a concept or program activity rather than an architectural structure. It is still necessary, however, that a certain area or areas be set aside for the conduct of the more specialized aspects of the program activities. The following recommendations are by necessity quite general and intended as guides for the physical therapist who must plan a new department within a residential facility. The important thing, as described earlier in the chapter, is to be thoroughly familiar with the resident population, the personnel and the programs since these will largely determine the kinds of space and equipment required. For the purpose of this manuscript we will assume a large institution—a full distribution of all ages, types and degrees of retarded individuals. Likewise, we will also assume a full spectrum of physical therapy services.

FACILITIES. A comprehensive physical therapy program will require the following room or area allocation: office, hydrotherapy, gymnasium or exercise room, small treatment room, and satellite treatment areas.

1. Physical therapy office. The office space required will naturally vary according to the number of personnel who will use the area. If there is an outpatient program, space must be allocated for a waiting room. Other area assignments may include a private office for the administrator or chief therapist, an area for the secretary-receptionist, including sufficient space for file cabinets, and a small conference room for case discussion between the chief and staff therapist and attending physicians. It is important that this office have easily accessible communication with all other treatment areas either by telephone or interoffice communication system.

2. Hydrotherapy. A separate *well-ventilated* room should be allocated for hydrotherapy. The ceiling should be covered with a soundproofing material and the floor should have a nonskid surface. The dressing area should be well screened and have good proximity to linen and swimsuit storage. An automatic locking safety gate should cover the entire entrance to hydrotherapy. This is particularly true if a swimming pool is located in this area. The swimming pool should include both a ramp and a step approach. A safety rail should extend around the entire inner edge of the pool. A parallel bar can be attached to this safety rail when the pool is used for therapeutic purposes such as early ambulation following orthopedic surgery, or the bar can be removed when the pool is being used for recreation purposes.

3. Physical therapy gym or exercise room. This room should be large enough to accommodate the size of the usual therapeutic gymnasium equipment and still allow room for gait training and

other gross motor activities. Ventilation must be good and an outdoor exit should be easily accessible. The room should be set up to accommodate large groups of children and young adults for physical fitness programs as well as small groups for mat work.

4. Small treatment room. This room may not be necessary in all programs as its use is primarily limited to specialized individual treatment such as the application of traditional physical therapy modalities or testing sessions. Hyperactive or easily distractible children, however, may require a less stimulating environment and a one-to-one treatment setting in order to derive full benefit from physical therapy services.

5. Satellite treatment areas. Each major dormitory, building, or group of cottages should have a group physical therapy room. It follows that the groups developed will come from the cottages or wards having the closest proximity. The groups, however, will be formed on the basis of age and functional level. The design and equipping of the room will also vary according to the age and functional level of the groups.

  a. Toddlers and young children group. This room may be obviously decorated for children and equipped with standing tables, walkers, crawlers, and a variety of children's toys.

  b. Teenage and young adults group. Decorated with the age of the group in mind, this room should have those gym and small equipment items necessary for a program of functional activities and physical fitness.

  c. Geriatric group. This program, like any other geriatric or nursing home program, will meet and handle the usual problems associated with old age—hip fractures, stroke, arthritis and other degenerative disorders. Because older retarded individuals are resistant to changes in routine, it may be better to carry out their program activities in the ward or cottage setting. Parallel bars can be set up in the day room and ambulation with walkers can be carried out in the same area. Transfer activities (bed to chair, chair to commode and return) are best done in the residential area. This is the setting in which these individuals will probably remain for the rest of their lives and functional activities should be planned accordingly.

EQUIPMENT. Into the following section, wherever possible, reference will be made to items of equipment which will require individual construction as well as those models which are commercially available. Description of function and/or use will be given only for the less traditional items.

1. Treatment tables. The standard length and height is recommended but a 36-inch width is preferable to the standard 29-inch table. To obtain this desired width, two standard tables may be fastened together. This added width is desirable because many of the current exercise regimes call for increased mobility on the part of the patient. With a very small child it is frequently more advantageous for the therapist to work at table height rather than on the floor, and the added width becomes a safety and convenience factor. Treatment tables should have at least a 1-inch foam mattress covered with a waterproof material.

2. Benches. Independent sitting is an important motor milestone for young children. Retarded children may acquire this skill anywhere between the age of six months and six years. (Indeed, many retarded children never acquire this skill.) Sitting should be practiced on a firm surface where both feet can touch the floor and both hands have room on the supporting surface to provide balance and support. Benches used for sitting balance exercises do not require a back rest. We suggest that benches be constructed out of wood with the following dimensions: 2' x 1' x 6', 2' x 1' x 8', 2' x 1' x 10' (See Fig. 10-13).

3. Chairs. Many children with cerebral palsy have difficulty sitting because of their inability to adequately flex at the hips. This, coupled with extensor spasms, causes the spastic child or the child with tension athetosis to slide down in his chair and sit on his lower spine. Commercially made cerebral palsy chairs are available, but the cost may be prohibitive for individual use (Figs. 10-16 and 10-17). Such chairs, however, have the advantage of being adaptable in size in several dimensions to accommodate a variety of children. When a number of children require this type of chair, it is probably a better plan to construct the chair, which can be done quite economically out of wood and can be made according to the size of each child. The chair then becomes the

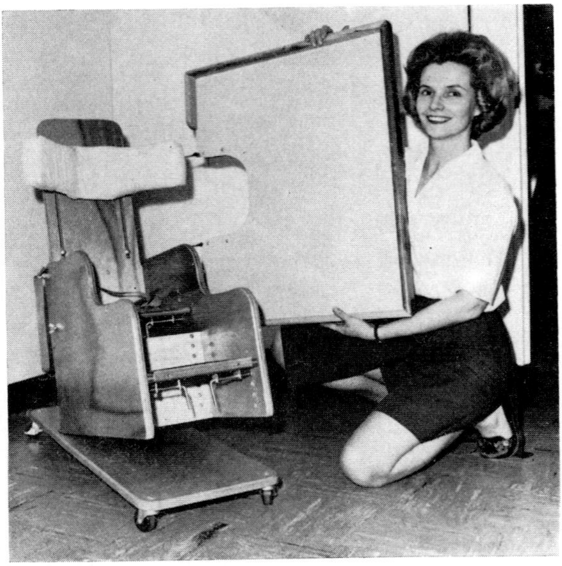

452 *Physical Therapy Services in the Developmental Disabilities*

Figure 10-16. Cerebral palsy chair. Can be adjusted to size of child and to desired tilt angle.

property of that child and is used at mealtime, during school, or any other time when a sitting position is required. One word of caution, however: because of the danger of joint contracture, no child should be left in any one sitting position for extended periods of time.

4. Wheelchairs. Each child who requires a wheelchair should have one chair which is assigned to him, and if necessary, is adapted to fit his need (Fig. 10-18). These adaptations should consider the angle between the seat and the back rest, the height of the back rest, the drive mechanism, the level of the tabletop and any other specialized equipment for functional activities (e.g. slings, feeders, etc.). It is frequently helpful for the cerebral-palsied individual to have a special tabletop which is used only for meals and has cut out inserts for dishes and a cup. Generally, an individual with cerebral palsy will require a tabletop which is a little higher than one used by other handicapped people.

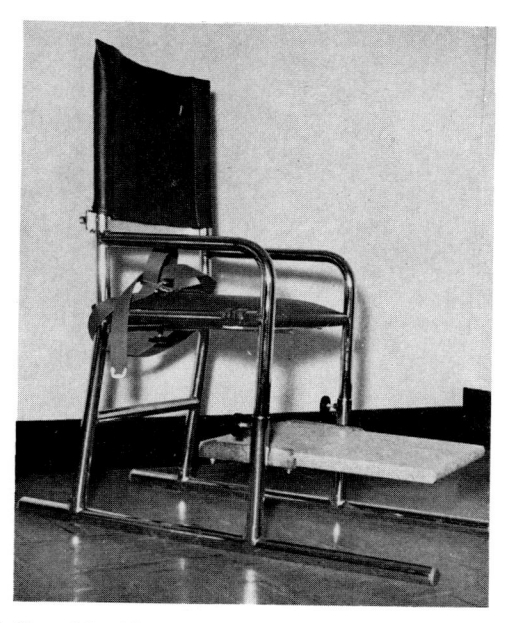

Figure 10-17. Adjustable kindergarten chair. This chair also can be fitted with a detachable tray.

5. Standing table and boxes. Although available commercially, these items provide good project work for volunteer groups. Most residential facilities will require both individual and group arrangements. Both types, however, should have provisions for varying the height and the interior dimensions of the box.

6. Walkers. Most institutions will require a variety of walkers, both in kind and in size. There is a walker commercially available for every age, beginning with the little canvas sling attached to an aluminum frame which allows an infant to scoot about on the floor. Also available are the so-called cerebral palsy or juvenile orthopedic walkers. These may be purchased with a rib belt and saddle seat for total support of the child, or with a balance ring for giving the child minimal support Fig. (10-19). Walkers are also available for adult or geriatric patients. Most therapists are already familiar with the walking aid or walkerette, as well as the large

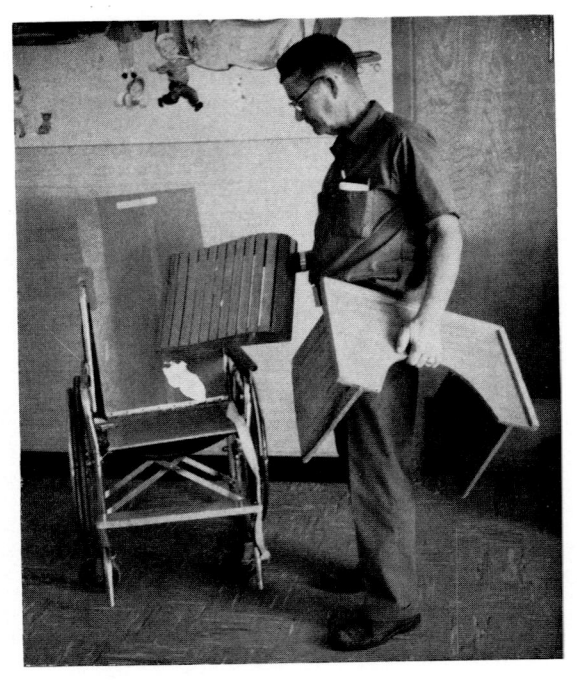

Figure 10-18. Wheelchair with various adapters and tray. (Photo courtesy of Winfield State Hospital and Training School.)

orthopedic walker which comes equipped with wheels, seat, and axillary crutches.

7. Scoot-about. Being able to move about at will on the floor is a very important part of early motor development. For reasons of hygiene or convenience, many institutionalized youngsters are denied this important experience. Because of his frail lower extremities and problems of incontinence, the child with meningomyelocele presents a hygiene problem to himself and to attending personnel. The infant or young child with a congenital hip dislocation requires many months of immobilization in plaster casts; in a residential institution, this may also mean confinement in bed. The multiple congenital anomalies frequently have an orthopedic component for which the therapeutic management

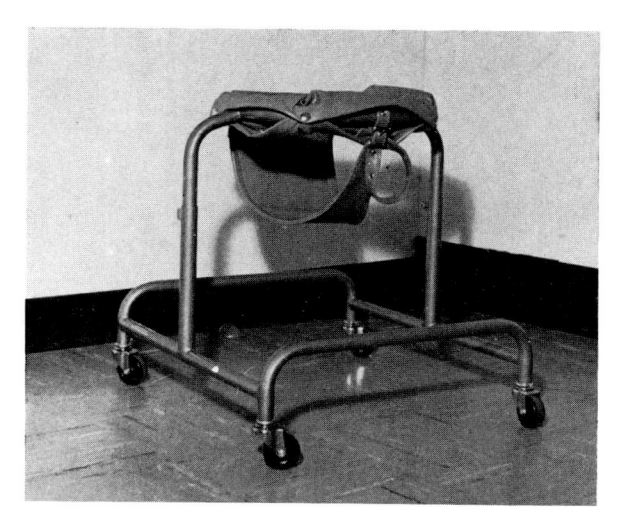

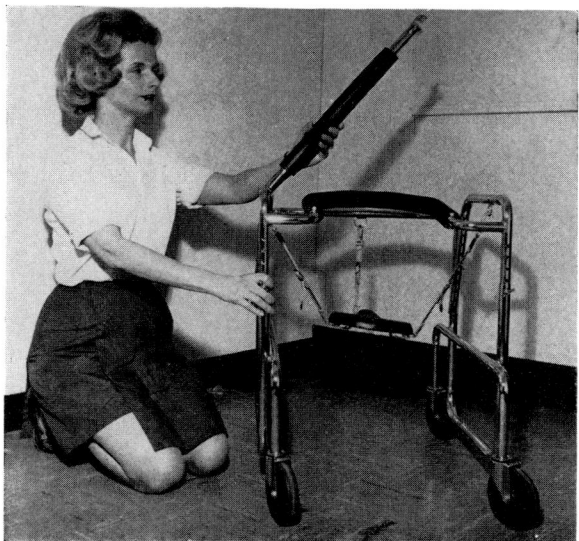

Figure 10-19. Variety of commercial walkers. *Lower,* the removable bar facilitates handling of heavy children who otherwise would have to be lifted into the balance ring.

entails frequent and prolonged periods in plaster casts. With only moderate hand function, these children can be placed on the "scoot-about" and have a modicum of independence while presenting no undue problems of safety or hygiene to themselves or their environment. A commercial model is available through suppliers of hospital and rehabilitation equipment; however, the cost may be prohibitive if an institution requires a large quantity. The homemade variety can be constructed for a total cost of approximately $2.50. This also is a good project for a volunteer group.

8. and 9. Parallel bars and stairs. These traditional items of equipment are available commercially; however, an institution having a well-equipped maintenance or engineering department will find it more economical to make them. Plans are available through the National Society for Crippled Children and Adults. Plans for other adaptive equipment are also available through this voluntary health agency.

10. Tilt table. The tilt table is used in the therapeutic regime for traumatic paraplegias and quadriplegics who generally are not found in residential institutions for the mentally retarded. There is a place for a tilt table, however, in institutions housing adult or geriatric residents. It is frequently necessary for this type of individual to build a tolerance to standing and for this purpose the tilt table is most useful.

11. Mat. The standard 4' x 6' mat will be satisfactory for individual work; however, it is suggested that a 9' x 9' mat be obtained for group work. A 6' bolster will accommodate several children on this larger mat, allowing them to participate either in group or individual activities. This arrangement is also very workable in a classroom where the teacher can join the group on the mat or sit on a low bench to present her educational materials. Many cerebral-palsied children who have limited hand control and/or hand function while sitting at a desk, show a surprising amount of both head control and hand function while lying in the prone position on a mat with the upper chest and arms over a bolster.

12. Large ball. The large beach balls are used to practice func-

tional activities and reflex-inhibiting patterns in much the same manner as the bolster is used. (See earlier discussion on the bolster.) The diameter of the ball will vary according to both the size of the child and the functional activity being carried out. A ball with a 12-inch diameter will be suitable for the practice of the four point or hands and knees position with a young child. An 18- to 20-inch diameter will be required for kneeling, sitting, rolling, or other gross motor activities.

13. Special therapeutic modalities. Need for the equipment associated with therapeutic modalities can best be determined by consulting the functional profile (refer to earlier discussion). An institution which houses a large number of fairly functional young people and employs them as resident workers, or facilities which operate a farm program or a vocational workshop can probably anticipate a significant number of industrial type accidents. Plans for physical therapy in these institutions should include at least a small program for the treatment of acute, traumatic conditions. This program would necessitate the purchase of equipment for several of the therapeutic modalities (e.g. electrical muscle stimulator, ultra sonilator, intermittent traction, diathermy, etc,). An institutional program for infants and young children should be developmental in nature and therefore should not require this type of equipment.

14. Hydrotherapy. The inclusion of a hydrotherapy program requires a tremendous financial outlay for installation and purchase of equipment as well as maintenance of the department. Careful examination of the resident functional profile must be carried out before the decision for or against a hydrotherapy program is made. A program with a developmental emphasis for infants and young children will probably have limited need for hydrotherapy. Consideration must be given for industrial type injuries associated with vocational workshop and farm programs, as well as the use of resident employees. Further consideration should be given to the amount of orthopedic surgery being carried out in the institution. The use of hydrotherapy following trauma or reconstructive surgery is well known and need not be elaborated here.

Some discussion has been given to the use of a swimming pool; however, several points need elaboration. The location of the swimming pool should be such that use during recreation does not disturb other areas of the institution. Provisions for safety are essential. Dressing rooms must provide privacy for patients and staff alike. The depth of the pool is an important factor, and here again the nature of the resident must be considered. If the population is very young or severely handicapped, the depth should vary from 1 foot at the shallow end to no more than 4 feet at the deep end. A more functional group of residents can safely be taught the proper behavior in and about a swimming pool and can accommodate themselves to a standard pool.

Conclusion

Regardless of the situation the therapist finds in a particular residential facility for the mentally retarded, it will require a different orientation and new approaches from that found in the usual physical therapy department of a hospital or rehabilitation center. Careful planning requires a knowledge of the patient population, the staffing pattern, the availability of volunteers, and the physical facilities. This must be combined with realistic goals and a dedication to the principle of maximum extension of the physical therapist's knowledge and skills through the training and utilization of other supportive personnel within the institution.

BIBLIOGRAPHY

Bensberg, F.J., Colwell, C.N., and Cassel, R.H.: Teaching the profoundly retarded self-help activities by behavior shaping techniques. *Amer J Ment Defic, 69:*51, 1965.

Bobath, K.: The Prevention of Mental Retardation in Patients with Cerebral Palsy. Presented at 5th International Congress of Child Psychiatry, 1962.

Bobath, K., and Bobath, B.: The neurodevelopmental treatment of cerebral palsy. *Phys Ther, 47:*11, November, 1967.

Bobath, K., and Bobath, B.: The very early treatment of cerebral palsy. *Develop Med Child Neurol, 9:* August, 1967.

Ethun, Carol A.: Physical management of the multihandicapped child. *GP, 34:*1, July, 1966.

Girardeau, F.L., and Spradlin, J.E.: Token rewards in a cottage program. *MR, 2:*6, 1964.

Koch, R., et al.: The predictability of Gesell Developmental Scales in mongolism. *J Pediat, 62:*93, 1963.

Rice, Harold K., et al.: Operant conditioning techniques. *Phys Ther, 48:*4, April, 1968.

Robins, Ferris, and Robins, Jennet: *Educational Rhythmics for Mentally Handicapped Children.* Ra-Verlag, Rapperswil, Zurich, Switzerland, 1963.

Robins, Ferris, and Robins, Jennet: *Educational Rhythmics for Mentally and Physically Handicapped Children.* Ra-Verlag, Rapperswil, Zurich, Switzerland, 1966.

Trotter, Ann B., and Inman, Douglas, A.: The use of positive reinforcement in physical therapy. *Phys Ther, 48:*4, April, 1968.

Watson, Luke S.: Applications of behavior shaping devices to training severely and profoundly mentally retarded children in an institutional setting. *MR,* December, 1968.

SUGGESTED READING

A Look to the Future. Monograph, United Cerebral Palsy Association, Inc., New York.

Robinault, Isabel: Using latest techniques for therapy. *A Look to the Future,* United Cerebral Palsy Association, Inc., New York.

Semons, Sarah: Modern techniques for therapy in cerebral palsy. *A Look to the Future,* United Cerebral Palsy Association, Inc., New York.

Mental Retardation: A Handbook for the Primary Physician. A report of the American Medical Association Conference on Mental Retardation, 1964.

Haynes, Una: *The Role of Nursing in Programs for Patients with Cerebral Palsy and Related Disorders.* United Cerebral Palsy Association, Inc., New York, 1962.

Zausmer, Elizabeth: Evaluation of strength and motor development in infants. *Phys Ther Rev, 33:*11, 12, November and December, 1953.

Haynes, Una: *A Developmental Approach to Casefinding.* U.S. Department of Health, Education, and Welfare, 1967.

Fisher, Ernst.: Neurophysiology a physical therapist should know. *Phys Ther Rev. 38:*11, 1958.

Masland, R., Sarason, S., and Gladwin, T.: *Mental Subnormality.* Basic Books, 1958.

Minimal Brain Dysfunction in Children. PHS No. 1415, U.S. Department of Health, Education, and Welfare, 1966.

Looking Ahead to Residential Care for the Cerebral Palsied: United Cerebral Palsy Association, Inc., New York.

Lemkau, Paul: The Influence of Handicapping Conditions on Child Development. United Cerebral Palsy Association, Inc., New York.

Curran, Patricia: A study toward a theory of neuromuscular education through occupational therapy. *Amer J Occup Ther, 14*:2, 1960.

Nunley, Rachael: The physical therapist at home with the mentally retarded. *Phys Ther, 47*:10, October, 1967.

The Child with Central Nervous System Deficit. Children's Bureau, Publication No. 432, U.S. Department of Health, Education, and Welfare, 1965.